The Midwifery Research

MIRIAD

A sourcebook of information about research in midwifery

Edited by
Carol Simms, Hazel McHaffie, Mary J Renfrew and Hazel Ashurst
Midwifery Research Programme, National Perinatal Epidemiology Unit, Oxford

Books for Midwives Press
Books for Midwives Press is a joint publishing venture between
Haigh & Hochland Publications Ltd and The Royal College of Midwives

Published by Books for Midwives Press, 174a Ashley Road, Hale, Cheshire, WA15 9SF, England

©1994, Crown Copyright. Published by permission of the Controller of Her Majesty's Stationery Office. No part of this publication may be reproduced in any form without the permission of the Department of Health.

First edition

ISBN 1-898507-18-X

British Library Cataloguing in Publication Data
A catalogue record for this book is available from the British Library

Printed in Great Britain by Cromwell Press Ltd.

Contents

Preface

.

Midwives in the UK are increasingly questioning their practice, and the traditional systems of care which have evolved over the years. The challenges which have arisen from the Winterton report, and the report on Changing Childbirth, have coincided with a continuing growth in research into midwifery. This research has the potential to influence and inform practice, and it demonstrates the development of a questioning approach among midwives as they strive to provide the best care for mothers, babies and their families.

The Midwifery Research Database, MIRIAD, provides a way of mapping this growth in research. The studies listed in this third MIRIAD report range from small studies done in an individual midwife's spare time, to very large randomized controlled trials; and they illustrate the wide range of interests and responsibilities of midwives. Antenatal education, epidurals, women's views of the care they receive, water birth, care of families from ethnic minority groups, care of babies in special care units, postnatal care in the community, pain relief and midwifery education are just some of the topics addressed in these studies.

There has been a notable increase in the number of studies examining the organisation of midwifery services, including continuity of care and team midwifery.

This report, in its new, easier-to-read format, is the only source of information about many of these studies. This is the first time that it has been published by a professional publishers; as a result, it will be accessible to a much wider audience than in the past.

I would like to congratulate the Midwifery Research Programme at the NPEU for producing this book and also those midwives who have endeavoured through their research to keep the focus on women centred care.

BARONESS CUMBERLEGE

Acknowledgements

Compiling this report has involved many people who have given generously of their time and expertise. Especially important have been the researchers who have provided us with details about their studies, and who have responded to our many requests for additional information. They have been very patient during the change in the format of the abstracts and during delays in the production of this report.

As always, our Steering Group members and advisers have been helpful and supportive. All of them contribute so much to the project; special thanks to Ann Thomson for chairing the group, and to Valerie Tickner and Joan Greenwood who have recently retired.

Malcolm Newdick of Update Software has provided the programming support for the database with skill and good humour.

Henry Hochland and his colleagues at Haigh and Hochland Publications Ltd have made possible the publication of this report by working to a seemingly impossible timetable.

Sue Hawkins, of the Midwives Information and Resource Service (MIDIRS) has used her expertise to compile the list of key words.

The Royal College of Midwives worked on the distribution of the 1991 report, and we are grateful for their help.

Our colleagues at the National Perinatal Epidemiology Unit have supported us in so many ways, as they always do. Jo Garcia was especially helpful throughout the last two years.

Our families have been a constant source of support, especially during the busy times. Jamie and Calum Renfrew had a special influence on MIRIAD, as their births were the main reason for the delay in producing this new report.

And finally, this report would not have been possible without the skill and commitment of Suzanne Williams, who has carried out all of the data entry, editing and word processing; in spite of the workload, she has been calm and cheerful throughout.

The Department of Health has funded the database since it was developed in 1988.

Staff and Steering Group members 1991-1994

Staff

Hazel Ashurst	Computer Co-ordinator
Hazel McHaffie	Midwife Researcher
Mary Renfrew	Midwife Researcher
Carol Simms	Database Administrator/Research Midwife
Kay Willbery	Secretary (from May 1994)
Suzanne Williams	Secretary (until April 1994)

Steering Group members

Hazel Ashurst	National Perinatal Epidemiology Unit
Elisabeth Clark	Royal College of Nursing
Joan Greenwood	Department of Health (retired 1994)
Sue Hawkins	Midwives Information and Resource Service
Jane Robinson	University of Nottingham (resigned 1993)
Jane Salvage	King's Fund (resigned 1991)
Rudi Singh	Department of Health
Jennifer Sleep	West Berkshire Health Authority
Ann Thomson	University of Manchester
Valerie Tickner	Royal College of Midwives (retired 1994)
Elizabeth Wilson	Department of Health (resigned 1992)
Kathryn Partington	Department of Health

Steering Group advisors

Hazel McHaffie	University of Edinburgh
Tricia Murphy-Black	Simpson Memorial Maternity Pavilion, Edinburgh
Sarah Robinson	King's College, London
Jane Salvage	World Health Organisation

Introduction

This is a time of great challenge for midwives across the UK. The 1991 report of the House of Commons Health Committee on the Maternity Services (House of Commons 1991), and 'Changing Childbirth', the report of the Expert Committee chaired by Baroness Julia Cumberledge, (Department of Health 1993), have suggested fundamental changes in the way in which maternity care is organised. The needs of women and their babies have been acknowledged to be central, and midwives are being supported in taking on a key role in providing care. The resultant changes in the organisation and content of maternity care are greater than any that have been seen since the move from home to hospital birth in the middle of this century.

In such a time of change, it is essential to question our practice, both old and new, and to generate evidence to help to guide that practice. The researchers whose studies are listed in this book have demonstrated this questioning approach, and have helped to generate some of the information that is needed. As a result, this book will be of interest and value to midwives, health service managers, maternity organisations, and researchers, as well as to childbearing women and their families.

Interest in research in midwifery has been growing over the past two or three decades. Although still relatively new, the field is developing quickly; this is demonstrated by the growth in the numbers of studies in this report.

This sourcebook is a unique compilation of information about research in midwifery. Since 1988, details about midwifery research studies in the UK have been collected on a computerised database run by the Midwifery Research Programme at the National Perinatal Epidemiology Unit in Oxford. Details of studies in clinical practice, midwifery education, the organisation of midwifery services and the history of midwifery are all included. This is the only source of information about much of this work - over a fifth of the studies are still in progress, and many of the completed studies have never been published elsewhere.

This is the third report of the information held on the database, which is known as MIRIAD. In the past we have published the report ourselves, and it has been distributed by the Royal College of Midwives. This is the first MIRIAD report to be published by Books for Midwives Press - as a result of this new arrangement, the book has been more professionally produced, and it will be much more widely available.

This report gives details of 267 midwifery research studies. To find those studies, we generated publicity about the database each year in professional and research journals, and at relevant conferences. Researchers were asked to contact us for a registration form. They then returned that form to the MIRIAD office, giving details about their study. If the criteria for entry to the database were fulfilled (see below) their studies were entered onto the computer, and examined for accuracy and completeness. A printout was then sent back to the researchers for checking.

Criteria for entry to MIRIAD

1. *All studies are or were carried out in the UK.*

2. *Each study is related to midwifery but the researchers may or may not be midwives.*

3. *Quality assurance/audit projects are not included.*

    Although quality assurance and research are sometimes closely related, the decision was made not to include quality assurance projects unless they involved directly some element of research.

4. *Studies are not generally included if they were done as part of a student project at lower than undergraduate level.*

    This is to exclude projects whose primary purpose was as a learning experience for the student, rather than as a research study. However, in exceptional cases, this criterion has been waived.

Once any study is completed, the entry will not be updated in the future, except for changes of address, and details about publications. If a study is in progress, we will update the entry to reflect progress made since the previous report.

The studies vary widely in scale, method, and quality. They have not undergone peer review unless they have already been published in refereed journals. Further investigation by the reader will be needed, including critical reading of any publications, or contacting the researchers involved, to assess the quality of the study. In addition, the studies reported here may not be the only relevant work - there may be important studies which are not listed here, and there may be studies in fields other than midwifery which are also important. All relevant work on a particular topic should be explored before implementing changes in practice. Ways of finding information about other work is outlined below:

Further information about published studies in midwifery can be obtained from the Midwives Information and Resource Service (MIDIRS), 9 Elmdale Road, Clifton, Bristol, BS8 1SL telephone 0272 251791 and from the Royal College of Midwives Library, 15 Mansfield Street, London W1M 0BE telephone 071 580 6523.

Other important sources of information include libraries, computerised indexes such as MEDLINE, and the computerised database of reviews of perinatal trials, 'The Cochrane Collaboration Pregnancy and Childbirth Database', edited by Murray Enkin, Marc Keirse, Mary Renfrew and James Neilson, issued on disk twice yearly by Update Software, Manor Cottage, Little Milton, Oxford OX44 7QB, telephone 0844 278887.

Those who have read the two previous reports (published in 1990 and 1991) will notice a number of changes in this one. The most obvious is the length - there are now almost 270 studies listed. The other important change is the way in which the information about each study is presented. Many of the studies were completed some time ago, and we have left those abstracts in the old format. About half the studies use the original, free text abstract. The other half use a new, structured format. These new abstracts have been structured under headings to guide the reader in identifying the relevant information, and assessing the type and quality of the study.

The database is continually updated. However, because of the time needed to produce the book from the information listed on the database, only studies submitted to MIRIAD before the end of 1993 have been included. Since this manuscript went to press, further studies have been submitted to us; these will be included in the next report, due to be published in 1995.

This present report will be the only volume in which details of all studies will be given in full. In future years, studies which are completed and unchanged from the previous year will only be listed in summary form; full details will of course be available from previous years' reports. Those who wish to have a complete record of all MIRIAD studies will therefore need a copy of each volume of the report.

It is important that we collect information about as many studies as possible, so that this book is really useful to the readers. Information about completed or ongoing studies in midwifery will always be welcome.

We rely completely on researchers sending us details of their research; if they do not, we cannot enter their study onto the database.

If you have a study which you would like to register, please contact the MIRIAD office, National Perinatal Epidemiology Unit, Radcliffe Infirmary, Oxford OX2 6HE, telephone number 0865 224122 and ask for Carol Simms or Kay Willbery.

References

Department of Health (1993). Changing Childbirth. 2 parts, London: HMSO.

House of Commons. Health Committee (1992). Second report, session 1991-2: Maternity services. 3 vols, London: HMSO.

Summary of information about midwifery research studies

Completed and ongoing studies

Of the 267 studies listed in this report, 209 have been completed, and 58 are ongoing. In next year's report, only limited information about completed studies will be given: this year's report is the only one in which full details of all studies will be available.

Categories of study

There are four main categories of study: Clinical, Educational, Management and Historical. MIRIAD staff allocate these categories according to the subject area(s) covered by each study. A study may fall into more than one category; for example, it may be about the effect of education on clinical practice. If this is the case, it will be listed in full in the most appropriate section, and summary details will appear in other relevant sections. Two hundred and five studies examine clinical questions, 42 look at education, 54 are concerned with management and organisational issues, and 2 are historical studies.

Details of all the studies are listed under these main headings in the next section of this report.

Keywords

Each study has been allocated a maximum of 10 keywords by the researchers or by MIRIAD staff. These have been used to compile the index, and to indicate the frequency with which topics occur.

Excluding the term 'midwifery', which is of course used in a very large proportion of studies, the keywords which were used most frequently in this report were:

Keywords used (including closely related keywords)	Number of entries
Breastfeeding	83
Midwifery education	81
Labour	62
Antenatal care	41
Women's experience	43
Perineal care	39
Consumer satisfaction	29
Midwife's role	26
Maternity services	19
Postnatal care	18
Continuity of care	14

Breastfeeding, labour, antenatal care and perineal care were the most frequently mentioned clinical topics in the two previous MIRIAD reports (1990 and 1991), and this remains the same this year. The topic of midwifery education has increased greatly since its 1991 total of 34 studies. Evidence of midwives' concern with women's views is shown in the frequency with which consumer satisfaction and women's experiences are listed. This concern, together with the obvious interest in the maternity services and continuity of care, demonstrates that midwives have been involved for some time in working to improve the services that women receive, as was recommended by the Cumberledge and Winterton reports.

Timing of studies

Table 1 shows when the studies were started. An important feature of previous reports was the registration of older studies, but that work seems now to have been replaced by keeping pace with new studies. There has been little change in the number of entries prior to 1990, indicating that almost all the new entries are for very recent studies.

Table 1. Starting date of studies (n=267)

Year	Number	Percent
1975 and before	2	1
1976 to 1980	21	8
1981 to 1985	39	14
1986 to 1990	121	45
1991 to 1993	84	31

Were studies carried out in work time?

Researchers were asked whether the person who carried out the study did so as part of a job, in her/his own time, or as part of a course. Table 2 gives the answers to this question. The responses are not mutually exclusive; for example, some researchers may have carried out a study which formed part of a course, as well as part of their job, and additionally have spent some of their own time working on it.

Table 2. Were studies carried out in work time? (n=267)

Study was conducted:	Number	Percent
As integral or additional part of a job	162	61
Outside work time	132	49
As part of a course	103	39
Other	27	10

It has not been possible accurately to differentiate between an integral and an additional part of a job, often because those carrying out the research themselves have difficulty deciding where the scope of their job ended. For example, some researchers used the clinical facilities in which they were working to carry out their study, but additionally used their own time outside their normal duties. Others carried out a study in their normal hours, but with an increased workload as a result. Full-time researchers, especially, had difficulty in differentiating between normal and additional parts of a job; the hours worked by researchers are not usually rigidly defined, and work is often done at home.

Table 3 shows the average amount of time principal researchers used outside their work hours throughout the study. This figure is hard for those involved in the research to estimate, for some of the reasons outlined above. In addition, research does not happen at a steady pace, and more time will be spent in some phases of a study than in others.

Table 3. Time spent by principal researchers outside their work hours (n=267)

Average number of hours per week	Number of principal researchers	Percent
Less than 2 hours	23	9
2 to 6 hours	49	18
7 to 12 hours	44	16
13 to 20 hours	24	9
More than 20 hours	16	6
None of their own time	111	42
Total who used their own time	156	58

These results indicate that being involved in research eats substantially into the majority of researchers' own time, with 40 (15%) spending more than an additional 12 hours a week on their studies.

Sources of funding

Questions about the way the study was funded are also difficult to answer. Does 'funding' include material support, such as stationery and photocopying, or time release from work? Researchers seemed to answer this question in a variety of ways, and as a result it is not possible to make any definitive statement about how studies were funded. Table 4 gives such information as is available about sources of funding: some studies had more than one source of funding, so the answers are not mutually exclusive. These figures probably underestimate funding, as they do not always include estimates of integral costs such as time allowed at work. In addition, many of the researchers who reported receiving support also funded parts of their own studies, in time or money. Those coded 'other source' were simply impossible to categorise in any straightforward way. Some of these researchers requested that we keep the source of funding confidential. Others found it hard to work out, for example, how much of an award for educational support was spent on their study.

Table 4. Source of funding for studies   (n=267)

Source of funding for studies	Number	Percent
Employer	127	48
Funding agency	104	39
Other source	47	18
No funding received	48	18
No response	1	1

Finding funds for research is always difficult, perhaps especially so in midwifery where there are few obvious sources of appropriate sums of money. Organisations which did contribute funds to studies registered on MIRIAD are listed on pages 349-360.

Updating studies

Keeping track of all MIRIAD researchers is not easy. Wherever possible, we have contacted the researcher and they have amended their own entries.

Studies which have not been updated by the researcher have been dealt with in one of three ways:

a)   Some studies which were virtually complete in previous reports have had their publications updated by MIRIAD staff.

b)   Where we have been unable to fully update the entries, the entries are marked, 'Not updated since 1991'. There are 23 such entries.

c)   A few studies listed in previous reports will not now be completed. It would have been surprising if there had not been some unfinished studies. The work involved between generating an idea for a study and completing it is often unpredictable, and greater than might have been anticipated. In addition, people's circumstances may change - such as their place of work, or where they live - and this accounts for a number of the studies which have not come to fruition. Researchers have told us of four such studies.

In addition, we have been unable to contact the researchers for full information about another nine studies for which preliminary details only were listed in previous reports. So as not to lose the important questions which they asked, we have listed their titles and study numbers at the end of the report (p 348). Details about the plans for these studies can be found in the two previous MIRIAD reports (1990 and 1991).

Studies with new structured abstracts

For studies with the new form of structured abstract (128 out of a total of 267), we have collected further details, which are described here.

Ethics committee approval

For those 128 studies, 76 reported that they had gained ethics committee approval; 52 had not. Many of these researchers asked permission from other sources, such as the Director of Midwifery Services, instead of applying to an Ethics Committee. Others felt that ethics approval was not needed for their study. In some studies this was because those being interviewed were health professionals. In other circumstances, it was not clear why the researcher felt that ethics committee approval was not required. For example, some researchers collected information from case notes, and others interviewed women individually and in groups, without having requested ethics committee approval.

Study design

Information was given about the study design. One question asked whether the study was descriptive or experimental. Thirty five researchers noted that their study was experimental, and 101 carried out a descriptive study; some studies combined both designs.

Research method

Table 5 gives details about the research method used by those who completed the new, structured abstract. More than one method could be used within a single study; some studies consisting of several interconnected parts involving different methods. Examples of methods used in the 'other' category include case note reviews, analysis of documents, and group discussions.

Table 5. New, structured abstracts - Research method used   (n=128)

Research method	Number	Percent
Survey	59	46
Ethnography	17	13
Case study	15	12
Historical study	5	3
Randomized controlled trial	27	21
Case control	1	1
Action research	6	5
Other	31	24
No response	1	1

Finally, many of the completed studies have not been published. It is understandable that many researchers, working under pressure, with scarce resources, and without good supervision, find it hard to find the time to finish a study. A survey of these researchers has been carried out to ascertain some of the reasons for this lack of publication; the results will be available in next year's MIRIAD report.

In conclusion

The work presented in this report demonstrates the growth of research in midwifery in recent years, and the variety of topics addressed.

This report also highlights a number of problems. Firstly, some researchers have not sought ethics committee approval even when this seemed to be appropriate. In addition, a number of studies have never been completed, possibly because of a lack of support and advice, or funding, or perhaps because inappropriate questions were asked. Finally, other studies have been completed but not published; we plan to clarify the reasons for this. These problems need to be addressed by the midwifery profession, by managers, researchers and funding bodies.

The questions being addressed in the research presented here are of importance to women, their babies and their families, as well as to midwives, and others working in the maternity services. Future volumes will demonstrate how this work has developed.

Listing of individual studies

Full details of all studies are given in this section under four main headings; Clinical, Educational, Management and Historical. Where studies appear under more than one heading the full record appears in the most appropriate category and is cross referenced to any other relevant category. Within each of these headings, entries are listed in order of their study number; this number was allocated chronologically, as studies were entered on the database.

The study number and title are listed first, followed by the dates during which the study was/is being carried out. The researchers names and job titles are next. The first name listed is usually that of the person who had/has principal responsibility for the study. The person who is willing to be contacted about the study is listed as the Contact, followed by their address. This address is usually the person's current address and is therefore not always the address of the institution where the study was carried out. We have not listed researchers' private addresses or telephone numbers. If no contact address is listed, please contact the MIRIAD office, 0865 224122 for further details. Job titles are also updated, and are therefore for current jobs, for the principal researcher (who is listed first), and the contact person. Collaborators' job titles are those which were current at the time of the study.

Funding details are then given, followed by the study abstracts. There are two forms of abstract. The original abstract form was unstructured, free text. Studies which were completed in the last (1991) report, or which were ongoing but have not been updated since then, remain in this format. New studies, and those which have been updated since 1991, are now in a structured form, with headings to differentiate parts of the abstract. These entries give fuller details about studies. Key words are listed next; these correspond to those listed in the key word index, and will assist in identifying studies of interest. Finally, any publications or reports are cited in full.

In a few cases, researchers indicated that they wished the abstract to remain confidential. If this is the case, the abstract is not reproduced here, and only the word 'Confidential' will appear. If you wish to know more about these studies, contact the researchers directly.

We have been unable to update some of the studies. Those entries are marked, "Not updated since 1991".

At the back of the report there is an author index and a keyword index, both listed alphabetically, to help you find studies of interest.

Note: MIRIAD is not intended to provide a direct basis for changing practice. Studies entered on MIRIAD have not undergone peer review unless they have been published in refereed journals. Further investigation by the reader will be required in all instances, to assess the quality of the study. In addition, the studies reported here may not be the only relevant work in the field, and it is important to explore all work on a particular topic before implementing change.

Title Index

STUDIES WHICH WILL NOT BE COMPLETED

STUDIES WHERE FULL DETAILS ARE NOT AVAILABLE

Clinical Studies

1. DEVELOPMENT OF FEEDING BEHAVIOUR IN BREAST- AND BOTTLE-FED INFANTS

January 1974–January 1978
Rosemary A Crow, Professor of Nursing, Director NPRU, Josephine Fawcett, Research Assistant, P Wright, Lecturer in Psychology. **Contact:** Rosemary A Crow, Department of Nursing & Midwifery, University of Surrey, Guildford, Surrey GU2 5XH. Tel: 0483 509772

Funded as integral or additional part of a job by Scottish Home and Health Department.

Abstract: This project was an observational study of the development of feeding behaviour in the breast- and bottle-fed human infant from birth to six months. The main aim was to explore the capacity of the infant to express satiety behaviourally. Naturally occurring behaviours were identified and categorised according to various objectively defined criteria during an initial period of observation on approximately sixty mother-infant pairs. A further sample of twenty mother-infant pairs was then used to examine more systematically a selected group of these behaviours. Each pair was visited at monthly intervals from birth to six months, and it is the data drawn from the results of these visits which forms the basis of the published papers.

In the exploration of the infant's capacity to express satiety, an attempt was first made to identify potential satiety signals. Behaviours which had this potential were observed in the neonate, but the nature of their expression was found to depend upon age and feeding technique. The value which the mother placed on these potential signals varied according to the feeding technique but not age. The differences found were described using the concept of control. Discussion brought out the possible influences which milk composition and the nature of mother control may have on the opportunities available for development in the infant's feeding behaviour.

The clinical implications for midwifery are two-fold; firstly, there is a need to understand that regulation of food intake involves both the amount consumed at the feed and the intervals between the feeds. If the mammary gland has reached its capacity to produce milk, then the only way breastfed infants can increase their intake is to feed more frequently. Any notion of an optimum feeding time-schedule would be counter-productive. Secondly, bottle-feeding mothers need to be educated about how their handling of the feed can affect the infant's feeding behaviour. Stimulating the infant to continue sucking is both unnecessary and disturbing.

Keywords: ARTIFICIAL FEEDING, ARTIFICIAL FEEDING BEHAVIOUR, BREASTFEEDING, BREASTFEEDING BEHAVIOUR, MILK INTAKE (REGULATION), SATIETY CUES

Fawcett J, Crow RA, Wright P. Hunger and its relation to sucking in early infancy. Proceedings of VI International Conference on the Physiology of Food and Fluid Intake, Paris, France 1977;23-4.

Wright P, Fawcett J, Crow RA. The development of feeding behaviour in human infants from birth to six months. Proceedings of the XV International Ethological Conference, Bielefeld, Germany 1977.

Wright P, Fawcett J, Crow RA. The development of differences in feeding behaviour of bottle- and breastfed human infants from birth to two months. Behavioural Processes 1980;5:1-20.

Crow RA, Fawcett J, Wright P. Maternal behaviour during breast- and bottle feeding. Journal of Behavioural Medicine 1980;3:259-77.

Crow RA. Infant feeding. In: Pearce E. A General Textbook for Nursing (20th edn). Faber and Faber Ltd. 1980: Chapter 2.

Wright P, Crow RA. Nutrition and feeding. In: Stratton P, Psychobiology of the Human Newborn. John Wiley and Sons Ltd. 1982: Chapter 13.

Crow RA. Development of breast- and bottle feeding in human infants. A thesis submitted for the degree of Doctor of Philosophy. University of Edinburgh 1978.

Crow RA. An ethnological study of the development of infant feeding. Journal of Advanced Nursing 1977;2:99-109.

2. THE WEST BERKSHIRE PERINEAL MANAGEMENT TRIAL
April 1982 - May 1983

Jennifer Sleep, Research Coordinator, Adrian Grant, Epidemiologist, Jo Garcia, Social Scientist, Diana Elbourne, Social Statistician, John Spencer, Registrar (Obstetrics and Gynaecology), Iain Chalmers, Director NPEU. **Contact:** Jennifer Sleep, Berkshire College of Nursing & Midwifery, Royal Berkshire Hospital, Craven Road, Reading, Berkshire RG1 5AN. Tel: 0734 877651

Funded as integral or additional part of a job. Over 20 hours/week of own time spent. Funded by employer and by funding agency(ies): Oxford Regional Health Authority, Maws/RCM Research Scholarship.

Abstract: The purpose of the study was to compare liberal and restrictive use of episiotomy for maternal indications in otherwise normal deliveries.

One thousand women were allocated at random to one of two perineal management policies, both intended to minimise trauma during spontaneous vaginal delivery. In one, the aim was to restrict episiotomy to fetal indications; in the other, the operation was to be used more liberally to prevent perineal tears. The resultant episiotomy rates were 10% and 51% respectively. An intact perineum was more common among those allocated to the restrictive policy. This group experienced more perineal and labial tears, however, and included four of the five cases of severe trauma. Overall, 69% of the women required suturing. There were no significant differences in terms of neonatal outcome based on Apgar scores at delivery and the number of babies admitted to S.C.B.U. The incidence of pain reported by mothers was very similar in the two groups both at ten days after delivery and at three months. Women allocated to the restrictive policy were more likely to have resumed sexual intercourse within one month postpartum, but there were no differences in the reported incidence of dyspareunia or of urinary symptoms three months following childbirth.

These findings provide little support for the liberal use of episiotomy for maternal indications in otherwise normal deliveries. Its use should, therefore, largely be restricted to fetal indications only.

Keywords: DYSPAREUNIA, EPISIOTOMY, MATERNAL MORBIDITY, PERINEAL CARE, PERINEAL TRAUMA, URINARY INCONTINENCE

Sleep J. The West Berkshire episiotomy trial. Research and the Midwife Conference Proceedings, Manchester 1983:81-95.

Sleep J. Episiotomy in normal delivery. RCN Research Society International Conference, Imperial College, London 1984:100. (abstract)

Sleep J, Grant A, Garcia J, Elbourne D, Spencer J, Chalmers I. The Reading episiotomy trial. 23rd British Congress of Obstetrics and Gynaecology, Birmingham. Royal College of Obstetricians and Gynaecologists, London 1984:24. (abstract)

Sleep J. Normal delivery. In: Alexander J, Roche S, Levy V, eds. Midwifery Practice, Vol 1. Basingstoke: Macmillan.

Sleep J, Roberts J, Chalmers I. Care during the second stage of labour. In: Chalmers I, Enkin M, Kierse MJNC, eds. Effective Care in Pregnancy and Childbirth. Oxford: Oxford University Press 1989:1129-44.

Sleep J. Physiology and management of the 2nd stage of labour. In: Bennet VR, Brown LK, eds. Myles Textbook for Midwives. Edinburgh: Churchill Livingstone 1989:192-208.

Sleep J. Episiotomy in normal delivery. Nursing Times 1984;80:29-30.

Sleep J. Management of the perineum. Nursing Times 1984;80:51-4.

Sleep J, Grant A, Garcia J, Elbourne D, Spencer J, Chalmers I. West Berkshire perineal management trial. British Medical Journal 1984;289:587-90.

Sleep J. Perineal care: A series of five randomised controlled trials. In: Robinson S, Thomson AM, eds. Midwives, Research and Childbirth. Vol 2. London Chapman and Hall. 1991:199-251.

Sleep J. Episiotomy. In: Faulkner A, Murphy-Black T, eds. Midwifery: Excellence in Nursing, the Research Route. London: Scutari Press. 7-8.

3. THE SOUTHAMPTON STUDY OF THE PREVALANCE OF INVERTED AND NON-PROTACTILE NIPPLES AMONGST ANTENATAL WOMEN WHO INTEND TO BREASTFEED
August 1987 - February 1989

Joanne M Alexander, Midwife Teacher, John K Dennis, Prof of Human Reproduction & Obstetrics, Michael J Campbell, Senior Lecturer in Medical Statistics. **Contact:** Joanne M Alexander, Midwifery Education Department, Princess Anne Hospital, Southampton, Hants SO9 4HA. Tel: 0703 796047

Abstract: The study was confined to women who expressed an intention to breastfeed. The prevalence of inverted and non-protractile nipples amongst 3006 women was examined and, on the basis of this, recommendations are made as to which women require antenatal examination and at what gestation it should be conducted.

The gestational age of the first examination depended on organisational constraints. The odds ratio for having a problematic nipple (inverted or non-protractile) decreases by 3% for each increasing week of gestation, this trend being present amongst both nulliparous and multiparous women. The trend is also confirmed using McNemar's test for longitudinal data from 325 women examined at least twice in the same pregnancy. In contrast to the findings of previous researchers, the cross-sectional data demonstrate that parity, of itself, does not influence the prevalence of 'unfavourable' nipples, but women who have not breastfed before are almost two-and-a-half times as likely to have a problem as women who have. The odds ratio for having a problematic nipple decreases by 6% for each increasing year of maternal age but, in fact, the relationship is not linear, the lower prevalence occurring in women in their middle twenties. All three influential variables exert an independent effect on prevalence.

It was also found that women were significantly more likely (p=<0.001) to have bilaterally protractile or non-protractile nipples than to have one of each; the same trend appears to be evident for inversion. It is suggested that women who have successfully breastfed before do not require antenatal examination of their nipples. Those who have not should no longer be examined at the first antenatal visit but early in the third trimester, thus allowing time for spontaneous improvement of nipple anatomy to occur whilst still permitting treatment if it is considered desirable.

As a result of this study, a randomized controlled trial of alternative treatments for such nipples was designed (Record No. 4).

Keywords: ANTENATAL EXAMINATIONS, BREASTFEEDING, NIPPLES (INVERTED), NIPPLES (NON-PROTRACTILE)

Alexander JM, Dennis KJ, Campbell MJ. The prevalence of inverted and non-protractile nipples amongst antenatal women who intend to breastfeed. Abstract from the proceedings of the 4th European Congress of Allied Specialists in Maternal and Neonatal Care. Bruges September 1989.

Alexander JM. The prevalence and management of inverted and non-protractile nipples in antenatal women who intend to breastfeed. Unpublished PhD thesis 1991.

Alexander JM. The Southampton randomized controlled trial of alternative methods of treating inverted and non-protractile nipples in pregnancy. Research and the Midwife Conference Proceedings 1990.

4. THE SOUTHAMPTON RANDOMIZED CONTROLLED TRIAL OF ALTERNATIVE TREATMENTS FOR INVERTED AND NON-PROTACTILE NIPPLES DURING PREGNANCY

August 1987 - November 1989

Joanne M Alexander, Midwife Teacher, John K Dennis, Prof of Human Reproduction & Obstetrics, Michael J Campbell, Senior Lecturer in Medical Statistics **Contact:** Joanne M Alexander, Midwifery Education Department, Princess Anne Hospital, Southampton, Hants SO9 4HA. Tel: 0703 796047

Funded as integral or additional part of a job and by Maws/RCM Research Scholarship, Iolanthe Trust. Formed part of a course. 12-20 hours/week of own time spent.

Abstract: Strategies used to treat inverted and non-protractile nipples antenatally in women who intend to breastfeed, have never been compared with a no-treatment group, and it is possible that the improvements claimed may have been due to the natural increase in nipple protractility that occurs progressively throughout pregnancy (Hytten and Baird 1958; Alexander, Dennis and Campbell 1989).

Nulliparous women who intended to breastfeed had their nipples examined for protractility when they visited the consultant unit clinic between twenty-five and thirty-five completed weeks of pregnancy. If found to have at least one inverted or non-protractile nipple and agreeing to enter the trial, they were randomly allocated to one of four groups (two by two factorial design) and the relevant instructions were given. The four groups were:

Group 1 - no special nipple preparation;
Group 2 - breast shells;
Group 3 - Hoffman's exercises;
Group 4 - breast shells and Hoffman's exercises.

Twenty four women were recruited to each group. Their nipples were re-examined shortly before the first breastfeed and in order to assess breastfeeding success a postal questionnaire was sent to them six weeks postnatally. The response rate to the questionnaire was 100%.

Results: Sustained improvement in nipple anatomy was more common in the untreated groups but the differences were not significant: 52% (25/48) shells v 60% (29/48) no shells; difference - 8% (95% confidence interval - 28% to 11%) and 54% (26/48) exercises v 58% (28/48) no exercises: - 4% (-24% to 16%)). 24 (50%) women not recommended shells and 14 (29%) recommended shells (21%;40% to 2%) were breast feeding six weeks after delivery (p=0.05), reflecting more women recommended shells both deciding to bottle feed before delivery and discontinuing breast feeding. The same number of women in exercise and no exercise groups were successfully breast feeding (0%; -20% to 20%). 13% of women approached about the trial (and planning to breast feed) did not attempt breast feeding.

Conclusions: Recommending nipple preparation with breast shells may reduce the chances of successful breast feeding. While there is no clear evidence that the treatments offered are effective antenatal nipple examination should be abandoned.

This trial was extended to other English and Canadian maternity units under the auspices of the National Perinatal Epidemiology Unit, which also assisted recruitment by the National Childbirth Trust via the latter's national network (Record No. 101).

Keywords: ANTENATAL EXAMINATIONS, BREAST SHELLS, BREASTFEEDING, GESTATION, HOFFMAN'S EXERCISES, INFANT FEEDING, NIPPLES (FLAT), NIPPLES (INVERTED), NIPPLES (NON-PROTRACTILE)

Alexander JM, Dennis KJ, Campbell MJ. The prevalence of inverted and non-protractile nipples amongst antenatal women who intend to breastfeed. Abstract from the proceedings of the 4th European Congress of Allied Specialists in Maternal and Neonatal Care. Bruges September 1989.

Alexander JM. The prevalence and management of inverted and non-protractile nipples in ante-natal women who intend to breastfeed. Unpublished PhD thesis 1991.

Alexander JM, Grant AM, Campbell MJ. Randomized controlled trial of breast shells and Hoffman's exercises for inverted and non-protractile nipples. British Medical Journal 1992;304:1030-2.

5. THIRD TRIMESTER PLACENTAL GRADING BY ULTRASONOGRAPHY AS A TEST OF FETAL WELL BEING
October 1982 - July 1987

Jean Proud, Sister in Charge, Obstetric Ultrasound, Adrian Grant, Epidemiologist.
Contact: Jean Proud, Midwifery Education, Lakeland college. Tel: 0524-583877

Funded as integral or additional part of a job. 2-6 hours/week of own time spent. Funded by employer and by funding agency(ies): East Anglian Regional Health Authority, Maws/RCM Research Scholarship.

Abstract: In a study of 2000 unselected pregnant women, the development of a placental appearance (grade 3) on ultrasonography by thirty-four to thirty-six weeks' gestation, observed in 15% of cases, was associated with maternal smoking, low parity, low maternal age, and being white. These women had an increased risk of problems during labour and their babies had an increased risk of low birthweight, poor condition at birth, and perinatal death.

The women were randomly allocated to two groups: in one group, the result of the placental grading was reported to the clinician responsible for care; in the second, the result was noted but not reported. There was a significant decrease in the risk of perinatal death in the group where the grading was known. This reduction was responsible for a difference in the principal outcome index, a heterogeneous group of measures of mortality and morbidity, but this difference was not significant.

This study alone does not justify routine late scanning, and further, larger trials are required. Nevertheless, the results do provide a basis for the reporting of placental grading when ultrasound examination is performed during the third trimester.

Keywords: OUTCOMES (PERINATAL), PLACENTAL GRADING, ULTRASOUND

Proud J. Placental grading as a test of fetal well being. In: Robinson S, Thomson AM, eds. Midwives, Research and Childbirth. Vol 1. London: Chapman and Hall 1989;5:95-116.
Proud J, Grant AM. Third trimester placental grading by ultrasonography as a test of fetal well being. British Medical Journal 1987;294:1641-4.

8. AN EXAMINATION OF THE CONTENT AND PROCESS OF THE ANTENATAL BOOKING INTERVIEW
April - October 1982

R C Methven, Senior Midwifery Tutor. **Contact:** R C Methven, Rawdon Drive, Rawdon, Near Leeds, West Yorkshire LS19 6HG.

Formed part of a course. Funded by funding agency(ies): Department of Health.

Abstract: This descriptive study assessed the content of information obtained, as well as the interview and interactive skills employed, by midwives undertaking a conventional antenatal booking interview. The purpose was to compare the type and quality of data recorded on the mother's obstetric record with that resulting from a nursing process assessment based on Orem's (1980) Self Care model.

Forty mothers, ten from each of four different maternity hospitals, were observed. A transcript of each conversation was then combined with the observation checklist, and analyzed for midwifery/obstetric content, interactive style and interview technique. Mothers' satisfaction was assessed by questionnaire and the midwives' perception of their role explored by interview.

The results showed that the quantity and quality of information obtained from the mother at booking were affected by the question technique used, the grade and experience of the midwife conducting the interview, and the dominance exerted by the obstetric records. The layout of the antenatal front-sheet of the mother's obstetric record was shown to dictate what questions were asked, the way they were asked, and the order in which they were asked. A large amount of otherwise untapped data relevant to midwifery care was obtained by using a semi-structured interview. This suggests that a nursing process style of assessment does provide a superior method of clinical data collection, and offers a more comprehensive framework for the delivery of midwifery care than that being used when the study was conducted.

It was concluded that the antenatal booking interview was viewed as a low status task, and that the organisation of clinics was counter-productive to the formation of an effective relationship between mother and midwife. The function and potential of the booking interview as a medium by which midwives may plan and provide antenatal care for mothers needs to be further explored and clarified.

Keywords: ANTENATAL BOOKING INTERVIEW, ANTENATAL CARE PLANS, COMMUNICATION, COMPUTERISATION (OBSTETRIC RECORDS), CONSUMER SATISFACTION, MIDWIFE'S ROLE, MIDWIFERY PROCESS, NURSING PROCESS, SELF CARE

Methven RC. The antenatal booking interview: Recording an obstetric history or relating with a mother-to-be? Parts 1 and 2. Research and the Midwife Conference Proceedings 1982;63-76:77-95.

Methven RC. Mother knows best. Nursing Mirror 1985:38-40.

Methven RC. Care plan for a woman having antenatal care based on OREM's self care model. In: Webb C, ed. Women's Health - Midwifery and Gynaecological nursing. London: Hodder and Stoughton 1986.

Methven RC. Recording an obstetric history or relating to a pregnant woman? - A study of the antenatal booking interview. In: Robinson S, Thomson AM, eds. Midwives, Research and Childbirth. London: Chapman and Hall 1989;1.

Methven RC. The antenatal booking interview. In: Waltham M, Alexander J, Levy V, Roch S, eds. Midwifery Practice. Vol 1. London: MacMillan 1990:42-57.

9. THE POLICY AND PRACTICE IN MIDWIFERY STUDY
January 1983 - December 1988

Jo Garcia, Social Scientist, Sarah Ayers, Administrator, Sally Garforth, Research Midwife. **Contact:** Jo Garcia, National Perinatal Epidemiology Unit, Radcliffe Infirmary, Oxford OX2 6HE. Tel: 0865 224170

Formed integral or additional part of a job. Funded by employer and by funding agency(ies): Department of Health, Birthright, Iolanthe Trust.

Abstract: The Policy and Practice in Midwifery Study is a study of policy and policy-making in midwifery care in English health authorities.

In 1984, a questionnaire survey of the heads of midwifery services in England was conducted. The survey covered many aspects of policy in normal intrapartum and postpartum care. Ninety-three per cent of districts participated. A second phase of the study, which involved a detailed exploration of the links between policy and practice in a small number of districts, was conducted during the first half of 1985. This was carried out by interviews with midwives and parents, and by observation of specific aspects of care.

Various aspects of midwifery care are explored in the main publications arising from the project. Marked variations were found between policies in different places and, in some cases, policies were at odds with research evidence about good care. Practice, where observed, did not always follow directly from the stated policies. The study provided information about the involvement of midwives in determining policies for normal labour and postnatal care.

Keywords: LABOUR (CARE), LABOUR (NORMAL), MIDWIFERY POLICIES, POLICY MAKING, POSTNATAL CARE, ROUTINES

Garcia J, Garforth S, Ayers S. Midwives confined? Labour ward policies and routines. Research and the Midwife Conference, Manchester 1985. Research and the Midwife Conference Proceedings 1986;2-30.

Garcia J, Garforth S, Ayers S. The policy and practice in midwifery study: introduction and methods. Midwifery 1987;3:2-9.

Garforth S, Garcia J. Admitting - a weakness or a strength? Routine admission of a woman in labour. Midwifery 1987;3:10-24.

Garcia J. The role and structure of the Maternity Service Liaison Committee. Health Trends 1987;19:17-19.

Chalmers I, Garcia J, Post S. Regulating labour and delivery. In: Chalmers I, Enkin M, Keirse MJNC, eds. Effective Care in Pregnancy and Childbirth. Oxford: Oxford University Press 1989;815-9.

Garforth S, Garcia J. Hospital admission practice. In: Chalmers I, Enkin M, Keirse MJNC, eds. Effective Care in Pregnancy and Childbirth. Oxford: Oxford University Press 1989;820-6.

Garcia J, Garforth S. Parents and newborn babies in the labour ward. In: Garcia J, Kilpatrick R, Richards M, eds. The Politics of Maternity Care. Oxford: Oxford University Press 1991;163-82.

Garcia J, Garforth S. Midwifery policies and policy making. In: Robinson S, Thomson A, eds. Midwives, Research and Childbirth. Vol 2. London: Chapman and Hall.

Garforth S, Garcia J. Breastfeeding policies in practice - "No wonder they get confused". Midwifery 1989;5:75-83.

Garcia J, Garforth S. Labour and delivery routines in English consultant maternity units. Midwifery 1989;5:155-62.

10. POSTNATAL CARE IN GRAMPIAN - OBJECTIVES, EFFECTIVENESS AND RESOURCE USE
July 1988 - July 1992

Charis Glazener, Wellcome Research Fellow Postnatal Care. **Contact:** Charis Glazener, University of Aberdeen, Health Services Research Unit, Drew Kay Wing, Polwarth Building, Foresterhill, Aberdeen AB9 2ZD. Tel: 0224 681818 Ex 53732.

Funded as integral or additional part of a job and by funding agency(ies): Wellcome Trust.

Abstract: (Not updated since 1991). Postnatal care (PNC) has remained fundamentally unchanged for thirty-five years and has been subject to very little research. We have embarked on an evaluation of PNC within the Grampian region that will describe the objectives and processes of PNC, the resources it consumes and its effectiveness in terms of professional criteria and patient outcomes. The study will focus on criteria for postnatal discharge, the effects of early discharge, breastfeeding, coping strategies and postnatal complications, treatment and support.

Data will be collected by interview and questionnaire surveys of consumers and providers of PNC and from the Aberdeen Maternity and Neonatal Databank. We will use this information to assess whether the current processes of care need to be changed. If so, we will work towards the implementation of such changes and design a subsequent study to evaluate them. The results will be analyzed by SIR and SPSSx. Piloting was carried out November 1989-March 1990, and the main period of data collection is May 1990-July 1991.

Keywords: BREASTFEEDING, DISCHARGE CRITERIA, OUTCOMES (POSTNATAL CARE), POSTNATAL CARE, POSTNATAL MORBIDITY, POSTNATAL SUPPORT

Evans, D. Acquiring parentcraft skills in Aberdeen. Health Services Research Unit student report No. 6. University of Aberdeen 1988.

Maclean, R. Breastfeeding in Aberdeen. Health Services Research Unit student report No. 8. University of Aberdeen 1989.

Van Wezel P. Postnatal issues in Grampian. Health Services Research Unit student report No. 10. University of Aberdeen 1990.

12. ACQUIRING PARENTCRAFT SKILLS IN ABERDEEN
July - August 1988

Isobel A MacPherson, Research Fellow, Donna E Evans, 3rd Year Medical Student.
Contact: Charis Glazener, University of Aberdeen, Health Services Research Unit, Drew Kay Wing, Polwarth Building, Foresterhill, Aberdeen AB9 2ZD. Tel: 0224 681818 Ex 53732.

Formed part of a course. Funded by funding agency(ies): Scottish Home and Health Department.

Abstract: The purpose of this study was to describe the sources from which mothers receive information about parentcraft, to explore the value that mothers gave to this information, and to relate their views to those expressed by providers of parentcraft instruction and postnatal care (PNC). One hundred and thirteen mothers were surveyed by a questionnaire: of these, twenty primigravid mothers were interviewed to explore in more depth their answers to the questionnaire. Data were also extracted from records. Six service providers were also interviewed (two postnatal ward sisters, two parentcraft sisters, a breast-care sister and a staff midwife).

The major source of parentcraft information was from books and magazines, although hospital staff, antenatal classes and family and friends also contributed. Most of the respondents, including all the providers of PNC, felt that parentcraft is something that needs to be taught, although some mothers thought that it could be learned 'on the job'. Conflicting advice caused problems. Gaps in information were identified by the mothers. Most respondents felt that information about looking after a baby should be given most appropriately before delivery and reinforced afterwards. Timing of antenatal classes should be more flexible.

Keywords: COMMUNICATION PROBLEMS, EDUCATION FOR PARENTHOOD, INFORMATION GAPS, INFORMATION SOURCES, NATIONAL CHILDBIRTH TRUST (NCT), POSTNATAL CARE

Evans D. Acquiring parentcraft skills in Aberdeen. Health Services Research Unit student report No. 6. University of Aberdeen 1988.

13. BREASTFEEDING IN ABERDEEN
July - August 1989

Charis Glazener, Wellcome Research Fellow Postnatal Care, Rhona Maclean, 3rd year medical student. **Contact:** Charis Glazener, University of Aberdeen, Health Services Research Unit, Drew Kay Wing, Polwarth Building, Foresterhill, Aberdeen AB9 2ZD. Tel: 0224 681818 Ex 53732.

Formed part of a course. Funded as integral or additional part of a job and by funding agency(ies): Wellcome Trust, Scottish Home and Health Department.

Abstract: The purpose of this study was to assess the incidence of problems with breastfeeding and their contribution to its success or failure. Specifically, we described factors influencing the decision to breastfeed, the timing of breastfeeding after delivery, the use of supplements of water or milk, the incidence of problems with breastfeeding, the reasons for giving it up and factors which contribute to giving it up. The data were gathered by three questionnaire surveys of fifty newly delivered women immediately after delivery, prior to discharge from the postnatal wards of the Aberdeen Maternity Hospital and two weeks after delivery at home. The data were analyzed by SPSSx. Sixty-eight per cent of breastfeeding women had problems in hospital and 35% continued to have these two weeks later at home. These included sore nipples, engorged breasts, difficulty latching on, cracked and bleeding nipples and baby feeding too often. Despite this, 81% of the respondents were still breastfeeding at two weeks after delivery. The use of milk supplements was significantly related to cessation of breastfeeding. Ninety-two per cent of the sample received help with breastfeeding in hospital and 74% continued to receive help at home.

Recommendations arising from these findings include: continuing to provide expert help with breastfeeding, particularly from women who have breast-fed themselves; improved attendance at antenatal classes on feeding methods; avoidance of milk supplements; more advice on prevention of breastfeeding problems; more flexibility; and fewer hard and fast rules about breastfeeding regimens.

Keywords: BREASTFEEDING, BREASTFEEDING (FAILURE), BREASTFEEDING (PROBLEMS), BREASTFEEDING (SUPPLEMENTS), BREASTFEEDING (SUPPORT)

Maclean R. Breastfeeding in Aberdeen. Health Services Research Unit student report No. 3. University of Aberdeen 1989.

14. RHONDDA KNOW YOUR MIDWIVES EVALUATION STUDY
September 1987 - June 1989

Carolyn Lester, Research Officer, Stephen Farrow, Senior Lecturer. **Contact:** Carolyn Lester, Research Team (UWCM), Ward 17, St David's Hospital, Cardiff CF1 9TZ. Tel: 0222 374818
For full details see under Management Studies (Record No. 14).

15. INFLUENCES UPON AND DURATION OF BREASTFEEDING
July 1989 - January 1990
C Newton, Midwife. **Contact:** C Newton, May Lodge Drive, Rufford Abbey Park, Newark NG21 9DE.

Formed an integral or additional part of a job. 6-12 hours/week of own time spent. Funded by employer: Nottingham City Hospital and by Osterfeed.

Abstract: This prospective study was undertaken from a consultant obstetric unit within the Trent region. The researcher intended to investigate the antenatal influences upon a mother to breastfeed, to establish how long the sample intended to breastfeed for, whether they achieved this aim, and finally what influenced the sample to discontinue breastfeeding.

The study yielded an 81% (n=202) response rate. It consisted of an initial structured interview with the mother whilst still in hospital. This was followed three months later by a postal questionnaire. Ethical clearance was sought and obtained, and the results were analyzed on computer using the SPSSx package at Nottingham University.

The results demonstrated that 87% (162) of the sample had decided to breastfeed their baby before attending antenatal clinic, which poses the question that attitudes in our society may be changing positively towards breastfeeding. If it were possible to identify how this change in socialisation towards breastfeeding has occurred it might be possible to expand it. Three months postnatally 44% (88) were still breastfeeding, though 47% (94) stated they felt a major disadvantage of breastfeeding was the demand on their time. Attitudes described in this study confirm Gunn's (1986) findings that a more positive response was given whilst the women were in hospital than later at home. Using a Wilcoxon matched pair signed rank test, the difference in these positive responses did reach statistical significance at the 0.05 level.

Keywords: BREASTFEEDING, BREASTFEEDING (DURATION), INFANT FEEDING (DECISIONS), PROSPECTIVE STUDY, SOCIALISATION

18. THE ROLE OF THE INTREPRETER/LINKWORKER IN THE MATERNITY SERVICE
September 1987 - September 1989
L Hayes, Midwifery Tutor. **Contact:** L Hayes, Rectory Close, Drayton Bassett, Tamworth, Staffordshire B79 3UH
For full details see under Management Studies (Record No. 18).

19. BASIC SUPPORT IN LABOUR: INTERACTION WITH AND AROUND LABOURING WOMEN
October 1979 - May 1987
M J Kirkham, Midwifery Sister. **Contact:** M J Kirkham, Albert Road, Sheffield S8 9QY.

Formed part of a course. 6-12 hours/week of own time spent. Funded by funding agency(ies): Department of Health.

Abstract: Much has been written in recent years expressing dissatisfaction with the care women receive during labour. This study endeavoured to look at what actually happens during labour. Data were gathered by means of participant observation. One hundred and thirteen labours were observed: ninety in a consultant unit, eighteen in rural GP Units and five home confinements. Interviews were also conducted with antenatal and postnatal women and with midwives. The role, activities and language of the four major participants, (patients, husbands, midwives and doctors), were examined and contrasted in the different settings. The pressures of the power structure in their setting were shown in the words and action of all involved. Who controlled the labour depended upon whose territory the patient laboured on. In the consultant unit the patient was processed as a work object by midwives with little autonomy. The consultant unit was definitely the doctors' territory. The GP Unit was the midwives' territory and the home the territory of those whose home it was.

All the patients stressed their need for information. Tactics used by patients and husbands to gain information were examined, as were the ways in which midwives dealt with this search for information, usually without meeting patients' needs. Actions with regard to pain and fear similarly showed staff acting to maintain the control appropriate to the setting rather than meet patients' perceived needs. Pressures upon patients and midwives were examined, particularly their lack of language and concepts appropriate to labour as they experienced it. Both were therefore reduced to actions not consistent with their own priorities or with their accurate view of each other's needs and values.

Keywords: COMMUNICATION, EXPERIENCE (WOMEN'S), INFORMATION GIVING, LABOUR, LABOUR (CONTROL OF), MIDWIFERY

Kirkham MJ. Admission in Labour: Teaching the patient to be patient? Midwives Chronicle 1983;Feb:44-5.

Kirkham MJ. Labouring in the dark - limitations on the giving of information to enable patients to orientate themselves to the likely events and timescale of labour. In: Wilson-Barnett J, ed. Nursing Research: Ten Studies in Patient Care. Chichester: John Wiley 1983.

Kirkham MJ. Basic supportive care in labour: Interaction with and around labouring women. Unpublished PhD thesis. Manchester University, Faculty of Medicine 1987.

Kirkham MJ. Midwives and information-giving during labour. In: Robinson S, and Thomson AM, eds. Midwives, Research and Childbirth. London: Chapman and Hall 1989;1:117-38.

20. VARIATION OF CERVICAL DILATATION ESTIMATION BY MIDWIVES, DOCTORS, STUDENT MIDWIVES AND STUDENT MEDICAL STUDENTS IN 1985: A SMALL STUDY USING SIMULATION CERVICAL MODELS

July - October 1985

S E E Robson, Midwife Teacher, Dept of Midwifery Education. **Contact:** S E E Robson, Lime Close, Syston, Leicester LE7 8AZ.

6-12 hours/week of own time spent.

Abstract: This study was a randomized research trial to determine the accuracy of obstetricians, midwives, medical students and student midwives in estimating cervical dilatation on simulation cervix models. Fifty people participated, working in four different consultant units within two Regional Health Authorities.

Five imitation cervices were made to specific 'dilatations'. One had 'bulging membranes' and suture lines with a posterior fontanelle on another. A 'vaginal wall' and 'introitus' assisted with realism and prevented the participants from 'peeping.' The participants performed 'vaginal examinations' and recorded their findings. Accuracy was calculated on a percentage basis. There are sixteen tables.

The conclusions were as follows: 1) the greater the cervical dilatation, the less accurate the estimation of that dilatation was; 2) the presence of bulging caused practitioners significantly to underestimate or overestimate cervical dilatation compared with the same dilatation on another model with 'absent membranes'; 3) there was minimal difference between the accuracy of qualified doctors and midwives, except for the model with bulging membranes where 78% of the midwives overestimated the dilatation compared with 58% of the doctors; 4) dilatation was significantly overestimated when suture lines and a fontanelle could be felt; 5) staff midwives and student midwives were inaccurate at estimating effacement of the cervix; 6) women doctors were more accurate at estimating cervical dilatation than male doctors; and 7) further work on the accuracy of vaginal examination in labour needs to be conducted.

Keywords: CERVICAL DILATATION, DOCTORS' SKILLS, MEMBRANES, MIDWIFERY SKILLS, SIMULATION MODELS, VAGINAL EXAMINATIONS

Robson SEE. Variation of cervical dilatation estimation by midwives, doctors, student midwives and medical students in 1985 - A small study using cervical simulation models. Research and the Midwife Conference Proceedings 1991:26-35.

21. EARLY POSTNATAL TRANSFER: DOES IT PROVIDE MOTHER AND BABY THE BEST START TOGETHER?

October 1989 - April 1991

Joanne Whelton, Regional Co-ordinator CESDI. **Contact:** Joanne Whelton, Dept of Epidemiology & Medical Statistics, London Hospital Medical College (at QMW), Mile End Road, London E1 4NS. Tel: 071 982 6979

Funded as integral or additional part of a job and by Maws/RCM Research Scholarship. Formed part of a course. 2-6 hours/week of own time spent.

Aims of the study: To explore the experience of mothers undergoing early transfer home following delivery, and to identify areas where improvements could be made.

Ethics committee approval gained: Yes

Research design: Descriptive – Qualitative and Quantitative – Survey

> **Data collection:**
> > **Techniques used:**
> > > Questionnaire.
> > **Time data were collected:**
> > > 36 weeks following delivery prior to transfer home, and 6 weeks postnatally.
> > **Testing of any tools used:**
> > > Questionnaires were piloted.
> > **Topics covered:**
> > > Women's experience of midwifery support and advice given to them about transfer home.
> > **Setting for data collection:**
> > > Hospital and community within inner city environment.

> **Details about sample studied:**
> > **Planned size of sample:**
> > > 150 women.
> > **Rationale for planned size:**
> > > To include range of experiences.
> > **Entry criteria:**
> > > Both primiparae and multiparae.
> > > No medical/obstetric complications - ie. only those women who could be identified as suitable for short stay.
> > **Sample selection:**
> > > Opportunistic.
> > **Actual sample size:**
> > > 120 women at early stages.
> > > 80 women at 3rd questionnaire stage.
> > **Response rate:**
> > > 80% at early stages.
> > > 56% at 3rd questionnaire stage.

> **Interventions, Outcomes and Analysis**
> > **Analysis:**
> > > Manual content analysis.

Results: A need was identified for improved communication, advice/information, re-assurance, individualised care planning, and appropriate education in parentcraft-skills.

Recommendations for further research: Repeat study of even shorter length of stay to see if women's needs are met.

Keywords: EARLY POSTNATAL TRANSFER, MIDWIFERY PRACTICE (CHANGES), POSTNATAL SUPPORT

Whelton J M. Early postnatal transfer, does it offer the mother and her baby the best start together? Research and the Midwife Conference Proceedings 1991:43-51.

23. THE SCOTTISH LOW BIRTHWEIGHT STUDY
September 1984 - December 1990

G M McIlwaine, Community Medicine Specialist, V Fletcher, Research Assistant, D Lloyd, Paediatrician. **Contact:** V Fletcher, Randolph Road, Broomhill, Glasgow G11 7LG.

Funded as integral or additional part of a job by funding agency(ies): Scottish Home and Health Department. 6-12 hours/week of own time spent.

Abstract: (Not updated since 1990). A follow-up study was undertaken of infants weighing less than 1750g at birth, who were born to women resident in Scotland in 1984. The outcome of these children at the age of two years was examined in relation to their pregnancies, their perinatal experience, subsequent illness and the environment in which they were reared. During 1984, there were 908 live-born infants eligible for inclusion in the study; 99% of them were included. Survival rate at two years was 71%. No child weighing less than 650g or born before twenty-four weeks' gestation survived to two years. Assessment carried out on 92% of the children at two years (81% by doctors and 11% by health visitors) did not detect any impairment in 69% of those seen. Nearly 9% of the children showed evidence of neuromotor impairment; 3% had visual impairment and 7% had squints; 3% were hearing impaired and 14% developmentally delayed. There were no significant differences between singleton and multiple births in these outcomes. Many of the children had significant medical problems resulting from their neonatal problems and required frequent hospital admission. Parents reported a number of problems in caring for their low birthweight infants, the most common being sleep disturbance.

Keywords: GEOGRAPHICAL STUDY, LOW BIRTHWEIGHT, NEONATAL PROGRESS, OUTCOMES (AGE 2 YEARS)

McIlwaine GM, Mutch L, Pritchard C, Fletcher DV. The Scottish low birthweight study. The pregnancies, neonatal progress and outcome at two years. Report of the Scottish Home and Health Department.
Fletcher DV. Low birthweight study F.O.C.U.S. (Scottish Health Visitors Association Magazine) Issue No.14, Spring 1989;10-14

24. SOME FACETS OF SOCIAL INTERACTION SURROUNDING THE MIDWIFE'S DECISION TO RUPTURE THE MEMBRANES
January - December 1984

Chris Henderson, Director of Research & Development. **Contact:** Chris Henderson, Birmingham & Solihull, College Midwifery, Sorrento Maternity Hospital, Thorne House, Anderton Park Road, Birmingham B13 9HE. Tel: 021 442 4477

Funded as integral or additional part of a job by employer and by funding agency(ies): West Birmingham Health Authority, Maws/RCM Research Scholarship. Formed part of a course. 12-20 hours/week of own time spent.

Abstract: This paper describes the findings of a study conducted in Birmingham in 1984 of women in normal labour. The main focus of the study was on the interaction between the midwife and woman when the decision to rupture the membranes is made during vaginal examination. Since it is impossible to dissociate other factors within the working environment which may affect the midwife's decision and degree of consultation with the woman, the study also looked at some of those influences which affected the outcome of the encounter. Twenty-eight women from social classes 3 and 4 were observed during vaginal examination and interviewed afterwards. Twenty-two midwives participated and were also observed during vaginal examination and interviewed afterwards. The hypothesis being tested, 'that the midwife performs rupture of the membranes without consulting the woman', was supported.

The results showed that although explanations were given, no discussion with the women took place and, in general, most women failed to obtain information because the midwives were only prepared to give it to those who questioned. The study also showed that on the majority of occasions (twenty-four) midwives did not seek consent from the women when performing a vaginal examination or rupturing the membranes. The women accepted without question whatever was done to them, and as there was no challenge the midwives accepted this as consent to go ahead. The midwives deceived themselves as to the reasons for their actions, thinking that they were using their own judgement when, in practice, they were unwittingly following a routine. Their decisions were either directly or indirectly influenced by medical staff, as indicated by several midwives who mentioned the existence of tension and sometimes conflict if the membranes were not ruptured.

Keywords: ACTIVE MANAGEMENT, ARTIFICIAL RUPTURE OF THE MEMBRANES, COMMUNICATION, DECISION MAKING, EXPERIENCE (WOMEN'S), HOSPITAL POLICY, LABOUR, MIDWIFERY PROCEDURES, VAGINAL EXAMINATIONS

Henderson C. Artificial rupture of the membranes. Unpublished dissertation. Held in the following libraries: ENB, RCM, Warwick University, Birmingham and Solihull College of Midwifery Education & Training.

Henderson C. Artificial rupture of the membranes. In: Alexander J, Levy V, Roche S, eds. Midwifery Practice, Vol 2 Intrapartum Care. Macmillan Education Ltd. 1990;42-57.

Henderson C. Artificial rupture of the membranes. Nursing Times 1987; 83:63-4.

25. SALIVA AND BLOOD PETHIDINE CONCENTRATIONS IN THE MOTHER AND THE NEWBORN BABY

January 1978 - December 1979

Stephen W D'Souza, Senior Lecturer & Consultant Paediatrician, Steven Freeborn, MSc Student, R T Calvert, Lecturer in Pharmacy, Thomas MacFarlane, Senior Registrar in Obstetrics, Patricia Black, Research Midwife. **Contact:** Tricia Murphy-Black, Research and Development Adviser, Simpson Memorial Maternity Pavilion, Lauriston Place, Edinburgh EH3 9EF. Tel: 031 229 2477 Ex 4357

Funded as integral or additional part of a job by funding agency(ies): North West Regional Health Authority.

Abstract: In a group of mothers who received pethidine intramuscularly during labour, drug concentrations were higher in saliva than in blood, and there was a significant correlation (p<0.001) between saliva and blood concentrations measured between one hour and four hours and twenty minutes after dosage. In newborn babies, the pethidine concentrations detected in pharyngeal aspirates were higher than those in umbilical arterial or umbilical venous blood, but there was no correlation. Pethidine was also detected in the saliva from babies for forty-eight hours after birth. Furthermore, the appreciably higher levels in breastfed babies suggest that such babies may receive a dose of pethidine in the milk.

Keywords: BREASTFEEDING, LABOUR, PAIN RELIEF (LABOUR), PETHIDINE

Freeborn SF, Calvert RT, Black P, MacFarlane T, D'Sousa SW. Saliva and blood pethidine concentrations in the mother and the newborn baby. British Journal of Obstetrics and Gynaecology 1980;87:966-9.

26. PELVIC FLOOR EXERCISES IN POSTNATAL CARE

January - July 1985

Jennifer Sleep, Research Co-ordinator, Adrian Grant, Epidemiologist. **Contact:** Jennifer Sleep, Berkshire College of Nursing & Midwifery, Royal Berkshire Hospital, Craven Road, Reading, Berkshire RG1 5AN. Tel: 0734 877651

Funded as integral or additional part of a job and by funding agency(ies): Oxford Regional Health Authority, ICI.

Abstract: The purpose of the study was to evaluate the extent to which a programme of more intensive pelvic floor exercises prevents urinary incontinence three months after delivery.

Eighteen hundred women recruited within twenty-four hours of vaginal delivery were randomly allocated to one of two pelvic floor exercise policies. Nine hundred women received instruction currently available to all postnatal women in the West Berkshire Health District, and 900 were encouraged to follow a more intensive regime endorsed by the use of a four-week exercise diary. When assessed on the tenth postnatal day, women in the intensive exercise group were more likely to have performed their exercises than women allocated to the normal policy (78% versus 68%). This difference was greater three months after delivery (58% versus 42%). The chi-square test was used to compare the frequencies of outcome measured in the two groups. At three months postpartum, one in five women admitted some degree of urinary incontinence, 5% needing to wear a pad for some or all of the time. Three per cent had faecal incontinence. These frequencies were very similar in the two groups allocated to the different regimes. Women in the intensive exercise group were less likely to report perineal pain at this time. However, there were no differences in dyspareunia or in the timing of resumption of sexual intercourse. Women in the intensive exercise group reported feeling less depressed, which may reflect the lower prevalence of perineal pain; alternatively, it may be a consequence of the greater 'social' support provided by the intensive programme.

This study provides no support for the hypothesis that a programme of more intensive postnatal exercise education prevents either urinary or faecal incontinence. It is possible that the substantial resources involved could be used more effectively. At the time when this study was designed there was considerable reluctance on the part of the physiotherapists to deprive women of any component of the standard exercise programme; in the light of these results, a more flexible approach is now possible which would make such a design both acceptable and desirable.

Keywords: DYSPAREUNIA, FAECAL INCONTINENCE, PELVIC FLOOR EXERCISES, URINARY INCONTINENCE

Sleep J, Grant A. Pelvic floor exercises in postnatal care. Midwifery 1987;3:158-64.
Grant A, Sleep J. Relief of perineal pain and discomfort after childbirth. In: Chalmers I, Enkin M, Keirse MJNC, eds. Effective Care in Pregnancy and Childbirth. Oxford: Oxford University Press 1989:800-26.
Sleep J. Perineal management and care. A series of five randomised controlled trials. In: Robinson S, Thomson AM, eds. Midwives, Research and Childbirth. Vol 2. London: Chapman Hall 1991;199-251.
Sleep J. Postnatal perineal care. In: Alexander J, Roche S, Levy V, eds. Midwifery Practice Series. Vol 3. Basingstoke: Macmillan Education Ltd. 1990;1-17.

27. A STUDY OF INFANT GROWTH IN RELATION TO THE TYPE OF FEEDING
January 1977 - December 1978

Stephen W D'Souza, Senior Lecturer & Consultant Paediatrician, Patricia Black, Research Midwife. **Contact:** Tricia Murphy-Black, Research and Development Adviser, Simpson Memorial Maternity Pavilion, Lauriston Place, Edinburgh EH3 9EF. Tel: 031 229 2477 Ex 4357

Funded as integral or additional part of a job by North West Regional Health Authority.

Abstract: A total of 133 breastfed newborn babies, and 106 bottle-fed babies, were selected and studied prospectively. Details taken of feeding practices have shown that by five to seven weeks of age bottle feeds had been introduced in about 50% of breastfed babies. Entirely breastfed babies received their first solid food later than breast- and bottle-fed or entirely bottle-fed babies when such babies were in social class I, II, or III, but in social class IV and V entirely breastfed babies were weaned at a similar age to those in the other two groups of babies. In the first five to seven weeks of life there was a significant negative correlation between the increase in skin-fold thickness and the skin-fold thickness at birth. The study has also shown that the present practice of feeding babies modified milks retards weight gain and the increase in subcutaneous fat in male babies.

Keywords: ARTIFICIAL FEEDING, BREASTFEEDING, INFANT FEEDING, INFANT WEIGHT GAIN, WEANING

D'Souza SW, Black P. A study of infant growth in relation to the type of feeding. Early Human Development 1979;3:245-55.

29. COMPARATIVE STUDIES IN THE THIRD STAGE OF LABOUR
March 1987 - February 1989

Cecily M Begley, Academic Tutor. **Contact:** Cecily M Begley, Faculty of Nursing, Royal College of Surgeons in Ireland, Dublin. Tel: 353 1 4780200 Ex 2113

Funded as integral or additional part of a job, by employer and by funding agency(ies): Coombe Hospital Research & Development Trust Fund, Jannsen Pharmaceuticals, Dublin.

Abstract: A randomized controlled trial of 1429 women was carried out to compare 'active' management of the third stage of labour, using IV Ergometrine 0.5 mgs, with a method of 'physiological' management, in women at 'low risk' of haemorrhage. In the 'active' management group, a higher incidence of the following complications was found: manual removal of placenta ($p < 0.0005$), problems such as nausea ($p < 0.0005$), vomiting ($p < 0.0005$), and severe after birth pains ($p < 0.02$), hypertension ($p < 0.0001$) and secondary postpartum haemorrhage ($p < 0.02$).

The incidence of postpartum haemorrhage (blood loss greater than 500 mls) and postnatal haemoglobin less than 10 gms/100 mls were higher in the 'physiological' group ($p < 0.0005$, $p < 0.002$). No difference was found in the need for blood transfusion in either group.

A separate sub-study, with 168 women in each of the two groups, examined the possible effects of Ergometrine on serum prolactin levels and the duration of breastfeeding. No difference was found in peak (post-suckling) serum prolactin levels taken from 126 women between forty-eight and seventy-two hours postnatally. Women who did not receive the drug Ergometrine were more likely to continue breastfeeding for longer than four weeks than those who did ($p < 0.05$). The routine use of IV Ergometrine 0.5 mgs during the third stage of labour in women at 'low risk' of haemorrhage does not appear to be necessary and has many adverse effects. Further studies comparing different methods of 'physiological' management are recommended in order to reduce to a minimum the incidence of postpartum haemorrhage and anaemia.

Keywords: ACTIVE MANAGEMENT, BREASTFEEDING, ERGOMETRINE, LABOUR, PHYSIOLOGICAL MANAGEMENT, POSTPARTUM HAEMORRHAGE, PROLACTIN LEVELS, THIRD STAGE

Begley CM. Comparative studies in the third stage of labour. Unpublished MSc. thesis 1989. Trinity College, Dublin.

Begley CM. A comparison of active and physiological management of the third stage of labour. Midwifery 1990;6:3-17.

Begley CM. The effect of Ergometrine on breastfeeding. Midwifery 1990;6:60-72.

Begley CM. Post-partum haemorrhage - who is at risk? Midwives Chronicle 1991;101:102-6.

Begley CM. The factors affecting duration of breast-feeding. Conference Proceedings 23rd International Congress of the ICM 1993;1:163-76.

30. A RETROSPECTIVE STUDY OF PERINEAL TRAUMA
December 1984 - May 1985
Cecily M Begley, Academic Tutor. **Contact:** Cecily M Begley, Faculty of Nursing, Royal College of Surgeons in Ireland, Dublin. Tel: 353 1 4780200 Ex 2113

2-6 hours/week of own time spent.

Abstract: A retrospective study was carried out to ascertain the episiotomy, laceration and intact perineum rates for 2,422 women who had singleton normal deliveries over thirty-seven weeks' gestation in one maternity hospital in Dublin. The overall episiotomy rate was 54% for primigravidae, 25% for 'para 1' and 5% for 'para 2 and greater'. The difference in midwives' practice when delivering primigravidae was found to be highly significant (p<0.001), with episiotomy rates ranging from 6% to 84% and 'no suture' rates from 57% to 10%. The presence of a consultant obstetrician at delivery had an effect (either positive or negative) on the midwife's decisions re episiotomy and/or the need for perineal suturing. It is recommended that episiotomy and laceration rates be monitored closely, and the indication for episiotomy be recorded in the delivery notes, in an effort to reduce unnecessary intervention.

Keywords: ACTIVE MANAGEMENT, EPISIOTOMY, INTERVENTIONS, LABOUR, MIDWIFERY PROCEDURES (INFLUENCES), PERINEAL TRAUMA, SECOND STAGE (MANAGEMENT)

Begley CM. Episiotomy - use or abuse? Nursing Review 1986;4:4-7.

31. A FOLLOW-UP STUDY OF PERINEAL TRAUMA
September 1986 - February 1987

Cecily M Begley, Academic Tutor. **Contact:** Cecily M Begley, Faculty of Nursing, Royal College of Surgeons in Ireland, Dublin. Tel: 353 1 4780200 Ex 2113

2-6 hours/week of own time spent.

Abstract: A retrospective study was carried out on 2,144 women to ascertain whether any change had taken place in episiotomy, laceration and intact perineum rates following the dissemination of results of a previous study (Record No. 30).

A six-month period elapsed between the two studies to allow midwives time to practise deliveries without the frequent use of episiotomy. Both studies were carried out on women who had singleton, normal deliveries over thirty-seven weeks' gestation in one maternity hospital in Dublin. A significant reduction in episiotomy rate had occurred in the primigravid group, from 54% to 34% ($p < 0.0001$), in the 'para 1' group from 25% to 7% ($p < 0.0001$), and in the 'para 2 and greater' group from 5% to 2% ($p < 0.0005$). No increase in lacerations requiring sutures was seen in the primigravid or 'para 1' group, and in the 'para 2 and greater' group a significant decrease was found ($p < 0.0001$). A significant difference in midwives' practice was still found in the primigravidae group ($p < 0.005$), with episiotomy rates varying from 12.5% to 64% and 'no suture' rates from 68% to 20%.
The practice of this group of midwives has changed considerably following dissemination of research findings. A further decrease in episiotomy rates and increase in 'no suture' rates is possible as midwives' practice still differs significantly.

Keywords: EPISIOTOMY, INTERVENTIONS, MIDWIFERY PRACTICE (CHANGES), PERINEAL TRAUMA

Begley CM. Episiotomy - A change in midwives' practice. Irish Nursing Forum and Health Services 1987;5:6:12-4,34.

32. A RANDOMISED CONTROLLED TRIAL TO EVALUATE THE USE OF SPONTANEOUS BEARING DOWN EFFORTS IN THE SECOND STAGE OF LABOUR
May 1989 - June 1991

Helen Spiby, Midwifery Research Sister, Catherine Molloy, Staff Midwife, Susan Alston, Staff Midwife. **Contact:** Helen Spiby, Maternity Unit, Northern General Hospital, Herries Road, Sheffield S5 7AU. Tel: 0742 434343 blp 162

Funded as integral or additional part of a job by employer: Sheffield Health Authority, Sheffield District School of Midwifery.

Abstract: (Not updated since 1991). The aim of the study is to assess the effects of spontaneous maternal bearing down efforts on: 1) the progress of the second stage of labour; 2) maternal well-being; and 3) perinatal outcome.

The method used will be a randomized controlled trial in which women will be allocated to one of two management groups, as follows: 1) conventional bearing down efforts directed by the midwife during the second stage of labour; 2) mothers will use only spontaneous expulsive efforts during the second stage of labour. A sample size of 400 is required. Analysis of the results will be on an 'intention to treat' basis.

Keywords: LABOUR, MATERNAL EFFORT, PUSHING (DIRECTED), PUSHING (SPONTANEOUS), SECOND STAGE

34. THE EFFECT OF THE PRESENT PATTERNS OF MATERNITY CARE UPON THE EMOTIONAL NEEDS OF MOTHERS, WITH PARTICULAR REFERENCE TO THE POST-NATAL PERIOD
October 1980 - December 1982

J A Ball, Lecturer/Self-employed consultant. **Contact:** J A Ball, Elm Close, Saxilby, Lincolnshire LN1 2QH.

Funded as integral or additional part of a job and by funding agency(ies): DHSS Nursing Research Scholarship.

Abstract: This longitudinal study of 279 women, based upon the coping process (Lazarus 1966), examined the degree to which maternal factors associated with vulnerability to depression, the processes and events of labour and the puerperium, and the patterns of care during the puerperium were associated with different levels of maternal emotional well-being six weeks after delivery.

Each woman in the three-cohort sample was followed from the 36th week of pregnancy until six weeks post-delivery. Data about each woman were obtained by interview and questionnaire involving both the mother and the midwives caring for her. Personality was assessed by using Eysenck's personality inventory. Emotional well-being and satisfaction with motherhood were measured by a self-administered questionnaire based upon the work of Pitt (1968), Beck et al (1961) and Klaus and Kennel (1972).

The results, which were consistent with other studies of postnatal depression, indicate that patterns of care in delivery suites and postnatal wards have a considerable impact upon the adaptation process, and that midwives have a major contribution to make in the reduction and early identification of stresses which may, if unresolved, lead to postnatal depression. Major recommendations are made for the conduct of labour suites and postnatal wards.

Keywords: CONFLICTING ADVICE, EXPERIENCE (WOMEN'S), MATERNITY SERVICES, POSTNATAL CARE, POSTNATAL DEPRESSION, POSTNATAL DEPRESSION (RECOGNITION), PSYCHOLOGY, STRESS (MATERNAL)

Ball JA. The effect of the present patterns of maternity care upon the emotional needs of mothers with particular reference to the postnatal period. Unpublished MSc. thesis, Department of Nursing, Manchester University.

Ball JA. Reactions to Motherhood: The Role of Postnatal Care. Cambridge: Cambridge University Press 1987.

Ball JA. Postnatal care and adjustment to motherhood. In: Robinson S, Thomson AM, eds. Midwives, Research and Childbirth, Vol 1. London: Chapman and Hall. 1989:154-75.

Ball JA. Moving forward in postnatal care - some aspects of a research project. Midwives Chronicle 1983;96:1145.

Ball JA. What happens now? Nursing Times 1984;8:18-24.

Ball JA. Psychological problems in the puerperium. Nursing: the add on Journal of Clinical Nursing 1986;3:55-9.

Ball JA. Mothers need nurturing too. Nursing Times 1988;84:29-31.

35. SMOKING IN PREGNANCY: THE EFFECTS OF THE TAR, NICOTINE AND CARBON MONOXIDE YIELDS OF CIGARETTES ON THE FETUS IN LABOUR, AT BIRTH AND IN THE NEWBORN PERIOD
October 1977 - October 1981

Stephen W D'Souza, Senior Lecturer & Consultant Paediatrician, Jean K McFarlane, Professor of Nursing, Bernard Richards, Professor of Computing, Thomas McFarlane, Senior Registrar Obstetrics, R F Jennison, Consultant Pathologist, Patricia Black, Research Midwife. **Contact:** Tricia Murphy-Black, Research and Development Adviser, Simpson Memorial Maternity Pavilion, Lauriston Place, Edinburgh EH3 9EF. Tel: 031 229 2477 Ex 4357

Funded as integral or additional part of a job by North West Regional Health Authority. 2-6 hours/week of own time spent.

Abstract: As the influence of maternal nutrition on the growth of retarded babies of smokers is not clear, the weight gain in pregnancy and maternal subcutaneous fat were studied in 367 mothers. Fetal condition during labour and at birth was studied and anthropometric measurements of the baby examined the effect of smoking on overall size and subcutaneous fat at birth. The clinical condition of newborn babies of smokers was compared with those of non-smokers. The total consumption of nicotine, tar and carbon monoxide during pregnancy was calculated separately and compared with the effects of the number of cigarettes smoked each day on birthweight. The extent to which the smokers were advised against smoking and the effect this had on their smoking habits was investigated.

The maternal weight gain of smokers in pregnancy was less than that of non-smokers but there were no differences in the subcutaneous fat measured by skin-fold thicknesses, indicating that it was not maternal nutrition that caused the poor weight gain of the smokers. The condition of the babies during labour and at birth showed no differences between smokers and non-smokers. The increases in some haematological values demonstrated in smokers suggested a compensatory mechanism to cope with long-term raised levels of carboxyhaemoglobin. Despite overall growth retardation of the babies of smokers, subcutaneous fat was not affected, supporting the hypothesis that maternal nutrition is not a factor in the reduced size of the babies. Clinical conditions in the newborn period showed no differences between the babies of smokers and non-smokers. There was a strong correlation between the total consumption of nicotine, tar and carbon monoxide during pregnancy and the number of cigarettes smoked each day on birthweight. It is recommended that pregnant women should not be advised to change to a low tar/low nicotine cigarette.

Keywords: LOW TAR CIGARETTES, MATERNAL WEIGHT GAIN, PREGNANCY, SMOK-ING

D'Souza SW, Black PM, Williams N, Jennison RF. Effects of smoking during pregnancy upon the haematological values of cord blood. British Journal of Obstetrics and Gynaecology 1978;85:495-9.

D'Souza SW, Black PM, Richards B. Smoking in pregnancy: associations with skinfold thickness, maternal weight gain and fetal size at birth. British Medical Journal 1981;282:1661-3.

Black PM. Smoking in pregnancy: the effects of the tar, nicotine and carbon monoxide yields of cigarettes on the fetus in labour, at birth and in the newborn period. Unpublished MSc. thesis, University of Manchester 1981. Held in RCM library, London and the Steinberg Collection, RCN.

Black PM. The effects of low tar cigarettes on birthweight. Research and the Midwife Conference Proceedings 1982:14-24. King's College, University of London.

Black PM. Smoking during pregnancy - are low tar cigarettes safer? Nursing Mirror 1983;156:24-7.

Black P. Who stops smoking in pregnancy? Nursing Times 1984;80:59-61.

Black T. Smoking in pregnancy revisited. Midwifery 1985;1:135-45.

36. A PROSPECTIVE STUDY TO IDENTIFY CRITICAL FACTORS WHICH INDICATE MOTHERS' READINESS TO CARE FOR THEIR VERY LOW BIRTHWIEGHT BABY AT HOME
October 1984 - July 1988

Hazel E McHaffie, Research Fellow. **Contact:** Hazel E McHaffie, Institute of Medical Ethics, Edinburgh University Department of Medicine, Royal Infirmary, Lauriston Place, Edinburgh EH3 9YW. Tel: 031 229 2477 Ex 3387

Funded as integral or additional part of a job by Scottish Home and Health Department.

Abstract: The purpose of the research was to identify the phases mothers of very low birthweight (VLBW) infants pass through; to identify the critical factors which indicate their readiness to take the baby home; and to determine those individuals who are supportive throughout the experience.

The method used was a prospective, descriptive investigation. Six in-depth interviews were held with mothers of singleton VLBW infants (weighing 1500g or less); one week and one month after delivery; the day before the baby's discharge; one week, one month and three months after discharge. Diaries were kept, and demographic data recorded. Analysis was done using Copeland Chatterson cards and by categorisation of qualitative data. Six phases were identified:

a) While baby in hospital: anticipatory grief; anxious waiting; positive anticipation

b) After baby's discharge: anxious adjustment; exhausted accommodation; confident caring

Women who were unready to take the baby home had difficulty making and maintaining relationships and held very inappropriate perceptions of the infant. Partners were largely supportive. Grandmothers rallied round at times of crisis, but were not generally supportive at other times. Other relatives did not know how to help. Health visitors were not seen as supportive following the infant's discharge.

The implications were that more attention needs to be paid to the needs of families of VLBW babies, particularly in the period after the VLBW baby has gone home. Mothers' perceptions are vital in deciding when to send a VLBW infant home. It is recommended that progress through the phases should be carefully monitored for each woman and care tailored to her individual need. Some continuity of care should be provided across hospital/community experience. Criteria for discharge should include the mother's perception of her own readiness to care for the baby at home. Research should be carried out on the role of the extended family and the role of the health visitor.

Keywords: COMMUNITY CARE, DISCHARGE CRITERIA, EXPERIENCE (WOMEN'S), VERY LOW BIRTHWEIGHT

McHaffie HE. A prospective study to identify critical factors which indicate mothers' readiness to care for their very low birthweight baby at home. Unpublished PhD thesis, University of Edinburgh 1988.

McHaffie HE. Mothers of very low birthweight babies: how do they adjust? Journal of Advanced Nursing 1990;15:6-11.

McHaffie HE. Mothers of very low birthweight babies: who supports them? Midwifery 1989;5:113-21.

McHaffie HE. Isolated, but not alone. Nursing Times 1987;83:73-4.

McHaffie HE. Caring for very low birthweight babies: mothers' perceptions of care. Midwives Chronicle 1987;100:14-16.

McHaffie HE. Caring for very low birthweight babies. Nursing Times 1989;85:60.

37. A STUDY OF SUPPORT FOR FAMILIES WITH A VERY LOW BIRTHWIEGHT BABY

January 1988 - June 1991

Hazel E McHaffie, Research Fellow. **Contact:** Hazel E McHaffie, Institute of Medical Ethics, Edinburgh University Department of Medicine, Royal Infirmary, Lauriston Place, Edinburgh EH3 9YW. Tel: 031 229 2477 Ex 3387

Funded as integral or additional part of a job by Scottish Office Home & Health Department.

Aims of the study: To provide information on both professional and lay support of families with very low birthweight babies.

Ethics committee approval gained: Yes.

Research design: Descriptive – Qualitative and Quantitative – Survey

Data collection:
Techniques used:
Questionnaires.
Time data were collected:
Doctors and Nurses - April 1988.
Parents and Grandparents - 1 month after delivery and 1 month after baby's discharge home.
Testing of any tools used:
Questionnaires to Doctors and Nurses -piloted in three other neonatal units.
Questionnaires to parents and grandparents - piloted in seven regional units throughout Scotland.
Topics covered:
Opinions of visiting policies.
Role of Grandparents.
Perception of support - nature and effectiveness.
Setting for data collection:
Regional Neonatal Units.
Community.

Details about sample studied:
Planned size of sample:
265 qualified nurses/midwives
63 doctors
All families of infants born in 12 calender months in seven regional units who conformed to inclusion criteria (122)
Rationale for planned size:
Total population in seven units.
One calendar year of deliveries of VLBW babies who met criteria for inclusion.
Entry criteria:
Staff: Qualified.
Employed in Regional Neonatal Unit.
Families: English Speaking.
No previous VLBW infant.
The baby must weigh 1,500g or less, be a singleton, have no congenital abnormality.
Sample selection:
Total population of qualified staff.
Convenience sample of families.
Actual sample size:
Nurses/midwives - 198
Doctors - 33
Families: eligible - 122

actual - 97 agreed to participate
- 93 participated

Response rate:
Nurses/midwives - 75%
Doctors - 54%
Families: eligible - 80% agreed to participate
actual - 76% particpated

Interventions, Outcomes and Analysis:
Analysis:
SPSSX
Chi-square
Student's t-Test

Results:

1. Both doctors and nurses were dissatisfied with visiting policies for grandparents in their units. Many rated working with grandparents as not enjoyable.

2. All groups of respondents considered the principal role of grandparents was to offer emotional support to the parents and to facilitate the parents being with the baby.

3. Parents considered it necessary to have some restrictions in the interests of the babies but thought that they should decide who would best support them. Blanket rules were felt to be inappropriate and not to take account of individual circumstances. Although professional support was rated highly, nurses were seen to have too little time properly to listen to family members. Parents wanted grandparents to stay on the sidelines and only come into action when asked to do so. Maternal grandparents were perceived as more supportive than paternal by both mothers and fathers.

4. Grandparents often felt excluded by professional staff but were less critical of the visiting policies than the parents. They recognised the need to take their cues from the parents and not impose what they wanted to do to help.

5. Fundamental differences exist between lay and professional perceptions - for example, far more parents wished grandparents to obtain information on their behalf than both doctors and nurses felt should. In the perceptions of the majority, parents should have a greater say in how their families are managed.

Recommendations for further research: An experimental study comparing different forms of support following discharge of very low birthweight babies.

Keywords: EXPERIENCE (PARENTS'), GRANDPARENTS' ROLE, HOSPITAL POLICY, NEONATAL UNITS, PERCEPTIONS, SUPPORT (FAMILY), SUPPORT (PROFESSIONAL), VERY LOW BIRTHWEIGHT

McHaffie HE. Collaborating in research: Beyond the call of duty? Midwives Chronicle 1990;103:253-354.
McHaffie HE. Their child - our patient. Paediatric Nursing 1990;2:23-4.
McHaffie HE. Extended family support for parents of VLBW babies. Proceedings of 10th Anniversary Conference, Society for Reproductive and Infant Psychology. Girton College, Cambridge 1990.

McHaffie HE. Grandparents in a neonatal intensive care unit: promotion or relegation? Research and the Midwife Conference Proceedings, University of Manchester 1990:83-95.

McHaffie HE. Extended family support for parents of VLBW babies. Journal of Reproductive and Infant Psychology 1990;8:255.

McHaffie HE. Neonatal intensive care support systems. Nursing Times Short Report 1991;87:54-5.

McHaffie HE. Neonatal intensive care units: visiting policies for grandparents. Midwifery 1991;7:193-203.

McHaffie HE. A study of support for families with a very low birthweight baby. Nursing Research Unit Report, Department of Nursing Studies, University of Edinburgh 1991.

McHaffie HE. Neonatal intensive care in Scotland: visiting policies and support systems. Association of Registered Nurses in Newfoundland, Canada. Access 1992;12:6-7.

McHaffie HE. Staff perceptions of family needs in neonatal units. Journal of Clinical Nursing 1992;1:49-50.

McHaffie HE. Social support in the Neonatal Intensive Care Unit. Journal of Advanced Nursing 1992;17:279-87.

McHaffie HE. Supporting families of very low birthweight babies. HSR News, West of Scotland Health Services Research Network. Institute of Public Health 1992;5:3.

38. A STUDY OF THE USE OF BABY WIPES
February - May 1988

Maureen Williams, Senior Nurse. Denise Cooper, Staff Midwife **Contact:** Denise Cooper, Special Care Baby Unit, Maelor General Hospital, Wrexham, Clwyd. Tel: 0978 291100 Ex 5023

Funded as integral or additional part of a job.

Abstract: Having noted a large number of babies developing sore and dry bottoms in a special care baby unit, it was decided that research was needed to find the possible cause. At the time, a brand of baby wipes was used to clean babies' bottoms at nappy changes. It was decided to ascertain if the use of these wipes was the cause, and the total cost of using them.

The study involved 100 babies, fifty babies having their bottoms cleaned with baby wipes and fifty cleaned with water and cotton wool. The first fifty admissions to the unit were allocated to the group using baby wipes. The next fifty babies had their bottoms cleaned with water only. The gestation and weight of each baby, the length of time the two methods were used, the symptoms if any that developed and the treatment given to resolve the symptoms were all recorded during the study. The survey showed significantly less sore and dry bottoms when using water and cotton wool. Babies between twenty-seven and thirty-three weeks' gestation appeared to develop more dry bottoms than sore. Babies from thirty to thirty-five weeks developed more sore bottoms than any other gestation. However, there were a greater number of babies of that gestation admitted to the unit. The length of time the baby wipes were used appeared to be of no significance. The total cost of using baby wipes on fifty babies including the necessary treatment when symptoms developed was £77.54. When using water and cotton wool it was £37.24. It could not be proved that any of the symptoms that developed were due to the use of baby wipes. However, the increased number of sore, dry bottoms that was apparent when using baby wipes in comparison to the results when using water and cotton wool must be significant.

As a result of this study the unit now uses water and cotton wool. The method is working well and appears to be an effective, cheaper and kinder method to use.

Keywords: BABY WIPES, COST EFFECTIVENESS, DRY BOTTOMS, EQUIPMENT (ECONOMICS), NEONATAL UNITS, SORE BOTTOMS

39. MATERNAL CONSIDERATIONS IN THE USE OF PELVIC EXAMINATION IN LABOUR
January - June 1984

Karl W Murphy, Senior Registrar, Obstetrics and Gynaecology, Valerie Grieg, Senior Sister, Jo Garcia, Social Scientist, Adrian Grant, Epidemiologist. **Contact:** Karl W Murphy, Department of Obstetrics and Gynaecology, Queen Mother's Hospital, Yorkhill, Glasgow, Scotland G3 8SH. Tel: 041 339 8888

Funded as integral or additional part of a job. 2-6 hours/week of own time spent.

Abstract: In a randomized controlled trial involving 307 women, maternal discomfort associated with a policy of rectal examinations for routine management in labour was compared with that associated with an alternative policy of using vaginal examinations. The women, irrespective of parity, showed a clear preference for the vaginal examination policy: 28% in the rectal examination group compared with only 11% in the vaginal examination group described their examinations as 'very uncomfortable'. Furthermore, there was no evidence that the vaginal examination policy was associated with an increased risk of maternal or neonatal morbidity. The continuing use of routine rectal examinations in labour should be reassessed and greater consideration given to maternal feelings.

Keywords: EXPERIENCE (WOMEN'S), LABOUR, RECTAL EXAMINATION, VAGINAL EXAMINATIONS

Murphy K, Grieg V, Garcia J, Grant A. Maternal considerations in the use of pelvic examinations in labour. Midwifery 1986;2:93-7.

41. POSTNATAL CARE AT HOME: A DESCRIPTIVE STUDY OF MOTHER'S NEEDS AND THE MATERNITY SERVICES
May 1986 - September 1989

Tricia Murphy-Black, Research Fellow, Ian Atkinson, Research Fellow. **Contact:** Tricia Murphy-Black, Research and Development Adviser, Simpson Memorial Maternity Pavilion, Lauriston Place, Edinburgh EH3 9EF. Tel: 031 229 2477 Ex 4357

Funded as integral or additional part of a job by employer: Scottish Home and Health Department.

Abstract: The experience of 645 mothers delivered in hospital was studied by questionnaire and interview when their babies were ten days, one and three months old.

The study sample comprised 1% of the births in Scotland in 1986 and was representative of the study hospital and the country for various obstetric and social variables. The response rate to the questionnaires was good with 490 mothers (75.9%) returning all the questionnaires. The mean length of postnatal hospital stay was 4.6 days. Over 80% of the mothers were 'quite happy' with the time they left hospital. Community midwives visited 96% of mothers within twenty-four hours of returning home and 83% were seen by two or more midwives. The number of midwives visiting reduced continuity of care and contributed to the problem of conflicting advice. The mothers' reports demonstrated that the midwives gave mainly physical care, which was dictated by the time of discharge.

Over 50% of the mothers started breastfeeding, but this percentage was reduced by 13.3% by the time the babies were three months old. The main reasons reported by the mothers for discontinuing breastfeeding were 'insufficient milk' and an 'unsatisfied' baby. The mothers' comments illustrated both their lack of understanding of lactation and inaccurate advice from midwives and health visitors. The Nottingham Health Profile, a measure of perceived distress in six areas, identified those mothers who were having difficulty breastfeeding, problems with their babies and waking at night.

The recommendations included suggestions to reduce conflicting advice, and provide more continuous care by a smaller number of midwives. There is a need to improve the knowledge base of lactation physiology in basic and post-basic education. A distance learning package could fulfil this need. The mothers identified as distressed might benefit from increased support in the immediate postnatal period. As this study was descriptive there is a need for a structured evaluation of postnatal care.

Keywords: BREASTFEEDING, HEALTH VISITORS, MIDWIFE'S CARE, NOTTINGHAM HEALTH PROFILE, POSTNATAL CARE

Murphy-Black T. The use of the Nottingham Health Profile with postnatal women. Research and the Midwife Conference Proceedings. King's College, University of London 1987:31-42.

Murphy-Black T. Postnatal care at home - the experience of some Scottish mothers. Proceedings of the 21st Congress of the International Confederation of Midwives, The Hague 1987:47-50.

Murphy-Black T. Postnatal care at home: a descriptive study of mothers' needs and the maternity services. Nursing Research Unit Report 1989. University of Edinburgh.

Murphy-Black T. Midwives role in postnatal care. Nursing Times Short Report 1989;49:54-5.

Murphy-Black T. Coping with the normal newborn: the role of the professional. Paper presented to the Third International Conference of Maternity Nurse Researchers. Gothenburg, Sweden June 1990.

43. MIDWIVES' CARE OF THE BIRTH MOTHER: A QUALITATIVE STUDY OF THE CARE OF MOTHERS PLACING THEIR BABIES FOR ADOPTION

February 1989 - June 1992

Rosemary Mander, University lecturer. **Contact:** Rosemary Mander, Department of Nursing Studies, University of Edinburgh, Adam Ferguson Building, 40 George Square, Edinburgh EH8 9LL. Tel: 031 650 3896

Funded as integral or additional part of a job by employer and by funding agency(ies): Iolanthe Trust. 6-12 hours/week of own time spent.

Abstract: (Not updated since 1991). The research questions to be addressed are: 1) what are the experiences of mothers relinquishing their babies? 2) to what extent are the experiences of birth mothers in the UK similar to those of birth mothers in other countries? 3) how, in midwives' views, does the care they give to birth mothers differ from that provided for other mothers without babies? 4) how are decisions made regarding midwives' care of birth mothers? 5) what knowledge is involved in making these decisions? and 6) how is this knowledge acquired?

A qualitative approach is being used, firstly, because of the need for a holistic, sympathetic approach to explore such a sensitive topic and, secondly, because of the absence of data on midwifery care. Fieldwork for Phases 1 and 2 is complete. Phase 3 is being negotiated. In Phase 1, the help of certain birth parents' groups was enlisted. Contact was made and interviews were recorded and transcribed with twenty-two birth mothers who had relinquished their babies between six months and forty years ago. The aim was to assess the relevance of other countries' literature on the long-term feelings about such a loss.

In Phase 2, midwifery managers facilitated access to a sample of midwives who have been qualified for two years or more. Forty midwives agreed to interviews which were recorded and transcribed. The aim was to explore the care provided by the midwife, and, in particular, whether the care she gives to a birth mother differs from that provided for another mother without a baby.

In Phase 3, the aim is to observe and then describe the experience of the birth mother using a prospective, longitudinal technique. Interviews with a small group of birth mothers will focus on their experience of giving birth while, at the same time, coping with their decision to relinquish their babies, and the extent to which midwifery care had helped them through their experiences.

All the interviews were semi-structured. Informants were able to introduce relevant issues. The questions were based on the literature available, the researcher's own experience and issues raised by earlier informants.

Data analysis for Phases 1 and 2 is progressing using analytic description. Certain issues are emerging as crucial to the experience of the birth mother. These include: secrecy, the perception of activity or passivity, information giving, comparison with current birth mothers, a perception of not being believed, hiding emotions, and errors in caring and support.

Keywords: ADOPTION, BIRTH MOTHER, EXPERIENCE (WOMEN'S), GRIEF, MID-WIFE'S CARE, RELINQUISHMENT

Mander R. Midwives' care of the relinquishing mother. Paper presented at the 9th International Congress of Psychosomatic Obstetrics and Gynaecology, Amsterdam May 1989.

Mander R. Midwives' care of the relinquishing mother: preliminary data. Paper presented at the 8th Annual Conference of the Society for Infant and Reproductive Psychology, Oxford September 1989.

Mander R. Midwifery support of the mother relinquishing her baby for adoption: midwives' perceptions. Midwives Chronicle 1991;104:275-80.

44. A RANDOMIZED STUDY OF THE SITTING POSITION FOR DELIVERY USING A NEWLY DESIGNED OBSTETRIC CHAIR
May 1984 - March 1986

Peter Stewart, Consultant in Obstetrics and Gynaecology, Helen Spiby, Midwifery Research Sister. **Contact:** Helen Spiby, Maternity Unit, Northern General Hospital, Herries Road, Sheffield S5 7AU. Tel: 0742 434343 blp 162

Funded as integral or additional part of a job and by funding agency(ies): Trent Regional Health Authority, Rocket of London Ltd.

Abstract: The effect on labour and delivery of the upright position using a prototype birthing chair was assessed over a twenty-three month period. Comparison with the conventional semi-recumbent position was achieved by randomisation of 304 women, parity 0-4, in spontaneous labour at term. Transfer to the birthing chair was effected at the onset of the second stage of labour. The chair was maintained at a 15-20 degree angle from the upright. Management of the second stage was at the discretion of the attending midwifery and medical staff. Assisted vaginal delivery was performed in the allocated delivery position.

Analysis of results was based on the 'intention to treat' basis. All multiparae achieved spontaneous vaginal delivery. More primigravidae in the chair group required operative delivery, but this difference did not achieve statistical significance. Duration of second stage was similar amongst chair and bed allocated women. Fewer episiotomies were performed for the chair-allocated multiparae, but this was not apparent amongst primigravidae. Mean blood loss at delivery was significantly greater in chair-allocated patients as was the incidence of postpartum haemorrhage.

Assessment of satisfaction with delivery position undertaken by questionnaire reflected a greater degree of comfort amongst chair delivered mothers. Most mothers allocated to the birthing chair expressed a preference for that position for a subsequent birth compared to bed delivered mothers who still wished to try the birthing chair rather than the bed next time.

This study failed to show any beneficial obstetric effects from the use of the upright position for the second stage of labour and delivery but, rather, reflected, in the higher blood loss, a cause for concern.

Keywords: BIRTH CHAIR, LABOUR, PERINEAL TRAUMA, POSITIONS (DELIVERY), POSITIONS (LABOUR), POSTPARTUM HAEMORRHAGE, SECOND STAGE

Stewart P, Spiby H. A randomized study of the sitting position for delivery using a newly designed obstetric chair. British Journal of Obstetrics and Gynaecology 1989;96:327-33.

45. THE EFFECT OF AMNIOTOMY ON THE USE OF ANALGESIA DURING NORMAL LABOUR
January - August 1987
Pamela Foley, Research Midwife. **Contact:** Pamela Foley, Antenatal Clinic, Maternity Unit, Bradford Royal Infirmary, Bradford, West Yorkshire BD9 6RJ. Tel: 0274 542200 Ex 4511

Funded as integral or additional part of a job. 6-12 hours/week of own time spent.

Abstract: (Not updated since 1991). A randomized controlled trial was carried out to determine whether routine amniotomy during normal labour increased the use of analgesia. Women in spontaneous labour at term after a normal pregnancy, with a cephalic presentation and intact membranes, were eligible for inclusion. One hundred and twenty-two women were randomly allocated, using sealed opaque envelopes, to two groups: sixty-two were given routine amniotomy and sixty amniotomy only if indicated.
Analysis is on-going.

Keywords: ARTIFICIAL RUPTURE OF THE MEMBRANES, PAIN RELIEF (LABOUR)

46. RESEARCH OR RITUAL? A SURVEY OF THE MIDWIFE'S MANAGEMENT OF THE SECOND STAGE OF LABOUR
February 1990 - July 1991
D Skidmore, Director of Midwifery Education. **Contact:** D Skidmore, Chaworth Road, Ottershaw, Surrey KT16 OPE.

Formed part of a course. Funded by employer: Frances Harrison College of Healthcare.

Abstract: This study was a survey of the midwife's management of the second stage of labour. The mother's position in labour, the pushing technique used and the length of the second stage are all reviewed in the light of the Apgar score of the infant.

A questionnaire was used to collect the data, but the sample size at twenty-eight was smaller than the expected fifty. Consequently, no statistical analysis was performed. However, the data form a review of practice suitable for inclusion in a quality assurance programme. The majority of women chose to adopt the conventional semi-recumbent position for both the first and second stages of labour. The closed-glottis technique of pushing was encouraged by many midwives, and the mean length of the second stage is longer at sixty-nine minutes than the textbook quotations of forty-five to sixty minutes (Sweet, 1989).

Despite recording the presence of fetal distress in 50% of cases, no Apgar score was lower than six at one minute. This questions the reliability of the Apgar score and/or the significance of so-called "fetal distress". Clearly, there is a need for further research in this area to ensure the best possible care is available to mother and infant.

Keywords: APGAR SCORES, LABOUR, OUTCOMES (NEONATAL), PUSHING (DIRECTED), PUSHING (RESTRICTED), SECOND STAGE, SECOND STAGE (MANAGEMENT)

47. ARTIFICIAL RUPTURE OF MEMBRANES IN SPONTANEOUS LABOUR AT TERM: SOME FACTORS WHICH MAY AFFECT THE DECISION
June 1988 - March 1989

P M Lupton, Midwifery Sister. **Contact:** P M Lupton, Clarendon Road, Broadstone, Dorset BH18 9HY.

Formed part of a course. 6-12 hours/week of own time spent. Funded by employer and by funding agency(ies): East Dorset Health Authority, Iolanthe Trust.

Abstract: This paper describes the findings of a study, conducted in Dorset in 1988, of women in spontaneous labour at term. The aim of the project was: 1) to determine whether or not amniotomy in early 'normal' labour was beneficial to mother or fetus/baby; and 2) to ascertain the views of the midwives caring for them.

The quasi-experimental aspect of the study involved twenty-six women, of whom eighteen were expecting first babies. Eleven had an early amniotomy (cervical dilatation 2-4cms), and fifteen had the membranes left intact at this stage. Data concerning length of first stage of labour, analgesic requirements, and condition of the infants at birth were obtained for each group. Six of the women were subsequently interviewed regarding their views on artificial rupture of membranes in spontaneous labour. Forty-seven midwives working in two consultant obstetric units responded to questionnaires regarding their opinions on amniotomy, and the views of the consultant obstetricians were also sought.

The hypotheses that early amniotomy shortened the duration of labour and increased analgesic requirements were not proved for nulliparae, although there did appear to be a link between amniotomy and timing of the first dose of pethidine. The hypothesis that the state of the membranes does not significantly affect the condition of babies at birth was supported by the findings. Two-thirds of midwives considered the membranes should be left intact in 'normal' labour, whereas the consultant obstetricians generally preferred early amniotomy. However, the hypothesis that midwives' views were influenced by experience was not supported. The interviews with newly delivered mothers confirm that prior to labour, women have very little information concerning amniotomy, and therefore rely on the advice of the midwife or doctor.

Although this was a very small study, and the findings cannot be generalised, in nulliparous women experiencing 'normal' spontaneous labour at term no significant benefit resulted from early amniotomy. The researcher therefore concludes that when there are no known obstetric problems, individual women should be enabled to make a choice regarding the state of the membranes.

Keywords: ACTIVE MANAGEMENT, ARTIFICIAL RUPTURE OF THE MEMBRANES, LABOUR (SPONTANEOUS), MIDWIFERY PROCEDURES

Lupton P. Artificial rupture of the membranes in spontaneous labour at term. Midwives Chronicle 1992;105:76-8.

Lupton P. Assessing membrane rupture in labour. Nursing Times 1992;88:55.

Lupton P. Artificial rupture of membranes in spontaneous labour at term: some factors which may affect the decision. 1989 Unpublished BSc.(Hons) dissertation, Dorset Institute (now Bournemouth University).

48. FAMILY PLANNING INFORMATION – THE CONTRIBUTION OF THE MIDWIFE
September 1988 - April 1989

U Byrne, Midwifery Tutor. **Contact:** U Byrne, Aughrim Street, Dublin 7, Ireland.

Formed part of a course.

Abstract: Confusion exists among midwives in Ireland about their role in providing family planning information. Little guidance is available for midwives from either their statutory regulatory body (An Bord Altranais) or their professional organisation (The Irish Nurses Organisation). In fact, these institutions add to the confusion by implying that the term 'family planning' refers to natural methods of family planning only. This confusion does not exist in other countries.

A review of the literature shows that the role of the midwife in relation to family planning has received little attention. The role that midwives adopt in different parts of the world varies greatly from one country to another. Legislation, health service structure and personnel, access to medical services and the role midwives wish to take are all influencing factors. Studies in Ireland looking at the provision of family planning information are in short supply. This may reflect the newness of our family planning legislation - 1979 and 1985. The studies which have been conducted reveal that many people have unmet needs in relation to family planning information. No study was located which looked specifically at the contribution of midwives in this area.

This study was a logical first step in filling in some of the gaps in available information. Thirty women who had recently given birth were interviewed. Whether these women's family planning needs were met during their contact with the Maternity Services was assessed. The midwife's contribution to meeting these needs was ascertained and the possible expansion of the midwives' role was explored. The study showed that almost one quarter of the women had unmet needs in relation to family planning. The postpartum in-hospital stage was the only time that midwives were involved in providing family planning information. Information provided did not always match information required. Potential for midwives to expand their role was identified. Suggestions for further research in this area are given.

Keywords: CONTRACEPTION, FAMILY PLANNING, MIDWIFE'S ROLE (EXTENDED)

49. MATERNITY SERVICES IN LOTHIAN – A SURVEY OF USERS' OPINIONS
January 1987 - June 1988

Claudia Martin, Senior Research Fellow, Lyn Jones, Senior Lecturer, Amanda Amos, Lecturer. **Contact:** Claudia Martin, The Local Government Centre, University of Warwick, Coventry CV4 7AL. Tel: 0203 524109

6-12 hours/week of own time spent. Funded as integral or additional part of a job by employer and by funding agency(ies): Distict Councils within the Lothian Region, University of Edinburgh, Lothian Health Board.

Abstract: This study was instigated by a pressure group in the Lothian Region of Scotland who were concerned about future developments in maternity services in the area.

The study, a survey of 'consumer' opinion, was carried out by researchers based at Edinburgh University. Information was obtained using a postal survey of all women who had given birth in the five maternity units in Lothian during a seven-week period. Questionnaire development was carried out in collaboration with mothers and hospital personnel (midwifery and obstetric). The questionnaire covered the following areas: antenatal care; antenatal admission; care during labour and delivery; postnatal care in hospital. Within each of the areas we asked about: preferences; choice(s); how far preferences were taken into account; accessibility and convenience of services; information and communication; and relationships with staff. We also asked questions relating to overall and specific satisfaction with various aspects of care. We received a response rate (after two reminders) of 79%.

The main findings related to the importance of information, good communication and continuity of care as determinants of satisfaction with care. The survey results have been/are being used in policy discussions in the Lothian Region.

Keywords: COMMUNICATION, CONSUMER OPINION, CONSUMER SATISFACTION, INFORMATION GIVING

Martin CJ. How do you count maternal satisfaction? A user-commissioned survey of maternity services. In: Roberts H, ed. Women's Health Counts. London: Routledge 1990.

Amos A, Jones L, Martin C. Maternity services in Lothian - a survey of users' opinions. Report produced by Department of Community Medicine, University of Edinburgh 1988.

51. A STUDY OF THE USE OF IN-LINE FILTERS WHENUSING INTRAVENOUS ADMINISTRATION SETS IN SPECIAL CARE BABY UNIT

January - December 1989

Maureen Williams, Senior Nurse, Kathryn Martin, Staff Midwife, Denise Cooper, Staff Midwife. **Contact:** Denise Cooper, Special Care Baby Unit, Maelor General Hospital, Wrexham, Clwyd. Tel: 0978 291100 Ex 5023

Abstract: (Not updated since 1991). We are in the process of a study using filters in intravenous administration sets for babies in a special care baby unit. The three main aims of the project are: 1) to assess total cost and compare costs with and without a filter; 2) to compare serum gentamycin results of babies given the drug via the filter with those results of babies given the drug without a filter; and 3) to compare the number of necrosed areas that develop at the infiltration site when an in-line filter is used with the number that develop when a filter is not used.

The brand of filter we are using can be left in situ for ninety-six hours; those administration sets without filters have to be changed daily. This is following DHSS guidelines. The filters are used in intravenous administration sets for the removal of microbial contaminants and the associated endotoxins and entrained air. To achieve the above we have made a record of each baby receiving intravenous fluids during the past year alternating with and without filters. For each baby we have calculated the total cost for the administration sets used, recorded the resulting serum gentamycin levels, and any necrosed areas that may have developed. Although our study will not be completed until the end of the year we have already shown that: 1) there is a great saving in cost when using the filters; 2) serum gentamycin levels do not appear to be affected by the filter; and 3) necrosed areas are not reduced, there being no difference in the incidence when using the filter.

Keywords: COST EFFECTIVENESS, EQUIPMENT (ECONOMICS), GENTAMYCIN LEVELS, INFUSION SITE, INTRAVENOUS DRUGS (NEONATE), INTRAVENOUS INFUSION (FILTERS), NEONATAL UNITS

53. FACTORS AFFECTING LABOUR PAIN

September 1981 - October 1985

Catherine Niven, Reader in Psychology, Karel Gijsbers, Lecturer in Psychology. **Contact:** Catherine Niven, Department of Psychology, Glasgow Caledonian University, Cowcaddens Road, Glasgow G4 0BA. Tel: 041 331 3000

Formed part of a course. Funded by employer, Stirling University Studentship, and by Nuffield Foundation.

Abstract: The purpose of the research was to assess levels of pain during the first and second stage of labour. This was then related to a number of obstetric variables including parity, duration of labour, ARM, degree of cervical dilatation, demographic variables, analgesic use, and psychological variables including antenatal training, husbands' presence at the birth, expectations and experience of birth, and coping strategies used. The relationship between previous pain experience and labour pain experience was a focus of attention.

One hundred women were included in the study. Labour pain was assessed during the active phase of the first stage of labour and again by recall twenty-four to twenty-eight hours after the birth. Duration of labour (first stage), parity, ARM and weight of the baby were significantly related to higher levels of labour pain, while desirability of pregnancy, positive and accurate expectations of birth, antenatal training and the presence of the husband when it was welcomed by his wife were related to lower levels of pain. Previous pain experience had a complex relationship with labour pain levels and with the use of coping strategies.

Keywords: EXPERIENCE (WOMEN'S), FIRST STAGE, LABOUR, PAIN ASSESSMENT, PAIN EXPERIENCE, SECOND STAGE

Niven C. Factors affecting labour pain. Unpublished PhD thesis. University of Stirling 1986.

Niven C. How helpful is the husband's presence at childbirth? Journal of Reproductive and Infant Psychology 1985:45-53.

Niven C. Labour pain. Research and the Midwife Conference Proceedings 1984:102-24.

Niven C. Pain in labour. In: Faulkner A, Murphy-Black T, eds. Excellence in nursing: The Research Route. Scutari Press 1990:19-33.

Niven C. Coping with childbirth. In: Robinson S, Thompson AM, eds. Midwives, Research and Childbirth. Vol.3. Croom Helm (in press).

Niven CA, Gijsbers KJ. Do low levels of labour pain reflect low sensitivity to noxious stimulation? Social Science Medicine 1989;29:585-8.

Niven C, Gijsbers K. Obstetric and non-obstretric factors related to labour pain. Journal of Reproductive and Infant Psychology 1984;2:61-78.

Niven C. Psychological Care for Families: Before, During and After Birth. Butterworth Heinemann, Oxford.1992.

54. LONG TERM RECALL OF LABOUR PAIN
June 1986 - September 1987

Catherine Niven, Reader in Psychology. **Contact:** Catherine Niven, Department of Psychology, Glasgow Caledonian University, Cowcaddens Road, Glasgow G4 0BA. Tel: 041 331 3000

Funded as integral or additional part of a job by employer: Glasgow College.

Abstract: Thirty-three women who gave birth three to four years previously described the nature and intensity of the pain experienced during that birth using structured pain assessment scales (McGill Pain Questionnaire and Visual Analogue Scales). This study was a follow-up to a study on Factors Affecting Labour Pain (Record No. 53). These assessments were compared with assessments made at the time of birth. The subjects' recall of labour pain was surprisingly accurate. A small number of subjects reported that they had experienced considerable negative effect when they spontaneously recalled their labour pain. The majority of subjects acknowledged that their experience of labour pain had given rise to some positive consequences. Most commonly they reported that it had increased their ability to cope with other kinds of pain and stress.

Keywords: EXPERIENCE (WOMEN'S), LABOUR, PAIN ASSESSMENT, PAIN EXPERIENCE (RETROSPECTIVE)

Niven C. Labour pain: long-term recall and consequences. Journal of Reproductive and Infant Psychology 1988;6:83-7.

Niven C. Psychological Care for Families: Before, During and After Birth. Butterworth Heinemann, Oxford.1992.

55. ATTACHMENT IN MOTHERS OF PRE-TERM BABIES
October 1987 - September 1988

Catherine Niven, Reader in Psychology, L Alroomi, Consultant Paediatrician, Catherine Wiszniewski, Student. **Contact:** Catherine Niven, Department of Psychology, Glasgow Caledonian University, Cowcaddens Road, Glasgow G4 0BA. Tel: 041 331 3000

Funded as integral or additional part of a job by employer: Glasgow College.

Abstract: Thirty mothers of pre-term babies were interviewed on average at six months postnatally. Feelings of attachment/bonding during pregnancy, immediately after birth, during the first postnatal days and during the remainder of the baby's stay in hospital were assessed. All mothers experienced difficulties in attachment during the baby's stay in hospital. In twenty-seven cases these were resolved once the baby went home. The remaining three cases demonstrated reduced levels of attachment due to lack of support and the long-term stressful effects of IVF treatment. Earlier attachment difficulties were related to shock, fear of baby's death and previous reproductive problems. Feelings of guilt, loss and that the baby was not really theirs were also articulated. There was no evidence of a total 'failure to bond'. These findings are probably applicable to all babies whose lives are at risk who remain in hospital for an extended period following birth.

Keywords: BONDING, EXPERIENCE (WOMEN'S), INVITRO FERTILISATION, NEONATAL UNITS, PREMATURITY, PSYCHOLOGY, RELATIONSHIPS

Niven C, Wiszwiewski C, Alroomi L. Attachment in mothers of preterm babies. Journal of Reproductive and Infant Psychology 1993.

Niven C. Psychological Care for Families: Before, During and After Birth. Butterworth and Heinemann, Oxford 1992.

57. REPORT OF A SURVEY MADE INTO THE CONTENT OF ADVICE GIVEN TO MOTHERS REGARDING INFANT FEEDING BY MIDWIVES AND HEALTH VISITORS WORKING WITHIN THE WEST GLAMORGAN HEALTH AUTHORITY, SWANSEA HEALTH DISTRICT

January - November 1975

G D Maclean, International Consultant of Midwifery Education. **Contact:** G D Maclean, Maple Grove, Sketty Road, Swansea SA2 OJY.

Funded as integral or additional part of a job by employer: West Glamorgan Health Authority. 12-20 hours/week of own time spent.

Abstract: The purpose of the research was to consider the problem, content and extent of conflicting advice regarding breast and artificial feeding so that some progress could be made in addressing these issues.

Two open-ended questionnaires were sent to all midwives and health visitors in the district. The response rates were 62% (88) and 70% (99) for breastfeeding and artificial feeding questionnaires respectively. The data were analyzed by hand and supported the hypothesis that advice was both variable and conflicting. For example, timing of the first feed ranged from two to twelve hours, though most stated this should be 'as soon as possible'. Whilst the majority considered the first feed should be of clear fluid, a significant minority did not. For engorged breasts the advice included hot bathing or fomentation, kaolin poultice, hot and cold bathing, spirit poultice, support, restricting fluids, expressing milk before and/or after feeds or that lactation should be stimulated. Dietary advice was given to nursing mothers by 97% but the conflict arose in the allowance or prohibition of certain foods. Demand feeding, complementary and supplementary feeding, position of mother, timing at the breast, feeding at night, how to prevent breast complications were all areas of conflicting advice. The advice regarding artificial feeding was equally controversial and included: selecting brands of milk, sterilization, vomiting and regurgitation, 'winding', demonstration of feed preparation, mixed feeding introduction and reasons for crying.

The main recommendation, which was implemented, was the formation of a multi-disciplinary team to formulate guidelines for professional staff. An examination of attitudes to infant feeding was also advocated.

Keywords: ARTIFICIAL FEEDING, BREASTFEEDING, CONFLICTING ADVICE (FEEDING), HEALTH VISITORS, INFANT FEEDING, MIDWIFE'S CARE

Maclean GD. An appraisal of the concepts of infant feeding and their application in practice. Journal of Advanced Nursing 1977;2:111-26.

Maclean GD. Whoever told you that? Midwives Chronicle Part 1 1977;90:101-4.

Maclean GD. Whoever told you that? Midwives Chronicle Part 2 1977;90:129-32.

Maclean GD. Whoever told you that? Midwives Chronicle Part 3 1977;90:167-9.

Feeding your baby. A booklet published by West Glamorgan Health Authority.

58. UPTAKE OF SIX WEEKS POSTNATAL EXAMINATION BY PUERPERAL WOMAN IN OLDHAM
September 1982 - May 1984

J Bowers, Midwifery Tutor/Senior Nurse, Joel Richman, Sociologist, Manchester Polytechnic. **Contact:** J Bowers, Bourne Parc, Maison Victor Hugo, Greve d'Azette, St Clement, Jersey Channel Islands.

Formed part of a course. 6-12 hours/week of own time spent. Funded by funding agency(ies): Maws/RCM Research Scholarship, Nurses War Memorial Fund.

Abstract: This exploratory and quantitative study of 210 mothers was undertaken in partial fulfilment of the requirements of a BSc in Nursing Studies. It sought to find out the uptake of the six weeks postnatal examination, the factors that influenced uptake, and to correlate the perspectives of women and their GPs. It involved a random sample of women in Oldham and all GPs on the obstetric list.

Methods used were non-participative observation, structured interviews and postal questionnaires; the results were analyzed manually. Group differences in uptake rates were evident between social classes, multiparous and primiparous women, but not apparent when looking at delivery type and ethnicity. It was clear that mothers' views did not always correlate with their GPs, especially in relation to infant feeding. Similarities were shown between morbidities expressed by mothers and those found by GPs, though episiotomy problems and depression were not always evident to GPs. Attendance rates were 88%, but expectations were not often met; some mothers would have preferred to be examined by their midwife. Some of the recommendations were: to look at the feasibility of midwives undertaking six-week postnatal examinations and making women more aware of their rights; to combine six-week postnatal/six-week baby assessment clinics; to encourage more GPs to keep a morbidity register and keep statistics of postnatal examinations and attendances; provision of better educational aids to prepare women for this examination, and more evaluation of postnatal examination by doctors and midwives.

Keywords: EXPERIENCE (WOMEN'S), GENERAL PRACTITIONERS, MIDWIFE'S ROLE (EXTENDED), POSTNATAL EXAMINATION, PUERPERIUM

Bowers J. Is the six week postnatal examination really necessary? The Practitioner 1985;8.

Bowers J. The six weeks postnatal examination. Research and the Midwife Conference Proceedings 1984;28-50.

59. SURVEY OF POSTNATAL RECOVERY FOLLOWING PERINEAL REPAIR BY MIDWIFE

September 1987 - October 1988

S G Doyle, Full time mother and housewife. **Contact:** S G Doyle, French Weir Avenue, Taunton, Somerset TA1 1XQ.

Funded as integral or additional part of a job by employer: Somerset Health Authority. 2-6 hours/week of own time spent.
Abstract: (Not updated since 1991). The purpose of this study was to follow up the new mothers who had had a perineal injury sutured by a midwife, and evaluate their comfort and satisfaction with the service given.

The method involved asking 500 mothers following suturing if they would take part in the survey. They were included if they had had a perineal injury following normal delivery sutured by a midwife, and were given the questionnaire before they left the labour ward. The questionnaire asked how much, if any, pain or discomfort was felt by the mother at different intervals up to six weeks; whether she was experiencing any discomfort in a variety of activities; what advice, if any, she was given for treatment and hygiene. It also included space for comments from the midwife and GP of the appearance of the perineum. If, at six weeks, mothers had any discomfort or problems they were contacted again at three months by phone or letter to find out whether they were comfortable and healed or still experiencing some form of problem. Analysis, findings, implications and recommendations to follow.

Keywords: EXPERIENCE (WOMEN'S), PAIN, PERINEAL HEALING, PERINEAL TRAUMA, POSTNATAL COMPLICATIONS, SUTURING

60. THE "THIRD DAY BLUES"

January 1982 - December 1984

Valerie A Levy, Midwifery Tutor. **Contact:** Valerie A Levy, IANE, Royal College of Nursing, 20 Cavendish Square, London. Tel: 071 409 3333

6-12 hours/week of own time spent.

Abstract: In order to establish whether the period of dysphoria that often follows childbirth (the 'maternity blues') is peculiar to the puerperium, a validated self-rating blues questionnaire was administered every day for the first postnatal/post-operative week to forty-two women following childbirth, and to twenty-five men and fifty women after surgery. Chi-square tests and Pearson's correlations indicated that a period of dysphoria, similar in many respects to the maternity blues, was experienced by women and to a lesser extent by men, post-operatively. In the search for the cause of the maternity blues it may be helpful to study the same parameters in post-operative dysphoria. Respondents were invited to comment on the perceived cause of the blues and how and by whom they thought they could best have been helped. Recommendations arising from these comments are offered.

Keywords: MATERNITY SERVICES, POSTNATAL DEPRESSION, POSTOPERATIVE CARE, THIRD DAY BLUES

Levy V. "The third day blues". Midwives Chronicle. November 1984, Professional Day Supplement XIV-XV.

Levy V. "The third day blues". Research and the Midwife Conference Proceedings 1985:31-45.

Levy V. "The maternity blues in postpartum and postoperative women". British Journal of Psychiatry 1987;151:368-72.

Levy V. "The maternity blues in postpartum and postoperative patients". In: Robinson S, Thomson AM, eds. Midwives, Research and Childbirth Vol 3. (in press).

61. THE MIDWIFE'S MANAGEMENT OF THE THIRD STAGE OF LABOUR

January 1980 - December 1982

V A Levy, Midwifery Tutor, J Moore, Senior Midwifery Tutor. **Contact:** Valerie A Levy, IANE, Royal College of Nursing, 20 Cavendish Square, London. Tel: 071 409 3333

Funded as integral or additional part of a job and by funding agency(ies): Locally organised research scheme. 2 hours/week of own time spent.

Abstract: This study was instigated because it was noticed there was a high local postpartum haemorrhage (PPH) rate of 7% and, at the same time, a divergence between classroom teaching and clinical practice regarding the management of the third stage of labour. Students were taught in the classroom to deliver the placenta by controlled cord traction (CCT) without awaiting signs of placental separation and descent.

This study surveyed a small number of midwives regarding their preferred practice and found that many preferred to teach students to await signs before applying CCT. Midwives cited the most reliable sign of separation and descent as lengthening of the umbilical cord and a trickle of blood per vaginam. Two methods of CCT were compared; the PPH rate was significantly less when signs of placental separation were awaited. The extra time spent awaiting signs did not appear to increase the risk of PPH.

The final part of the study was an experiment to demonstrate fallibility in blood loss estimation; amounts of blood under 300ml were fairly accurately estimated but larger amounts were progressively underestimated. Neither seniority nor length of experience on delivery suite affected the accuracy with which blood loss was estimated.

It is stressed that this was a relatively small study and further research is needed before confident recommendations can be made. However, the recommendations arising from this study were that signs of placental separation and descent should be awaited before applying CCT, and blood loss estimates over 500ml should be doubled to give a more accurate assessment.

(**NB:** the blood loss experiment can be easily repeated, using coloured water to represent blood, to demonstrate to students their fallibility in estimating blood loss).

Keywords: BLOOD LOSS ESTIMATION, LABOUR, MIDWIFERY POLICIES, MIDWIFERY PRACTICE, POSTPARTUM HAEMORRHAGE, THIRD STAGE

Moore J, Levy V. Further research into the management of the third stage of labour and the incidence of postpartum haemorrhage. Research and the Midwife Conference Proceedings 1982;96-114.

Levy V, Moore J. The midwife's management of the third stage of labour. Nursing Times 1985;81:47-50 (occasional paper).

63. INCEST SURVIVORS' EXPERIENCES OF OBSTETRICS AND GYNAECOLOGY

January 1988 - October 1989

J Kitzinger, Research Officer. **Contact:** J Kitzinger, Southpark Avenue, Glasgow G12 8LF. Tel: 041 339 8855 Ex 6686

12-20 hours/week of own time spent.

Abstract: This research into experiences of obstetrics and gynaecology is part of a wider exploration of adult women's experiences of surviving childhood sexual abuse.

In-depth, semi-structured interviews have been completed with thirty-nine women. Over half of these women reported that obstetric and gynaecological intervention, including routine internal examinations, could traumatically recall or re-enact their childhood abuse. Some women avoid screening or treatment because of this or find that medical encounters leave them feeling dirty, violated and fearful. Childbirth may be a particular crisis point for survivors of childhood abuse because it combines medical treatment with the transition to motherhood. A survivor of childhood abuse may be fearful for her own child and distrustful of the child's father; she may even fear that she herself will abuse the child and therefore be wary of any intimate physical contact such as breastfeeding or washing her infant. Health care workers need to be aware of the impact of sexual violence on women's experience of obstetric and gynaecological events. We need to explore how medical encounters and hospitalisation can reinforce a woman's sense of inadequacy and powerlessness, and develop ways of conducting examinations and supporting women through childbirth so as to counteract the disempowering effects of childhood assault.

Recommendations from the women themselves include details of the type of information they would have liked, the choice of position for examination, and the attitude they appreciated from staff.

Keywords: CERVICAL SMEARS, POSTNATAL DEPRESSION, SEXUAL ABUSE (CHILDREN), VAGINAL EXAMINATIONS

Kitzinger J. The impact of gynaecological and obstetric events on adult recall of childhood sexual abuse. Journal of Psychosomatic Obstetrics and Gynaecology 1989;10:180.

Kitzinger J. Recalling the pain: Survivors of childhood sexual abuse and the role of the health worker. Nursing Times 1990;86:38-40.

Kitzinger J. The internal examination. The Practitioner 1990;234:698-700.

64. CONTINUITY AND FRAGMENTATION IN MATERNITY CARE
October 1979 - June 1985
R Currell, Research Midwife. **Contact:** R Currell, St. Thomas's Way, Great Whelnetham, Bury St Edmunds, Suffolk IP30 0TP.

For full details see under Management Studies (Record No. 64).

65. FACTORS ASSOCIATED WITH AND PREDICTIVE OF POSTNATAL DEPRESSION
January 1986 - January 1991
Valerie A Levy, Lecturer. **Contact:** Valerie A Levy, IANE, Royal College of Nursing, 20 Cavendish Square, London. Tel: 071 409 3333

Funded as integral or additional part of a job by employer and by funding agency(ies): Iolanthe Trust, Cornwall and Isles of Scilly Health Authority. 12-20 hours/week of own time spent.

Abstract: The purpose of this longitudinal study was to identify factors associated with perinatal depression.

A sample of 102 women was interviewed and asked to complete questionnaires in late pregnancy, the first ten days postnatally, six, twelve and twenty-four weeks postnatally. Biographical, medical and obstetric details were recorded. Eysenck's Personality Questionnaire was administered to assess traits of neuroticism and psychoticism. Using focused interviews, qualitative and quantitative data were obtained regarding stress, social support and aspects of motherhood. Current depression scores were measured by the Edinburgh Postnatal Depression Score (EPDS) (Cox JL et al 1987).

Quantitative data were processed by computer, using factor analysis (oblimin rotation) and the chi-square test. Qualitative data were subjected to content analysis. The incidence of depression over the study period varied from between 8% and 14%. Throughout the study, variables associated with depression included high stress levels, poor social support and high neuroticism and psychoticism scores. Variables were also identified associated more specifically with depression in late pregnancy, and six weeks and six months postnatally. These are similar to those variables associated with depression in the general population of women; few were directly related to childbirth. It appeared that childbirth added to an already stressed situation, but was not in itself a primary cause of depression. A small, atypical sub-group of women was noted to whom the above comments do not apply.

Recommendations included that all women should be actively screened for depression in late pregnancy and postnatally, preferably by means of the EPDS. Other recommendations were also made and it is hoped to publish a detailed account of these and other aspects of the study in due course.

Keywords: PERINATAL DEPRESSION, POSTNATAL DEPRESSION, POSTNATAL DEPRESSION (RISK FACTORS), SOCIAL SUPPORT, STRESS (MATERNAL)

Levy V. Factors associated with non-psychotic perinatal depression. Research and the Midwife Conference Proceedings 1990:64-71.

66. THE BRISTOL THIRD STAGE TRIAL: ACTIVE VERSUS PHYSIOLOGICAL MANAGEMENT OF THIRD STAGE OF LABOUR
January 1986 - January 1987

Walter J Prendiville, Consultant Obstetrician/Senior Lecturer, Walter J Prendiville, Lecturer/Senior Registrar, Joanna Harding, Research Midwife, Diana Elbourne, Social Statistician, Gordon Stirrat, Professor. **Contact:** Joanna Harding, School of Midwifery, Princess Anne Wing, Royal United Hospital, Combe Park, Bath, AVON BA1 3NG. Tel: 0225 428331 Ex 4674

2 hours/week of own time spent. Funded as integral or additional part of a job by funding agency(ies): World Health Organisation.

Abstract: The purpose of the study was to compare the effects on fetal and maternal morbidity of routine active management of the third stage of labour and physiological management, and in particular to determine whether active management reduced the incidence of postpartum haemorrhage (PPH).

The method of research was a prospective randomized controlled trial of women delivering at Bristol Maternity Hospital of active management versus physiological management of the third stage of labour. For analysis we used chi-square and t-test plus odds ratio and 95% confidence intervals where appropriate. Most of these analyses were done on statistical package SPSSx.

Our results showed PPH occurred in 5.9% of women in the active management group, compared with 17.9% in the physiological management group. This contrast was reflected in other indices of blood loss (Hb, PCV and blood transfusion). In the physiological group the third stage was longer (median fifteen mins versus five mins), and more women needed therapeutic oxytocics (29.7% v 6.4%). When women allocated to and receiving active management were compared with those who actually received physiological management, active management still produced a lower rate of PPH. Women having a 'physiological' first and second stage of labour (defined as low risk, spontaneous onset of labour, no augmentation or epidural and labour <12 hrs and normal delivery) also had higher incidence of PPH in the physiological group than the active group.

The conclusion we have drawn from our study is that the policy of active management as practised in this trial reduced incidence of PPH, shortened third stage and resulted in reduced neonatal packed cell volume. Our recommendations are that further research is needed into the components of active management and physiological management, the feasibility of oxytocics in the third world and replication of the Bristol third stage trial in a country where physiological management is the norm for mothers and midwives.

Keywords: ACTIVE MANAGEMENT, BLOOD LOSS, LABOUR, OXYTOCICS, PHYSIOLOGICAL MANAGEMENT, POSTPARTUM HAEMORRHAGE, SYNTOMETRINE, THIRD STAGE

Prendiville WJ, Harding JE, Elbourne DR, Stirrat GM. The Bristol third stage trial: Active versus physiological management of third stage of labour. British Medical Journal 1988;297:1295-300.

Harding JE, Elbourne DR, Prendiville WJ. Views of mothers and midwives participating in the Bristol randomized, controlled trial of active management of the third stage of labour. Birth 1989;16:1-6.

Elbourne D, Harding J. The Bristol third stage trial. Manchester Research & the Midwives Conference Proceedings. November 1989:19-31.

Prendiville W, Elbourne D. Care during the third stage of labour. In: Chalmers I, Enkin M, Kierse MJNC, eds. Effective Care in Pregnancy and Childbirth. Oxford: Oxford University Press 1989:1145-69.

Prendiville W, Elbourne D, Chalmers I. The effects of routine oxytocic administration in the management of the third stage of labour: An overview of the evidence from controlled trials. British Journal of Obstetrics and Gynaecology 1988;95:3-16.

Elbourne D, Prendiville W, Chalmers I. Choice of oxytocic preparation for routine use in the management of the third stage of labour: An overview of the evidence from controlled trials. British Journal of Obstetrics and Gynaecology 1988;95:17-30.

Elbourne D, Harding J. Management of third stage of labour. Midwives Chronicle 1989:130.

Elbourne D, Harding J. Hair colour and blood loss. Midwives Chronicle 1988:363.

67. EVALUATION OF PREPARATION FOR PARENTHOOD CLASSES FOR COUPLES ADOPTING A BABY
September 1987 - May 1988

Jenny Fraser, Midwifery Sister, David Howe, Lecturer (University). **Contact:** Jenny Fraser, Parenthood Education Department, Maternity Unit, Norfolk and Norwich Hospital, Norwich NR1 3SR. Tel: 0603 287239/287244

2-6 hours/week of own time spent. Funded by funding agency(ies): Norfolk & Norwich Hospital.

Abstract: The purpose of the study was to compare the experiences of adopters of babies who had attended special Parenthood Education Classes taught by a midwife, with adopters of babies who had no formal preparation for parenthood.

Twenty couples were interviewed. The couples were interviewed on tape in their own homes, using a semi-structured schedule. The taped interviews were subjected to content analysis. In our findings the parents who had attended the special preparation for parenthood classes noted four major benefits: 1) the waiting time between approval and placement was given structure and purpose; 2) practical advice about caring for a baby was given; 3) there was the chance to meet other adopters who had also had the taxing experience of infertility testing and the adoption assessment, and with whom there was a strong bond; and 4) there was support, both before and after placement, by the midwife who ran the classes.

The implications and recommendations from this study are that classes tailor-made and exclusively for first-time baby adopters help them prepare practically for the arrival of their baby. Continuity of care both before and after placement of their baby is of immense value. The opportunity to meet and gain emotional support from other approved adopters is always welcome. Classes give shape and purpose to the difficult time between approval and placement.

Keywords: ADOPTION, EDUCATION FOR PARENTHOOD, MIDWIFE'S ROLE (EXTENDED)

Howe D, Fraser J. Approval vs preparation: adoptive parents' views of the adoption process. Adoption and Fostering 1988;12:29-34.
Fraser J, Howe D. Baby adoptions, midwives and health visitors. Midwife, Health Visitor and Community Nurse 1989;25:70-4.

68. TREATMENT OF UMBILICAL CORDS: A RANDOMISED CONTROLLED TRIAL TO ASSESS THE EFFECT OF TREATMENT METHODS ON THE WORK OF MIDWIVES
April 1983 - July 1986

Isobel Waterhouse, Director of Nursing Services (Midwifery), Miranda Mugford, Economist, Ann Medd, Trial Clerk (part-time), Malinee Somchiwong, British Council Research Fellow (NPEU). **Contact:** Miranda Mugford, National Perinatal Epidemiology Unit, Radcliffe Infirmary, Oxford OX2 6HE. Tel: 0865 224187

2 hours/week of own time spent. Funded as integral or additional part of a job by employer: Department of Health, British Council Fellowship.

Abstract: The national code of practice for midwives practising in England and Wales defines duties during the postnatal period for the care of mothers and their babies. This period is a minimum of ten days, and up to twenty-eight days. Visits after the tenth day are at midwives' discretion, but a survey of heads of midwifery services suggests that most midwives would extend postnatal care beyond the tenth day if the baby's umbilicus was not healed. Methods used for routine treatment of the umbilical cord in the newborn babies vary widely. Previous studies suggest that the rate of healing depends on the method of treatment used. This, in turn, can affect the workload of midwives responsible for the care of newborn babies.

Babies born in the Royal Berkshire Hospital in the summer of 1984 (n=781) were randomly allocated to have their cords treated by one of four dusting powders, one of three cleansing methods and one of two frequencies of treatment, in a trial with a factorial design. The effect of treatment on the time of separation of the cord and the number of midwives' visits was estimated. It was found that the treatment methods used could significantly affect the healing process and therefore the number of visits made by midwives after the tenth day, and that the choice of cord powder could significantly affect the midwifery workload in the district. The difference would be enough to account for the work of one whole-time equivalent community midwife for every 3000-5000 births.

Keywords: CORD CARE, CORD SEPARATION, ECONOMICS, MIDWIFERY SERVICES, MIDWIFERY (CODE OF PRACTICE), NEONATAL CARE, POSTNATAL VISITS

Mugford M, Somchiwong M, Waterhouse IL. Treatment of umbilical cords: a randomised controlled trial to assess the effect of treatment methods on the work of midwives. Midwifery 1986;2:177-86.

Mugford M. Ster-Zac Advertisement. Letter to the Midwives Chronicle 1993:350-7.

69. THE EFFECT OF OXYTOCIN IN INDUCED LABOUR ON NEONATAL JAUNDICE

January 1977 - December 1978

Stephen W D'Souza, Senior Lecturer & Consultant Paediatrician, Patricia Black, Research Midwife, Thomas MacFarlane, Senior Registrar (Obstetrics), Bernard Richards, Professor of Computing. **Contact:** Tricia Murphy-Black, Research and Development Adviser, Simpson Memorial Maternity Pavilion, Lauriston Place, Edinburgh EH3 9EF. Tel: 031 229 2477 Ex 4357

Funded as integral or additional part of a job and by funding agency(ies).

Abstract: A prospective study of 180 mothers and babies examined the effects of oxytocin in induced labour on plasma bilirubin levels in cord blood, as well as on the incidence of neonatal jaundice. Raised plasma bilirubin levels in cord blood, probably enhanced by breakdown of fetal red cells, appeared to be a dose-dependent effect of oxytocin. Commensurate with this was the finding that a larger proportion of babies in the induced group manifested a greater severity of jaundice.

Keywords: ACTIVE MANAGEMENT, JAUNDICE, LABOUR, LABOUR (INDUCTION), OXYTOCIN

D'Souza SW, Black P, MacFarlane T, Richards B. The effect of oxytocin in induced labour on neonatal jaundice. British Journal of Obstetrics and Gynaecology 1979;86:133-8.

70. PSYCHOLOGICAL ASPECTS OF FETAL MONITORING: MATERNAL REACTION TO THE POSITION OF THE MONITOR AND STAFF

January - December 1978

Stephen W D'Souza, Senior Lecturer & Consultant Paediatrician, Judith E Jackson, MSc Student, Margaret Vaughan, Lecturer in Psychology, Patricia Black, Research Midwife. **Contact:** Tricia Murphy-Black, Research and Development Adviser, Simpson Memorial Maternity Pavilion, Lauriston Place, Edinburgh EH3 9EF. Tel: 031 229 2477 Ex 4357

Funded as integral or additional part of a job by North West Regional Health Authority.

Abstract: Thirty mothers, one day postpartum, were given a questionnaire about their reaction to fetal monitoring during labour. An attempt to manipulate the amount of information about the monitor given to the women shortly before the induction of labour was unsuccessful. As a group the women found monitoring reassuring rather than worrying, although worry seemed to increase slightly with longer labours. Most of the women preferred to be able to see the front of the monitor, and those who had seen the front recalled more about the monitor. The amount of reassurance evoked by the monitor and staff behaviour was significantly greater in women who had seen the front of the monitor during labour, when the husband was present during labour, and in women who had attended antenatal classes.

Keywords: ANTENATAL EDUCATION, EXPERIENCE (WOMEN'S), FETAL MONITORING, LABOUR

Jackson JE, Vaughan M, Black P, D'Souza SW. Psychological aspects of fetal monitoring: Maternal reaction to the position of the monitor and staff behaviour. Journal of Psychosomatic Obstetrics and Gynaecology 1983;2:97-102.

72. TANGLED WEBS: FAMILY NETWORKS AND ACTIVITY EXAMINED IN ONE INNER-CITY AREA OF NEWCASTLE UPON TYNE

October 1987 - October 1989

J M Davies, Community Midwife. **Contact:** J M Davies, Rectory Terrace, Newcastle Upon Tyne NE3 1YB.

Formed part of a course. 6-12 hours/week of own time spent. Funded by employer: Newcastle Health Authority.

Abstract: The purpose of the study was to describe the social context of women living in an inner city area with rates of unemployment and low income well above the city average.

The research was basically anthropological, using mapping as a means of conveying information. The mapping had originally been conceived as a way to collect data, and was made of the whole area using details from the Housing Department. Each household was marked. Information from the questionnaires was then put onto the map, and patterns of networks developed. A potential sample of 180 women who had had babies between 1983 and 1987 were identified. Those who had left the area, of whom there were seventy-six, were excluded. Of the rest, twenty-four were not interviewed - mainly because of time constraints. This left a sample of eighty women. The study method was a semi-structured interview, which was developed from a pilot study. Each interview lasted about an hour. As there was a lot of information already known through clinical contacts, it was a question of clarifying family relationships within the estate. Questions about health and the perception of problems were also included.

The main recommendation arising from this study was that midwives support women in their most important 'rite of passage', which is fundamentally a social rather than a medical act, and that they do not medicalise this act.

Keywords: ANTHROPOLOGY, CHILDBIRTH (SOCIAL FACTORS), FAMILY MAPPING, INNER CITY PROBLEMS, MEDICALISATION, MIDWIFE'S ROLE

Davies JM. "Tangled webs": family networks and activity examined in one inner-city area of Newcastle upon Tyne. Dissertation for MSc. degree 1989. Available at Newcastle-upon-Tyne Polytechnic Library.

73. A STUDY OF SINGLE ADMINISTRATION PRO-PIROXICAM IN POST-EPISIOTOMY PAIN RELIEF
November 1988 - March 1990

A A Spence, Professor of Anaesthesia, Ian Power, Lecturer, Ann Whitfield, Consultant, Valerie Morgan, Research Midwife. **Contact:** Valerie Morgan, Department of Anaesthetics, Royal Infirmary, Edinburgh EH3 9YW. Tel: 031 229 2477 Ex 4327

Funded as integral or additional part of a job and by Chiesi-Farmaceutici, Milan, Italy.

Abstract: (Not updated since 1991). This randomized, double-blind study aims to investigate the analgesic effect of a single administration of Pro-Piroxicam in women who have undergone episiotomy for vaginal delivery. Three dose levels of Pro-Piroxicam are being compared with aspirin 600mg, the medication being given within the first twenty-four hours after delivery. One hundred and twenty women who met the pre-specified entry criteria, who agreed to participate and who delivered while the trial was in progress, agreed to take part (thirty in each of the four treatment groups). Baseline assessment of pain and pain relief achieved and further assessments in the twenty-four hours following treatment were carried out by the women themselves using visual analogue scales. Scores for pain and pain relief were also made by the nurse observer at the same times. Pulse, blood pressure and respirations were also recorded in the first eight hours after treatment. Analysis is ongoing.

Keywords: ANTI-INFLAMMATORY DRUGS, EPISIOTOMY, NON-STEROIDAL DRUGS, PAIN RELIEF (PERINEUM)

Morgan V, Whitfield A. Unpublished interim report on the progress of the study (undated).
Unpublished report (Jouhar study monitor for pharmaceutical company. Chiesi-Farmaceutici, Milan, undated).

74. THE ROLE OF THE MIDWIFE IN THE DOMICILIARY CARE OF WOMEN WITH HIGH-RISK PREGNANCIES

January 1983 - December 1988

Charlette Middlemiss, Midwife Manager, Andrew Dawson, Lecturer in Obstetrics & Gynaecology, Nigel AJ Gough, Senior Electronics Technician, Eileen M Jones, Midwifery Research Sister, Edward C Coles, Senior Lecturer in Medical Statistics. **Contact:** Charlette Middlemiss, Princess of Wales Hospital, City Road, Bridgend, Mid-Glamorgan, S Wales CS31 1RQ. Tel: 0656 662166 blp 2308

Funded as integral or additional part of a job by employer and by funding agency(ies): Iolanthe Trust, Welsh Scheme for Development of Health & Social Research, Spastics Society, Jane Hodge Foundation, British Telecom.

Abstract: A preliminary randomized study has been made of a domiciliary management scheme which is intended to make better use of midwifery and obstetric resources for selected women with high-risk pregnancies. The scheme incorporates telephonic fetal heart rate monitoring. Anxiety ratings and patterns of hospital admission were compared between two groups of women with identified high-risk pregnancies.

Sixty-five women were eligible for study. Five refused randomization in preference to hospital care and sixty were randomized 2:1 to domiciliary care or conventional groups, with forty domiciliary and seventeen hospital records finally available for analysis. Weekly Zung depression ratings and STAI 'trait' levels of anxiety conducted at weekly intervals were similar in both groups while STAI 'state' levels were 34.05 (SD 9.24) and 41.05 (SD 9.93) in the domiciliary and conventional care groups. In the domiciliary group twenty-one (53%) avoided hospital admission altogether, the admission rate was more than halved, and the mean proportion of time spent in hospital was reduced from 50% to 16% of the observation period. The observed differences in STAI 'state' levels of anxiety were probably due to the greater security of home environment and individual support from the midwife, with a confirmation of the expected reductions in numbers and duration of hospital admissions.

Keywords: ADMISSIONS, ANXIETY (MATERNAL), COMMUNITY CARE, DEPRESSION, FETAL HEART RATE, HIGH RISK PREGNANCY, MIDWIFERY SUPPORT, TELEPHONE MONITORING

Dawson AJ, Middlemiss C, Coles EC, Gough NAJ, Jones ME. A randomized study of a domiciliary antenatal care scheme: the effect on hospital admissions. British Journal of Obstetrics and Gynaecology. 1989;96:1319-22.

Middlemiss C, Dawson AJ, Gough N, Jones EG, Coles EC. A randomised study of a domiciliary antenatal care scheme: maternal psychological effects. Midwifery 1989;5:69-74.

75. A STUDY OF THE RELATIONSHIP BETWEEN THE DELIVERY TO CORD CLAMPING INTERVAL, AND THE TIME OF CORD SEPARATION

May 1985 - July 1990

Elaine Healey, Midwifery Tutor, Carolyn Armstrong, Midwife, Kay Greenish, Community Midwife, Joanne M Alexander, Midwifery Tutor, Margaret Washington, Parentcraft Sister, Sarah Ayers, Computer Programmer. **Contact:** Elaine Healey, Oxford Midwives Research Group, c/o School of Midwifery, John Radcliffe Hospital, Headley Way, Oxford OX3 9DU. Tel: 0865 817804

Funded as integral or additional part of a job. 2-6 hours/week of own time spent.

Abstract: The primary purpose of the study was to examine the effect of the delivery to cord clamping interval on the time of cord separation. It was also planned to ascertain whether there were any differences in paediatric or maternal outcome as a result of varying the time of cord clamping.

The study was a randomized controlled trial. Allocation was to one of two groups - early or late cord clamping. Early clamping was done as soon as possible after delivery. Late clamping was done at three minutes after delivery or when the cord stopped pulsing, whichever was sooner. After giving informed consent, women were enrolled to the study on admission either in labour or for planned induction. Allocation was carried out prior to delivery by opening a sealed, opaque envelope. Envelopes were prepared using random number tables and all envelopes were numbered and opened sequentially. A total of 554 women were entered into the two groups. Data sheets were filled in by midwifery staff, firstly on delivery suite, secondly on the postnatal ward and thirdly, by the community midwife.

The data were entered onto a mainframe computer, and analysis was carried out using SPSSx. Cross tabulations, chi-square and Student's t-test were used to compare groups. Results are available in second publication listed below.

Keywords: BREASTFEEDING, CORD CLAMPING, CORD SEPARATION, JAUNDICE, LABOUR, OUTCOMES (MATERNAL), OUTCOMES (PAEDIATRIC), THIRD STAGE (MANAGEMENT)

Houston MJ, Weatherston L. Creating change in midwifery: integrating theory and practice through practice-based research groups. Midwifery 1986;2:65-70.

Oxford Midwives Research Group. A study of the relationship between the delivery cord clamping interval and the time of cord separation. Midwifery 1991;7:167-76

77. PSYCHOLOGICAL AND SOCIAL ASPECTS OF SCREENING DURING ROUTINE ANTENATAL CARE

March 1989 - February 1992

J M Green, Senior Research Associate, Martin Richards, Reader in Human Development, Helen Statham, Research Associate, Claire Snowdon, Research Associate. **Contact:** J M Green, Maternity Services Research Group, Centre for Family Research, University of Cambridge, Free School Lane, Cambridge CB2 3RF. Tel: 0223 334512

Funded as integral or additional part of a job and by funding agency(ies): Health Promotion Research Trust.

Abstract: Screening for fetal abnormalities has become an integral part of antenatal care for most women. The majority will now expect to have at least one ultrasound scan during the course of their pregnancy, and blood tests to measure the level of alpha feto-protein are also the norm in many hospitals. Women who are identified as being at high risk on the basis of these screening tests, or on the basis of their age, race or previous history, are likely to be offered amniocentesis which can offer a more definitive diagnosis.

The screening that a particular woman experiences will depend on the hospital at which she is booked. Hospitals may differ with respect to the frequency and timing of ultrasound scanning, the availability of alpha feto-protein testing and the age at which amniocentesis is suggested. Some women will receive written information and counselling before deciding to undergo these procedures, while others will not.

Previous research has focused on the anxiety levels of 'high risk' women at different stages of pregnancy. It is evident that some women find the screening process very distressing, even if they are subsequently able to receive reassurance about the health of their baby. Women who had not considered themselves to be at risk initially are particularly likely to find the process stressful. Beyond this, very few researchers have tackled the question of why some women find that screening creates anxieties while others are reassured. In addition, little is known about the feelings of the majority of screened women: those who are not identified as being at high risk.

This study, funded for three years from March 1989 by the Health Promotion Research Trust, examined the experiences of an unselected group of women at hospitals with different screening policies. Women completed four postal questionnaires: prior to booking, at twenty-two weeks, at thirty-five weeks and six weeks after the birth. One thousand eight hundred and twenty-five women were recruited. A linked study, focusing on Sickle Cell Screening, recruited a further 500 women in the Midlands. The questionnaires monitored changes in womens' knowledge and attitudes with regard to screening during pregnancy. These were considered relative to other aspects of their lives, including: reproductive history; experiences during their pregnancy; perception of their own risk of fetal abnormality; attitudes towards abortion; attitudes towards medical care; the desire to obtain information; and hospital practice.

Anxiety about fetal abnormality was examined in the context of other sources of anxiety and the women's general predisposition to being anxious. The study yielded rich data on the emotions of pregnant women in the context of their everyday lives. Relationship with partner was found generally to deteriorate during pregnancy and to be an important indicator of emotional well-being.

Pre-natal screening tests (unless giving positive results) were found to have little impact on women's anxieties. Those who had had AFP screening were no less anxious about their baby than women in hospitals where the test was not offered.

Further research on the best ways to implement screening programmes for Downs Syndrome is needed since it appears to cause considerable anxiety and confusion.

Keywords: ALPHA FETO-PROTEIN, AMNIOCENTESIS, ANTENATAL CARE, ANTE-NATAL SCREENING, FETAL ABNORMALITY, ULTRASOUND

Green JM, Statham HE. Psychological and social aspects of screening during routine antenatal care. Paper presented to BSA Medical Sociology Conference, Manchester September 1989.

Green JM. Calming or harming? A critical review of psychological effects of fetal diagnosis on pregnant women. Galton Institute Occasional Papers, Second Series No. 2. March 1990.

Green JM. Commentary: Prenatal screening and diagnosis: some psychological and social issues. British Journal of Obstetrics and Gynaecology 1990;97:1074-6.

Green JM. Women's experiences of prenatal screening and diagnosis. In: Abramsky L and Chapple J (eds), The Human Side of Prenatal Diagnosis. London: Chapman and Hall. 1994.

Green JM, France-Dawson M. Women's experiences of routine screening during pregnancy: the sickle cell study. Proceedings of a symposium entitled "Targetting health promotion: reaching those in need". Kings Fund Centre, London, 24 June 1992.

Green JM, Snowdon C, Statham H. Pregnant women's attitudes to abortion and prenatal screening. Journal of Reproductive and Infant Psychology 1993;11:31-9.

Green J, Statham H. Testing for fetal abnormality in routine antenatal care. Midwifery 1993;9:124-35.

Green JM, Statham H, Snowdon C. Screening for fetal abnormality: attitudes and experiences. In: Chard T and Richards MPM, (Eds). Obstetrics in the 1990s: Current Controversies. Mackeith Press. 1992.

Green JM, Statham H, Snowdon C. Women's knowledge of prenatal screening tests. 1: Relationships with hospital screening policy and demographic factors. Journal of Reproductive and Infant Psychology 1993;11:11-20.

Green JM, Statham H, Snowdon C. Pregnancy: A testing time. Report of the Cambridge Prenatal Screening Study. Centre for Family Research, University of Cambridge.

Richards MPM, Green JM. Attitudes towards prenatal screening for fetal abnormality and detection of carriers of genetic disease: a discussion paper. Journal of Reproductive and Infant Psychology 1993;11:49-56.

Statham H. Professional understanding and parents' experience of termination. In: Brock DJ, Rodeck CH and Ferguson Smith MA (Eds). Prenatal Screening and Diagnosis 1993:697-702. London: Churchill Livingstone.

Statham H. Women's experiences of termination of pregnancy for fetal abnormality. In: Abramsky L & Chapple J (Eds) The Human side of Prenatal Diagnosis. London: Chapman and Hall 1994.

Statham H, Dimavicius J. How do you give the bad news to parents? Birth 1992;19:103-4.

Statham H, Green J. The effects of miscarriage and other 'unsuccessful' pregnancies on feelings early in subsequent pregnancy. Journal of Reproductive and Infant Psychology 1994 (in press).

Statham H, Green J. Issues raised by serum screening for Down's syndrome: some women's experiences. British Medical Journal 1993;307:174-6.

Statham H, Green J, Snowdon C. When is a fetus a dead baby? Lancet 1991.

Statham H, Green J, Snowdon C. Psychological and social aspects of screening for fetal abnormality during routine antenatal care. Proceedings of 'Research and the Midwife' Conference. November 1992.

Statham H, Green J, Snowdon C. Mothers' consent to screening newborn babies for disease. British Medical Journal 1993;306:858-9.

Statham H, Green J, Snowdon C, France-Dawson M. Choice of baby's sex. Lancet 1993;341:564-5.

Green JM, Murray D. The use of the EPDS in research to explore the relationship between antenatal and postnatal dysphoria. In: Cox JL and Holden J,(eds). Prevention of Depression after Childbirth: Use and Misuse of the Edinburgh Postnatal Depression Scale. London: Gaskell Press. 1994.

Green JM, Statham H, Snowdon C. EPDS by post. British Journal of Psychiatry 1991;158:865.

Green JM. Ethics and late termination of pregnancy. Lancet 1993;342:1179.

79. SHOULD OUR MOTHERS KNOW MORE ABOUT BREASTFEEDING?

March - July 1989

L A Swanwick, 3rd Year Undergraduate in BN Nursing Studies. **Contact:** L A Swanwick, Hormare Crescent, Storrington, West Sussex RH20 4QX.

Formed part of a course. 2-6 hours/week of own time spent.

Abstract: The purpose of the study was to investigate whether or not information-giving increased the success of breastfeeding in early infancy, and to assess the amount of health education mothers receive on infant feeding.

The study was a small survey, using a semi-structured questionnaire posted to the participants at home six weeks after the birth of their baby. Half of the participants (study group) would have received previously an information sheet on latching their baby to the breast the day they arrived on the postnatal ward. All participants were primiparous women over the age of eighteen (n=30: control group n=15, study group n=15). The control and study groups were compared as to their breastfeeding duration. This was then compared to other factors. At six weeks postpartum, 50% of all mothers had ceased breastfeeding, the information sheet not seeming to have made any noticeable difference in prevalence, although the small numbers involved did not yield any significant results. None of the mothers had given solids and complementary feeding was not popular. Mothers in the youngest age group (eighteen to twenty-two years) fared worst with breastfeeding, only 10% still breastfeeding at six weeks. Mothers who had attended an antenatal class which had discussed breastfeeding thoroughly fared better, as did those whose husbands were keen for them to breastfeed. Half of the mothers received conflicting advice.

This study provides information which justifies further research into the effects of maternal age, antenatal class attendance and support on breastfeeding duration. It may be beneficial to have a mother who has succeeded and one who has failed at breastfeeding to talk at antenatal classes. A comprehensive set of easy to read articles and information sheets on breastfeeding could be given to mothers with plenty of encouragement early in pregnancy, and infant feeding practices could be constantly reassessed.

Keywords: BREASTFEEDING (DURATION), BREASTFEEDING (INCIDENCE), BREASTFEEDING (INFORMATION), BREASTFEEDING (SUPPORT), COMMUNICATION PROBLEMS, CONFLICTING ADVICE, INFANT FEEDING (DECISIONS), MATERNAL EDUCATION

81. COMPARISON OF MANAGEMENT AND OUTCOME OF LABOUR UNDER TWO SYSTEMS OF CARE
January - December 1986
D Walsh, Staff Midwife Postnatal & Antenatal ward. **Contact:** D Walsh, Darthorpe Avenue, Western Park, Leicester LE3 OUQ.
For full details see under Management Studies (Record No. 81).

83. A SURVEY OF TRANSITIONAL CARE
January 1984 - February 1989
C A Whitby, Midwife Manager, Jean F Boxall, Hon Research Fellow, University of Exeter, Clive Lawrence, Lecturer, University of Exeter, John Tripp, Senior Lecturer, University of Exeter. **Contact:** C A Whitby, Neonatal Unit, Rosie Maternity Hospital, Robinson Way, Cambridge CB2 2SW. Tel: 0223 245151
For full details see under Management Studies (Record No. 83).

85. A PRELIMINARY STUDY OF NEONATAL NURSES'/MIDWIVES' PERCEPTIONS OF NEONATAL PAIN WITH PARTICULAR REFERENCE TO THE LOW BIRTHWEIGHT INFANT
January - December 1990
V Fletcher, Research Midwife, Neonatal Unit. **Contact:** V Fletcher, Randolph Road, Broomhill, Glasgow G11 7LG.

Funded as integral or additional part of a job by employer: Glasgow Royal Maternity Hospital. 12-20 hours/week of own time spent.

Abstract: The purpose of the study was to explore the behavioural and physiological signs that neonatal midwives interpret as suggesting the possibility of pain in the neonate. In addition, neonatal midwives were asked to describe nursing interventions currently practised or known about which would reduce pain and discomfort in infants.

The study was descriptive, combining qualitative and quantitative approaches. The research instrument used was a previously tested general information and pain sensitivity questionnaire. The questionnaire asked neonatal midwives to identify those physiological and behavioural signs that suggest the possibility of pain and discomfort in the infant. The questionnaire was distributed to the five neonatal units in the City of Glasgow. A total of 109 neonatal midwives were invited to participate who had more than six months' experience of neonatal intensive care nursing. Ninety-two (84%) questionnaires were returned. These data, identified only by a unique study number, were analyzed using combined computer and hand methods. Ninety-nine per cent of neonatal midwives questioned felt infants under their care suffered pain and discomfort irrespective of period of gestation. Main reasons given for this included insufficient medical knowledge with respect to pain control (74, 80.4%), and insufficient nursing knowledge with respect to pain control (63, 68.4%).

Over half (52%) of midwives felt that insertion of a chest drain was the most painful procedure experienced by the infants. Despite this, seventy-four (80.4%) of the midwives stated analgesia was never/rarely given in their experience for this procedure. Over three-quarters (72, 78.2%) of the neonatal midwives questioned correctly identified the main behavioural and physiological measures previously validated as indicating pain and distress in infants. Despite this high level of awareness only fifty-four (58.6%) described or identified nursing interventions which may help to reduce pain and distress in the infants in their care.

Keywords: LOW BIRTHWEIGHT, MIDWIVES (NEONATAL), NEONATAL UNITS, NURSING INTERVENTION, PAIN (NEONATAL)

Fletcher V. A study of neonatal nurses' and midwives' perceptions of pain and discomfort in the neonate. Unpublished report, Neonatal Unit, Glasgow Royal Maternity Hospital March 1990.

86. PERCEPTIONS OF FIRST TIME MOTHERS DURING THE FIRST THREE POSTPARTUM MONTHS
January 1987 - December 1991

Pearl Herbert, Assistant Professor. **Contact:** Pearl Herbert, School of Nursing, Memorial University of Newfoundland, St John's, Newfoundland, Canada A1B 3V6. Tel: 0101 709 737 6755

Formed part of a course. Funded by funding agency(ies): Medical Research Council of Canada, UK Universities overseas research student award.

Abstract: This study collected prospective data from first-time mothers who previously had not had the responsibility of caring for a young baby, regarding their perceptions during the first three postpartum months.

The women who participated had partners, were aged eighteen years or older, and had given birth vaginally to a well baby who was being discharged from hospital at the same time as the mother. They were recruited into the study during the first three postpartum days, while they were still in hospital. Information regarding the study and how their names would be protected was given to them and if they agreed to participate a consent form was obtained. A questionnaire was completed to obtain demographic information and to ensure that they met the criteria for the study. At this time they were given a diary, with instructions for its completion over the next three months. There were forty-seven mothers who met the criteria to participate, of whom fifteen refused, eight withdrew, and twenty-four completed the four interviews (twenty-two kept a diary for three months). They were then visited at home for a semi-focused audio-tape-recorded interview four times during these three months. During these visits the pages of their diary were collected. The instruments had been tested prior to the main study.

The consistently, striking perception that mothers had of being a mother was that the experience was tiring, and resulted in irritable and difficult situations. They considered that they were tired because of the physical healing which was occurring, and changes in their sleep routine as they had to wake to care for their baby. When the babies did sleep at night they were awake during the day and requiring attention which prevented the mothers from resting. The mothers were worried if they perceived that something was wrong with the baby. They were reassured if the baby gained weight and compared favourably with other babies. The mothers organised their life around the baby and this aided them to get to know their baby for whose safety they felt responsible. The mothers perceived that there were many changes happening to their bodies and that becoming a mother is an ongoing process.

Recommendations arising out of this study are that further research is needed to discover the perceptions of mothers who have a disability or have a baby requiring prolonged hospitalization and to investigate how men perceive becoming a father.

Keywords: ADAPTATION TO MOTHERHOOD, BODY IMAGE, CONCERNS (WOMEN'S), EXPERIENCE (WOMEN'S), MATERNAL TASKS, PERCEPTIONS OF MOTHERHOOD (WOMEN'S), PRIMIGRAVIDAE

Herbert P. The perceptions of first time mothers during the neomaternal period. In: International Confederation of Midwives 23rd Triennial Congress, Proceedings 1993;2:832-48.

89. INNOVATIONS FOR ANTENATAL BOOKING
January - September 1988

Susan Williams, Mary Thompson Research Fellow. **Contact:** Susan Williams, Glasgow College, Cowcaddens, Glasgow G4 OBA. Tel: 041 332 3731 Ext 4

Funded as integral or additional part of a job by employer: Ayrshire & Arran Health Board.

Abstract: (Not updated since 1991) CONFIDENTIAL

Keywords: ALCOHOL, ANTENATAL BOOKING INTERVIEW, ANTENATAL EDUCATION, DIET, INFORMATION GIVING, PREGNANCY, SMOKING

90. AN INVESTIGATION INTO MIDWIVES' ATTITUDES TO MIDWIFERY PRACTICE AND THE ROLE OF WOMEN
September 1988 - September 1989

J Rogers. **Contact:** J Rogers, Court Cottage, Salwarpe, Droitwich, Worcs WR9 OAH.

Own time spent. Formed part of a course. Funded by employer and by Iolanthe Trust.

Abstract: This research project consists of a multi-strategy approach combining interview and questionnaire data on midwives working in a West Midlands health district. The purpose of the study was to explore midwives' perceptions of their role with regard to: 1) desire for responsibility; 2) response to the medicalisation of maternity care; and 3) attitudes to the role of women.

A variety of social factors including length and type of qualification, age, designation, duty and location of work, educational level, maternal status, and possession of additional midwifery qualifications were correlated with attitude constructs. In addition, factors such as level of voluntary midwifery activity and experience or desire for involvement in innovative midwifery projects were included in the correlations. The strongest correlations occurred between attitudes to the role of women and the midwife's perception of her role as facilitator or authoritarian. The desire for responsibility was also related to the midwives' conceptual models of pregnancy, as well as their perceptions of their role and their attitudes towards the role of women. Social factors were not strong indicators of overall attitude scores, though they did differentiate groups of respondents on individual statements.

The study also attempted to assess the level of support among midwives for changes to midwifery practice as suggested by their professional organisations. There was overwhelming support for these proposals. The major stumbling block to their implementation, however, was perceived to be medical resistance to losing control of responsibility in maternity care.

Keywords: MEDICALISATION, MIDWIFE'S ROLE, MIDWIFERY, VOLUNTARY PROFESSIONAL ACTIVITY, WOMEN'S ROLE

92. A CONFIDENTIAL ENQUIRY INTO THE RELIEF OF PAIN IN LABOUR
June - July 1990

G Chamberlain, Professor of Obstetrics & Gynaecology, Ann Wraight, Survey Co-ordinator. **Contact:** Ann Wraight, Department of Obstetrics & Gynaecology, St George's Hospital Medical School, London SW17 ORE. Tel: 081 672 9944 Ex 53670

2-6 hours/week of own time spent. Funded by funding agency(ies): The National Birthday Trust.

Abstract: The aims of this descriptive, prospective study were: 1) to determine methods of pain control (non-pharmacological as well as pharmacological); 2) to identify how the couple was prepared to cope with the pain of labour; and 3) to compare the woman's assessment of her relief with those who cared for her in labour. The study consisted of three parts: 1) a profile of the maternity unit; 2) a profile of the woman, her labour and pain control (assessments of the effectiveness of the methods used were made by herself, her supporter and the professionals who provided her care; a paediatric assessment was made on the baby); and 3) a random sample of 10% of the women who participated completed a follow-up questionnaire when their babies were six weeks old.

All maternity units in the UK (ie, the NHS, Armed Services and Independent Units) were invited to take part in this national study. Eighty-eight per cent agreed to participate. Data were collected from postal questionnaires completed by everyone involved in the birth of a baby during the week commencing 25 June 1990. This included home confinements.

The results of the study are summarised in the following paragraphs.
A wide variety of pain relieving methods are available in the UK and most women use some form of pain relief in labour. The major determinents of the use of pain relief are the method the women planned to use and the duration of labour. Only a small number of women used alternative methods of pain relief.
Entonox and pethidine are widely used. Pethidine has side effects on mother and baby which make it less than ideal. It was associated with a reduction in the proportion of babies who successfully established breast feeding.
Epidural analgesia was available in only 63% of maternity units. Couples need to be made aware in pregnancy about the availability of epidurals.
Pain associated with perineal repair is often severe and women assess the analgesic methods used as inadequate.

Recommendations arising out of this study are that further research is needed into ways of reducing the side effects of pethidine and improved methods of pain relief for perineal repair.

Keywords: ANTENATAL EDUCATION, EXPERIENCE (PARENTS'), EXPERIENCE (WOMEN'S), LABOUR (SATISFACTION), PAIN ASSESSMENT, PAIN EXPERIENCE, PAIN RELIEF (LABOUR)

Wraight A. Happy birthdays. (National Birthday Trust Fund to ask midwives to participate in a nationwide survey of pain relief in labour). Nursing Times 1990;86:22-3.

94. ASIAN ANTENATAL CARE PROGRAMME
November 1989 - March 1992
Judy Dance, Research Nurse, Shams Un Nihar, Linkworker, Ratna Alom, Linkworker, Nasim Altaf, Linkworker, Farah Diba, Linkworker, Rekha Sarkar, Linkworker.
Contact: Judy Dance, Room 06 : Community Offices, Yardley Green Unit, East Birmingham Hospital, Yardley Green Road, Birmingham B9 5PX. Tel: 021 766 6611 Ex 2306

Funded as integral or additional part of a job by employer: East Birmingham Hospital.

Aims of the study: To evaluate the introduction of an Asian Linkworker Programme with specific reference to perinatal mortality rates and the number of low birthweight infants in the Asian community.

Ethics committee approval gained: Yes.

Research design: Experimental – Quantitative – Case Study

    Data collection:
        Techniques used:
            Case note review
        Time data were collected:
            During pregnancy, specifically:
            18 weeks, 25 weeks and 33 weeks for women booking less than 18 weeks.
            25 weeks, 30 weeks and 35 weeks for women booking more than 18 weeks.
            Plus any other time of contact.
            Postnatally, 4-10 days; 7/8 weeks.
        Testing of any tools used:
            None needed.
        Topics covered:
            Mortality.
            Analgesia during labour.
            Episiotomy rates.
            Length of labour.
            Breast feeding.
            Attendance for postnatal examination.
        Setting for data collection:
            Community.

Details about sample studied:
Planned size of sample:
Approximately 200 women per year.
Rationale for planned size:
Based on feasibility calculation.
Entry criteria:
Inclusion:

Primigravidae Asian women.

Multigravidae having their first "British birth".

Exclusion:

Those with a history of low birthweight infant or perinatal death unless it was associated with:

i) multiple pregnancy.

ii) elective Caesarean Section.

iii) gross congenital abnormality

All women booking later than 24 weeks gestation.
Sample selection:
Inclusive sample.
Actual sample size:
464 women in experimental group.

221 women in "control" group.

Interventions, Outcomes and Analysis
Interventions used:
In addition to routine antenatal care, Asian women received a minimum of three home visits and two phone calls from an Asian Linkworker who spoke their mother tongue. The Linkworker's role was to provide basic health education/information and social support.
Main outcomes measured:
Death.

Analgesia in labour.

Requirement for episiotomy.

Length of labour.

Breast feeding - inclination and duration.

Attendance for postnatal examination.
Analysis:
Chi-square.

Results: Women included in the Programme had an improved perinatal mortality rate (12.9 per 1000) compared with women not included in the Asian Linkworker Programme (19.2). They also had a lower rate of low birthweight infants (8.1% compared with 11.3%).

Comparison of other factors indicated that those in the Programme:

- had fewer low birth weight perinatal deaths.
- required less analgesia during labour.
- required less episiotomies.
- had shorter labours.

- were more inclined to breast feed.
- breast fed for longer.
- were more likely to attend for postnatal examination.

Recommendations for further research: Asian Antenatal Care Programme - ongoing.

Keywords: ANTENATAL CARE PLANS, ANTENATAL EDUCATION, ASIAN WOMEN, BIRTHWEIGHT, ETHNIC GROUPS, LINKWORKERS, LOW BIRTHWEIGHT, OUTCOMES (PERINATAL)

Dance J. Evaluation of Asian Linkworker Programme. East Birmingham Health Authority Antenatal Care Services Review: 1989-1992:12-22.

95. A STUDY OF THE EFFECT OF LATERAL ASYMMETRIES ON BREASTFEEDING SKILL AND OF THE INTERVENTIONS USED BY MIDWIVES TO OVERCOME UNILATERAL BREASTFEEDING PROBLEMS
April - November 1989
D Stables, Midwife Teacher. **Contact:** D Stables, Cranham Gardens, Upminster, Essex RM14 1JQ.

Formed part of a course. 2-6 hours/week of own time spent.

Abstract: Midwives are aware of unilateral breastfeeding problems and use intervention holds to help. This problem may be caused by lateral asymmetries in mother or infant.

Three lateral asymmetries - handedness, maternal preferred holding side and neonatal preferred head-turning - were examined in a sample of sixty first-time breastfeeding women, who were divided into two groups: experimental (n=32) who had a unilateral breastfeeding problem, and controls (n=28) with no problem.

The two groups of mothers did not differ significantly in their age, social class, marital status, baby's weight or sex. Multiparous women were less likely to have a unilateral breastfeeding problem and to report a preferred feeding side and more likely to be breastfeeding at six weeks. Hand preference was examined using Bryden's (1982) modification of the Edinburgh handedness inventory and hand performance by a test which combined speed with accuracy of placing dots in circles. Neither test differentiated between women with or without a unilateral breastfeeding problem, the degree of difficulty, preferred feeding side or breastfeeding at six weeks. When the mother's dominant hand was different from her preferred holding side, she was more likely to have a problem feeding side and a preferred feeding side. Neonatal head-turning preference was associated with the unilateral breastfeeding problem. All three lateral asymmetries were associated with the development of a unilateral breastfeeding problem, and having a problem was associated with reporting a preferred feeding side.

This last lateral asymmetry was the only one significantly associated with failure at six weeks.

The midwives' intervention holds were not associated with breastfeeding success; it could, therefore, be important to try to minimise the effects of the three lateral asymmetries researched by antenatal interventions.

Keywords: BREASTFEEDING, BREASTFEEDING BEHAVIOUR (INFANT), BREASTFEEDING BEHAVIOUR (MATERNAL), BREASTFEEDING (PROBLEMS), BREASTFEEDING (UNILATERAL), HAND PREFERENCE, LATERAL ASYMMETRIES, MIDWIFERY SKILLS

98. INDICATORS OF BREASTFEEDING SUCCESS: TOWARDS A SOCIOLOGY OF BREASTFEEDING
January 1988 - December 1995
Louise Silverton, Lecturer/Practitioner. **Contact:** Louise Silverton, Queen Charlotte's College of Health Studies, Hammersmith Hospital, Du Cane Road, London W12 OHS. Tel: 081 740 3213

Formed part of a course. Own time spent.

Abstract: (Not updated since 1991) CONFIDENTIAL.

Keywords: BREASTFEEDING, BREASTFEEDING (DURATION), BREASTFEEDING (SUPPORT), FAMILIES

99. INFLUENCING BREASTFEEDING SUCCESS
January - October 1983
Louise Silverton, Lecturer in Midwifery. **Contact:** Louise Silverton, Queen Charlotte's College of Health Studies, Hammersmith Hospital, Du Cane Road, London W12 OHS. Tel: 081 740 3213

Formed part of a course. Funded by employer: Lothian Health Board.

Abstract: The research involved developing an antenatal programme to prepare mothers for breastfeeding. The programme was planned to involve detailed teaching of physiology and management of breastfeeding. The content of this programme was based on a thorough literature review. Hayward's work on information-giving and the work of Helsing and Gunther was most important in designing the teaching programme. The mothers in the education group were to be compared with a matched controlled group as regards length of feeding, reasons for discontinuing and knowledge base. Because this was part of an MSc. degree and due to the time scale of the study, the educational programme and questionnaires were developed and piloted with a group of twelve women but the full project was never undertaken. Some aspects have now been incorporated in the author's PhD studies.

Keywords: ANTENATAL EDUCATION, BREASTFEEDING, BREASTFEEDING (DURA-TION)

Silverton LI. Breastfeeding yesterday and today. Midwifery 1985;1:162-6.
Silverton LI. Influencing breastfeeding success. Unpublished MSc thesis, University of Edinburgh.

100. PARENTCRAFT AS EDUCATION
October 1986 - August 1988

A L Wainwright, Midwifery Tutor, L Chisholm, Lecturer Supervisor. **Contact:** A L Wainwright, Kingsway, Wembley, Middlesex HA9 7QR.

Formed part of a course. Funded by funding agency(ies): St Bartholomew's Hospital, The Royal Free Hospital.

Abstract: This descriptive study was concerned with the attendance of pregnant women at parentcraft classes, and their effectiveness as viewed by the consumers (primiparae); and the professionals involved with this education.

The sample populations were drawn from the two groups already mentioned with the research extending over a period of two months. As there were no figures available concerning the patterns of attendance, the pilot study was of considerable value in this respect. A different semi-structured interview schedule was used with each group, allowing for quantitative and qualitative data to be collected. During the first week of the field work all primiparae were interviewed on the third/fourth day postpartum. This 100% sampling enabled the proportion of full attenders, partial attenders and non-attenders at parentcraft classes to be identified. An estimate was then made of the total number of each group over the two-month period. It was discovered that the partial attenders were the largest group. In order to achieve approximately the same number in each group, it was decided that 100% samples would be taken of the full attenders and non-attenders; and a systematic sample of one in two was applied, retrospectively, to the partial attender respondents in the first week. Eighty-two primiparae and fourteen professionals participated with 100% response rate.

The completed questionnaires were coded and data entered into data files in a Nanostat package on the Compaq computer. Descriptive statistics were obtained from all variables. The overall view was one of optimism, with 74% of the women attending classes fully or in part, and general satisfaction was felt with the provision by both the consumers and the professionals. However, the research did suggest four main problem areas: attendance patterns, communication, competency to teach, and finally knowledge and control. Recommendations were made concerning these issues.

Keywords: ANTENATAL EDUCATION, EDUCATION FOR PARENTHOOD, EDUCATION FOR PARENTHOOD (ATTENDANCE), EDUCATION FOR PARENTHOOD (TEACHERS), EDUCATION (GENERAL), EXPERIENCE (WOMEN'S)

101. THE MULTICENTRE RANDOMISED CONTROLLED TRIAL OF ALTERNATIVE TREATMENTS FOR INVERTED AND NON-PROTRACTILE NIPPLES IN PREGNANCY

February 1988 - September 1993

Mary J Renfrew, Director, Midwifery Research Programme, Adrian Grant, Epidemiologist, Joanne M Alexander, Midwife Tutor, Rona McCandlish, Research Midwife, Ellen Hodnett, Associate Professor, Paula Mastrilli, Project Director. **Contact:** Rona McCandlish, National Perinatal Epidemiology Unit, Radcliffe Infirmary, Oxford OX2 6HE. Tel: 0865 224332

Funded as integral or additional part of a job by employer and by funding agency(ies): Department of Health, The Hospital for Sick Children Foundation, Toronto.

Aims of the study: To assess the effects of Hoffman's nipple stretching exercises, breast shells and the combination of Hoffman's exercises and breast shells on the duration of breastfeeding in women with inverted and non-protractile nipples.

Ethics committee approval gained: Yes

Research design: Experimental – Qualitative and Quantitative – Randomized Controlled Trial

Data collection:
Techniques used:
Completion of trial entry form.
Self-completed questionnaire.
Time data were collected:
Entry data - between 25 and 35 completed weeks of pregnancy.
Postal questionnaire - 6-8 weeks postnatally.
Testing of any tools used:
All documents piloted with local midwives and NCT branches.
Topics covered:
Entry data:
Basic demographic information;
state of nipples;
previous breastfeeding experience.
Postnatal data:
Duration and experience of breastfeeding;
problems with breastfeeding;
introduction of other infant feeding;
infant weight gain.
Setting for data collection:
Entry data: Community and hospital antenatal clinics in 10 hospital centres in UK and 6 hospital and 1 public health unit in Ontario, Canada. Also via 20 National Childbirth Trust coordinators.
Postnatal data: Participants' own homes.

Details about sample studied:
    Planned size of sample:
        600
    Rationale for planned size:
        To permit accurate assessment of the effect on breastfeeding of either one, the other or both interventions on breastfeeding rates at 6 weeks (80% power, 2 tailed alpha = 0.05)
    Entry criteria:
        One or both nipples inverted or non-protractile.
        Singleton pregnancy.
        Intending to breastfeed.
        Between 25 and 35 completed weeks of pregnancy.
        Not previously breastfed for longer than 7 days.
        Not planning to give baby up for adoption.
        No history of surgery to the nipple or areola.
        Not already using breast shells or nipple stretching exercises.
    Sample selection:
        Random allocation using pre-prepared, sealed opaque envelopes, to one of four groups.
    Actual sample size:
        463
    Response rate:
        95%

Interventions, Outcomes and Analysis
    Interventions used:
        Breast shells.
        Hoffman's nipple stretching exercises.
    Main outcomes measured:
        Duration of breastfeeding during first 6 weeks after birth.
    Analysis:
        SPSS
        Student t-test
        Chi-square
        Rates differences
        Odds ratio

Results: One hundred and three (45%) women allocated to breast shells and 104 (45%) women not allocated to shells were breastfeeding at six weeks after delivery. One hundred and seven (46%) women allocated Hoffman's nipple stretching exercises and 100 (44%) women not allocated to Hoffman's nipple stretching exercises were breastfeeding six weeks after delivery.

In the light of the results from this and a previous single centre trial (Alexander et al 1992) there is no basis for recommending the use of either breast shells or Hoffman's nipples stretching exercises as antenatal preparation for breastfeeding for women with inverted and non-protractile nipples.
See also MIRIAD Study No. 3.

Keywords: ANTENATAL CARE, BREAST SHELLS, BREASTFEEDING, BREASTFEEDING (DURATION), HOFFMAN'S EXERCISES, MULTICENTRE, NIPPLES (INVERTED), NIPPLES (NON-PROTRACTILE), RANDOMIZED CONTROLLED TRIAL

Renfrew MJ, McCandlish R. With women: new steps in research in midwifery. In: Robert H, ed. Women's Health Matters 1992:81-98. London: Routledge.

McCandlish R, Renfrew MJ. Development of the multicentre randomised controlled trial of alternative treatments for inverted and non-protractile nipples in pregnancy: the MAIN Trial. Research and the Midwife Conference Proceedings 1991:21-4.

McCandlish R, Renfrew MJ. Trial and Tribulation. Nursing Times 1991;87:40-1.

McCandlish R, Renfrew MJ. Antenatal treatments for inverted or flat nipples. Nursing Times 1991;87:15.

McCandlish R, Renfrew MJ, Ashurst H, Bowler U. Getting results: the processes involved in organising and analysing data from the MAIN trial. Research and the Midwife Conference Proceedings 1992:17-25.

102. HOW LONG SHOULD A BREASTFEED LAST?
January 1978 - July 1979

Peter W Howie, Professor of Obstetrics, Mary J Houston, Research Sister (Midwifery), Ann Cook, Research Sister, Lesley Smart, Medical Student, Teresa McArdle, Medical Student, Alan S McNeilly, Research Scientist. **Contact:** Mary J Renfrew, National Perinatal Epidemiology Unit, Radcliffe Infirmary, Oxford OX2 6HE. Tel: 0865 224876

Funded as integral or additional part of a job. Funded by employer. MRC Reproductive Biology Unit.

Abstract: The amount of milk taken by normal birthweight breastfed babies was studied in fifty mothers and babies on days five to seven postpartum. No information was previously available about this; management of breastfeeding by midwives and paediatricians was often based on results of routine test-weighing, or on the amount of time babies fed for. Standard feeding times were recommended for all mothers and babies. Test-weighing using accurate electronic scales was carried out by the mothers themselves at five-minute intervals during two consecutive feeds. Prolactin levels were measured by blood samples taken from an indwelling cannula at specified intervals from the start of the feed until two hours later.

In line with recommended feeding routines in place in the study hospital, women were asked to feed either for ten minutes on each breast, or on an alternating regime of five minutes on one breast and five on the other, five on the first and five on the other. This latter regime increased the amount of milk taken in the first ten minutes, but did not influence the final milk intake or the suckling induced prolactin release. There was a marked variation of breastfeeding patterns between mothers in respect of the duration of the feed (range seven to thirty minutes) the initial rate of milk flow (range 1-14 g/min) and the final milk intake (range 42-125 g/min).

The standard advice to breastfeed for twenty minutes was inappropriate for the majority of women: feeding time was fifteen minutes or less in 75% of feeds. Other babies took up to thirty minutes before they were satisfied. As a result of this study, it is recommended that the duration of a breastfeed should be determined by the infant's response and not by an arbitrary time schedule, and midwives and others supporting breastfeeding women should become more aware of the need to encourage mothers to respond to their own babies.

Keywords: BREASTFEEDING, BREASTFEEDING (DURATION), BREASTMILK, BREASTMILK INTAKE, PROLACTIN LEVELS

Howie PW, Houston MJ, Cook A, Smart L, McArdle T, McNeilly AJ. How long should a breastfeed last? Early Human Development 1981;5:71-7.

103. THE MEASUREMENT OF BREAST MILK INTAKE
January 1978 - January 1979
Mary J Houston, Midwife Researcher, Peter W Howie, Consultant Obstetrician, Alan S McNeilly, Research Scientist. **Contact:** Mary J Renfrew, National Perinatal Epidemiology Unit, Radcliffe Infirmary, Oxford OX2 6HE. Tel: 0865 224876

Funded as integral or additional part of a job by employer: MRC Reproductive Biology Unit. Formed part of a course. 2 hours/week of own time spent.

Abstract: The purpose of this study was to develop and test a technique for the accurate measurement of breastmilk intake by babies in the early days of life. This technique was intended for further studies to assess potential problems and the effects of routine hospital practices on breastfeeding.

A convenience sample of eighteen women and their babies who met pre-established entry criteria (intending to breastfeed, babies >2500g, thirty-eight weeks' gestation or more, and agreement to participate) were recruited from the Simpson Memorial Maternity Pavilion, Edinburgh. Nine were recruited antenatally, nine within the first twenty-four hours after delivery. Ten women were primiparous, eight were multiparous. In order to achieve the maximum accuracy possible, test-weigh measurements were carried out using a Mettler integrated electronic balance (Gallenkamp and Co. Ltd., London). This balance gave readings which were reproducible to within 2g, even if the baby moved vigorously during weighing. Minimal disturbance was caused to the baby as the cot itself was placed on the scales.

Using these scales, women measured the milk intake of their babies at each feed throughout the day for the duration of the study period (which continued until they were discharged). A total of sixty-three completed days of measurement, from Day 1 to Day 9, were recorded. Intake at 366 breastfeeds was measured.

The actual intakes over each twenty-four hour period were then compared with two estimated intakes. One estimate was based on each infant's intake at one feed (multiplied by the number of feeds in that twenty-four hour period) and the second estimate was based on intake at two consecutive feeds. These estimates compared well (correlation coefficient of 0.896 on the basis of one feed, 0.948 on the basis of two feeds) with actual intakes.

The results suggest that using this accurate technique, a close estimate of breastmilk intake can be gained from measurement of one or two breastfeeds in twenty-four hours. This technique could be used in research studies, but not for the routine test-weighing of breastfed infants, as the test-weigh conditions in this study were strictly controlled, and the scales were highly accurate.

Keywords: BREASTFEEDING, RESEARCH TECHNIQUE, TESTWEIGHING

Houston MJ. Requirements for successful breastfeeding. 1982 Unpublished PhD thesis, MRC Reproductive Biology Unit/CNAA/University of Edinburgh.
Houston MJ, Howie PW, McNeilly AJ. Measurement of breastmilk intake in the first week of life. Early Human Development 1983;8:49-54.
Houston MJ. Successful breastfeeding: the need for support. Proceedings of the Research and the Midwife Conference, 1980; London & Glasgow.

104. EXAMINATION OF THE PROBLEMS ENCOUNTERED BY, & CARE OFFERED TO, BREASTFEEDING WOMEN
January 1980 - December 1981

Mary J Houston, Midwife Researcher, Peter W Howie, Obstetrician. **Contact:** Mary J Renfrew, National Perinatal Epidemiology Unit, Radcliffe Infirmary, Oxford OX2 6HE. Tel: 0865 224876

Funded as integral or additional part of a job by employer MRC Reproductive Biology Unit. Formed part of a course. 2-6 hours/week of own time spent.

Abstract: The purpose of this study was to describe in detail the problems encountered by breastfeeding women, and the care offered to them both by professional sources and by family/friends/voluntary groups.

One hundred and five women (thirty-five consecutive admissions to each of the three postnatal wards from the study hospital in Edinburgh, who were planning to breastfeed) were recruited to the study. Data were gathered from hospital records and during an extensive interview at home at twelve to sixteen weeks postpartum. The interview was semi-structured; it was designed for this study and extensively tested. It yielded both quantitative and qualitative information. Quantitative analysis was performed using the SPSS package. Other material was examined, sorted and categorised according to type and timing of problems or advice.

The findings were extensive. In summary: breastfeeding mothers encountered many problems which led them to give up breastfeeding against their own expressed wishes; secondly, mothers most often gave physical problems (a crying baby, or 'insufficient milk') as the main reason for premature discontinuation.

Detailed analysis showed that problems were many and varied, and that a solution based on solving 'insufficient milk' would be a major over-simplication. Related problems were especially troublesome about week two; the most common were tiredness, and a crying baby. A further peak of problems occurred around weeks seven to eight for mothers in lower social class groups. Social class was strongly related to success in breastfeeding, but was relatively unimportant in the enjoyment of breastfeeding, or in the number of problems reported. This suggests that it may not be the problems, but the ability to overcome them, that is the important factor. Social class based on paternal occupation was more discriminating than that based on maternal occupation. This suggests that it may be environmental factors, and not simply inherent maternal factors, that are important. Other variables were important and these may provide a picture of the 'at risk' factors such as previously unsuccessful breastfeeding mothers, and those who decided to breastfeed later in pregnancy. Mothers did not often find the help offered to them to be useful. There was no positive discrimination in distribution of care directed towards those most at risk.

Keywords: BREASTFEEDING, CONFLICTING ADVICE (FEEDING), POSTNATAL CARE, SUPPORT, SUPPORT (FAMILY)

Houston MJ. Successful breastfeeding: the need for support. Proceedings of the Research and the Midwife Conference, 1980: London & Glasgow.
Houston MJ. Requirements for successful breastfeeding. Unpublished PhD thesis, 1982 MRC Reproductive Biology Unit/CNAA/University of Edinburgh.
Houston MJ, Howie PW. The difficulties of breastfeeding and the care offered to breastfeeding mothers at home. Nursing Mirror Midwifery Forum 2 1983;156:1-7.
Houston MJ, Howie PW. Infant feeding. Nursing Mirror Midwifery Forum 4 1983;1-4.
Houston MJ. Home support for the breastfeeding mother. In: Houston MJ, ed. Maternal & Infant Health Care: Recent Advances in Nursing Series. Edinburgh: Churchill Livingston. 1984

105. EXTRA FLUID INTAKE BY THE BREASTFED BABY AND DURATION OF BREASTFEEDING
January - December 1980

Mary J Houston, Midwife Researcher, Peter W Howie, Obstetrician. **Contact:** Mary J Renfrew, National Perinatal Epidemiology Unit, Radcliffe Infirmary, Oxford OX2 6HE. Tel: 0865 224876

Funded as integral or additional part of a job by employer: MRC Reproductive Biology Unit. Formed part of a course. 2 hours/week of own time spent.

Abstract: The purpose of this study was to investigate the relationship between extra fluid intake by breastfed babies in the early puerperium with duration of breastfeeding. Three different regimes of giving extra fluid were monitored: that is, three postnatal wards in one hospital practised demand feeding, but differed in their use of extra fluids. In Ward A, extra fluids were given infrequently. In Ward B, extra fluids (Hartmanns, dextrose 5% or formula) were offered after every breastfeed in the first six days. In Ward C, extra fluids were offered fairly liberally but not as a strict routine.

The study included all seventy-eight breastfeeding mothers and their babies admitted to the three postnatal wards during the three-week study period. Mothers with multiple births and those whose babies were immediately admitted to SCBU were excluded. Data on feeding practices were gathered from the mothers' own records for the duration of their stay in hospital. Other data were gathered from the hospital records. A follow-up home interview (two weeks postpartum) was carried out to obtain information on breastfeeding duration. Seventy-seven out of seventy-eight women were interviewed.

The results provided no evidence that giving extra fluids to breastfed babies was necessary: all three groups had a similar duration of breastfeeding. There was no difference in jaundice levels. There was a marked difference in duration of feeding relating to the social class of the women in each of the three wards: women in social classes I and II continued for longer than women in social classes III, IV and V.

Keywords: BREASTFEEDING, EXTRA FLUIDS

Houston MJ. Successful breastfeeding: the need for support. Proceedings of the Research and the Midwife Conference 1980: London & Glasgow.

Houston MJ, Howie PW, McNeilly AS. The effect of extra fluid intake by breastfed babies in hospital on the duration of breastfeeding. Journal of Reproductive and Infant Psychology 1984;1:42-8

Houston MJ. Requirements for successful breastfeeding. Unpublished PhD thesis 1982 MRC Reproductive Biology Unit/CNAA/University of Edinburgh.

106. AN EXPERIMENTAL APPROACH TO HOME SUPPORT FOR THE BREASTFEEDING MOTHER
January 1979 - December 1980

Mary J Houston, Midwife Researcher, Peter W Howie, Consultant Obstetrician, Ann Cook, Research Sister, Alan S McNeilly, Research Scientist. **Contact:** Mary J Renfrew, National Perinatal Epidemiology Unit, Radcliffe Infirmary, Oxford OX2 6HE. Tel: 0865 224876

For full details see under Management Studies (Record No. 106)

107. EARLY MILK TRANSFER AND THE DURATION OF BREASTFEEDING
January 1979 - January 1980

Mary J Houston, Midwife Researcher, Peter W Howie, Consultant Obstetrician, Alan S McNeilly, Research Scientist. **Contact:** Mary J Renfrew, National Perinatal Epidemiology Unit, Radcliffe Infirmary, Oxford OX2 6HE. Tel: 0865 224876

Funded as integral or additional part of a job by employer: MRC Reproductive Biology Unit. Formed part of a course. 2 hours/week of own time spent.

Abstract: The purpose of this study was to investigate whether or not breastmilk intake by the baby on the third postpartum day was reflected in the subsequent duration of breastfeeding. In addition, it was planned to compare the clinical feeding practices of mothers who were giving larger amounts of milk on the third postpartum day with those who were giving lesser amounts of milk. Could we predict women who might develop problems with breastfeeding? If so, this might assist us in planning the provision of care.

Forty-seven breastfeeding women and their babies who met pre-established selection criteria (baby >2500g, gestation thirty-eight weeks or more, not jaundiced on the third postnatal day, agreed to participate) were recruited to the study. All women who met these criteria and who could be recruited within the constraints of the researcher's hours of work were recruited. Breastmilk intake was measured on day three postpartum according to a technique previously described by the researcher (Record No. 103). More women in the 'high' (>200g/24hrs) and 'medium' (50-200g/24hrs) intake groups continued to breastfeed at six weeks than women in the 'low' (<50g /24hrs) intake group (p<0.01 high v.low, p<0.05 medium v. low). Significant differences were found between these groups in their baby's weight loss at six days, the number of breastfeeds on each day postpartum (mothers in the 'high' group fed most often) and the volume of extra fluid given (the 'high' group gave least extra fluid). No difference was found in the timing of the first feed. Association was also found between social class and duration of breastfeeding, independently of intake on day three.

This study suggests that the outcome of breastfeeding may be affected and assessed as early as the third postpartum day. This has implications for the care given by midwives in the early days after birth.

Keywords: BREASTFEEDING, BREASTFEEDING (FREQUENCY), BREASTFEEDING (INCIDENCE), EXTRA FLUIDS, SOCIAL CLASS

Houston MJ. Requirements for successful breastfeeding. Unpublished PhD thesis, CNAA/MRC Reproductive Biology Unit/University of Edinburgh. 1982

Houston MJ, Howie PW, McNeilly AS. Measurement of breastmilk intake in the first week of life. Early Human Development 1983;8:49-54.

Houston MJ, Howie PW, Smart L, McArdle T, McNeilly AS. Factors affecting the duration of breastfeeding. Early Human Development 1983;8:55-63.

108. DELIVERIES - MOTHERS OR MIDWIVES? - A STUDY OF COMMUNICATION STYLES IN MIDWIFERY
November 1986 - May 1987
M E Adams, Head Midwifery and Womens Health Faculty. **Contact:** M E Adams, Meadway Drive, Horsell, Woking, Surrey GU21 4TF.

Formed part of a course. Funded by employer and by funding agency(ies): Maws/ RCM Research Scholarship.

Abstract: Communication was highlighted as long ago as 1960 as being an important therapeutic tool in the care of mothers and babies. Very little research has been carried out on this interaction skill, which is used by midwives for at least one-third of their working time.

This study was conducted by observation, with the use of video recordings, of the second stage of childbirth with the researcher having free access to this normally private event. Eleven video recordings were used to enable transcripts of speech and activities to be recorded in writing on a minute-to-minute basis, and the following categories of midwives' communication appeared from the data: innovating, encouraging, directing, educating, questioning, socialising and professional discussion. Calculations were made of the total and the pattern of each category during the second stage of labour. Three main categories emerged, with overlap between two of them which were combined as educating/encouraging, and this was compared to the directing category. The results of the interviews with the mothers indicated that they felt most satisfied with midwives who had a higher ratio of education/encouragement style of communication than those of the directive style. Two models of midwifery communication were identified: the education/encourager, who passed on her knowledge at intervals and allowed the mother more control over her own delivery, and the directing midwife, who retained her knowledge and therefore controlled the woman's behaviour by constant repetition of directions.

The reasons for these differences were explored, and recommendations made for the following: 1) better education towards the acquisition of improved communication skills; 2) the increased opportunity for midwives to train as 'direct entrants' could minimise the tendency for them to use nursing language usually spoken when caring for the sick, which is inappropriate in midwifery; and 3) to establish an organisation of care that provides more personal links between the midwife and the mother, so enabling them to communicate on a more social as well as professional level in order that the social significance of childbirth will be increased.

Keywords: COMMUNICATION, COMMUNICATION SKILLS, EXPERIENCE (WOMEN'S), LABOUR, OBSERVATIONAL STUDY, SECOND STAGE

Adams ME. Providing a service - supplement on parentcraft. Nursing Mirror 1977;29:12-3.

Ward ME, Adams ME. A masters degree in midwifery. Midwives Chronicle 1979;37-8.

Prince J, Adams ME. Minds, Mothers and Midwives - A psychology of childbirth. Churchill Livingstone Edinburgh, New York, Melbourne. 1978).

Adams ME. Neonatal abilities. Nursing 1980:913-5.

Beischer N, Mackay. Obstetrics and the newborn. 2nd Ed. Midwifery Notes - section 14. London: Bailliere Tindall 1986:715-42.

Prince J, Adams ME. The psychology of childbirth. 2nd edition of Minds, Mothers' and Midwives. Churchill Livingstone, Edinburgh, New York, Melbourne. 1987.

Smith VS, ed. Midwifery Questions Answered. London: Faber & Faber 1988

Adams ME. Baillière Midwives Dictionary. 7th Edition. London: Baillière Tindall 1983

Adams ME, Parsons B, Morgan B. Preparing for labour. In: Harvey D, ed. A New Life, Pregnancy Birth and Your Child's First Year. Marshall Cavendish. 1979;86.

Adams ME, Lee B. Labour and birth. In: Harvey D, ed. A New Life, Pregnancy, Birth and Your Child's First Year. Marshall Cavendish. 1979:72.

109. WHY DON'T MOTHERS BREASTFEED?
September 1988 - September 1990
R Moss, Health Visitor. **Contact:** R Moss, Ballynoe Road, Antrim BT41 2QX.

Formed part of a course. 6-12 hours/week of own time spent.

Abstract: (Not updated since 1990.) The purpose of the study was to investigate the reasons for particularly low rates of breastfeeding in the Antrim and Ballymena areas of Northern Ireland.

The methods were qualitative: twenty-eight semi-structured interviews of sixty to ninety minutes' duration were carried out in the clients' own home at six to eight weeks after birth. Only first-time mothers (selected on an opportunistic basis) were interviewed. Topics covered in the interview were: pregnancy, labour, the influence of relatives and friends, support by professionals, embarrassment, pain and milk supply. Analysis is currently in progress.

Keywords: BREASTFEEDING, BREASTFEEDING (INCIDENCE), BREASTFEEDING (PROBLEMS), NORTHERN IRELAND

110. WHY DON'T WOMEN BREASTFEED?
October 1976 - September 1978
Ann Thomson, Lecturer. **Contact:** Ann Thomson, School of Nursing Studies, University of Manchester, Coupland III Building, Coupland Street, Manchester M13 9PL. Tel: 061 275 5342

Funded as integral or additional part of a job. Formed part of a course. Funded by employer: Scottish Home and Health Department, Nursing Research Training Fellowship.

Abstract: The purpose of this study was to pinpoint when, in relationship to pregnancy, primiparous women living in a stable union made the decision on how to feed their baby. A prospective survey using semi-structured questionnaires was used to follow twenty-five women from booking for antenatal care until six weeks post delivery. To assess the possibility of the Hawthorne effect, forty-one women were recruited at the follow-up antenatal clinic and followed up until six weeks post delivery. The data were analyzed using SPSSx, and the chi-square test was used to assess differences between groups of women where appropriate.

Twenty-one (84%) of the women recruited at the booking clinic had made a decision on how they were going to feed their baby, and eighteen (72%) were within the first trimester of pregnancy. Only three had had a discussion on baby feeding with a member of the health professions prior to attending the booking clinic. As in previous studies, women who were older, came from the higher social classes and had a higher level of education opted to breastfeed. Of the total sample of sixty-six, forty-two (64%) intended to breastfeed. At six weeks post delivery eighteen (27%) were breastfeeding. The breastfeeding policy at the hospital where the study was undertaken was not based on the physiology of lactation. Until those women who want to breastfeed can be helped to be successful there is no point in encouraging more to breastfeed. To encourage women to breastfeed, health education should begin in schools before the decision is made. As husbands were found to be significant in the decision to breastfeed the teaching should be to boys as well as girls.

Keywords: ANTENATAL EDUCATION, BREASTFEEDING, BREASTFEEDING (FAILURE), INFANT FEEDING (DECISIONS)

Thomson AM. Why don't women breastfeed? 1978 unpublished report to Scottish Home and Health Department, Edinburgh.

Thomson AM. Why don't women breastfeed? In: Robinson S, Thomson AM, eds. Midwives Research and Childbirth. Vol 1. London: Chapman and Hall. 1989

111. A PILOT STUDY OF A RANDOMISED CONTROLLED TRIAL OF PUSHING TECHNIQUES IN THE SECOND STAGE OF LABOUR
September 1987 - September 1991

Ann Thomson, Clinical Lecturer/Midwife. **Contact:** Ann Thomson, School of Nursing Studies, University of Manchester, Coupland III Building, Coupland Street, Manchester M13 9PL. Tel: 061 275 5342

Funded as integral or additional part of a job by employer: University of Manchester.

Abstract: A literature review demonstrated no evidence to support routine directive pushing in the second stage of labour (Thomson, 1988). A pilot study for a randomized controlled trial of pushing techniques has been undertaken. Thirty-two primiparae aged eighteen years or over, with a term pregnancy where there was no maternal or fetal condition affecting management of labour, were randomly allocated to either a directed pushing (control) group or a spontaneous pushing (experimental) group. To ensure reliability of group allocation and in an attempt to increase the body of knowledge of behaviour in spontaneous second stage, the second stage of labour was observed.

The women in the two groups were found to be comparable on a range of variables, but there was an increased use of Pethidine, and the length of the first stage of labour was longer in the experimental group. There was no difference between the two groups in the outcomes of estimated blood loss, type of delivery, and condition of the baby at delivery. The length of the second stage was significantly longer in the experimental group. As women in the experimental group had a significantly longer mean first stage, and there was a significant positive correlation between the length of the first stage and the length of the second, the increased length of the second stage in the experimental group cannot necessarily be attributed to the pushing method. The pH of the venous cord blood at delivery was adversely affected the longer the second stage in the control group. There was no such association in the experimental group. When pushing spontaneously, women do not 'take a deep breath', but appear to use both open and closed glottis breathing. Reliability of group allocation was achieved in this study, but informal conversations with midwives suggest that reliability of group allocation to the experimental group may be a problem in the main study.

Keywords: LABOUR, PUSHING (DIRECTED), PUSHING (SPONTANEOUS), SECOND STAGE, SECOND STAGE (MANAGEMENT)

Thomson AM. Management of the woman in normal second stage of labour: a review. Midwifery 1988;4:77-85.

Thomson AM. A comparison of pushing techniques in the second stage of labour: a pilot study of a randomised controlled trial. Unpublished MSc thesis, University of Manchester, 1990.

Thomson AM. Pushing techniques in the second stage of labour. Journal of Advanced Nursing 1993;18:171-7.

Thomson AM, Hillier V. A re-evaluation of the effect of pethidine on the length of labour. Journal of Advanced Nursing (in press).

112. GREAT EXPECTATIONS: A PROSPECTIVE STUDY OF WOMEN'S EXPECTATIONS AND EXPERIENCES OF CHILDBIRTH
October 1986 - August 1988

J M Green, Senior Research Associate, Vanessa Coupland, Research Assistant, Jenny Kitzinger, Research Assistant, Martin Richards, Reader in Human Development. **Contact:** J M Green, Maternity Services Research Group, Child Care & Development Group, University of Cambridge, Free School Lane, Cambridge CB2 3RF. Tel: 0223 334512

Funded as integral or additional part of a job and by funding agency(ies): Nuffield Provincial Hospital Trust.

Abstract: Approximately 800 women booked for delivery in six hospitals in the south east of England completed three lengthy postal questionnaires, two before the birth and one six weeks after. Antenatal questions covered a wide range of attitudes, preferences and expectations, including obstetric interventions, pain and pain relief, and social/behavioural aspects of labour. The postnatal questionnaire established the events of labour and also assessed women's satisfaction, fulfilment, emotional well-being and perceptions of their babies. Expectations were found to be significantly related to a number of events of labour and also to satisfaction and emotional well-being, with optimism being associated with positive outcomes. Feeling in control, both of your own behaviour and of what is done to you, was consistently associated with all psychological outcome measures, as was a perceived lack of information and not being able to adopt the most comfortable positions during labour.

Most of these findings were more significant for multiparous women; first-time mothers were less satisfied and more negative about their babies, whatever their experiences.

Keywords: CONSUMER SATISFACTION, EXPERIENCE (WOMEN'S), INFORMATION GIVING, LABOUR, LABOUR (CONTROL OF), MIDWIFERY SERVICES (EVALUATION), PERCEPTIONS OF CHILDBIRTH (WOMEN'S), PSYCHOLOGY

Green JM, Coupland VA, Kitzinger JV. Great expectations: a prospective study of women's expectations and experiences of childbirth. Child care and development group, 1988.

Green JM, Kitzinger JV, Coupland VA. Choice and control in childbirth. In: The needs of parents and infants: a symposium on the health needs of parents and infants. Health Promotion Research Trust, Cambridge, 1989.

Green JM, Coupland VA, Kitzinger JV. Expectations, experiences and pychological outcomes of childbirth: a prospective study of 825 women. Birth. 1990;17:15-24.

Green JM, Kitzinger JV, Coupland VA. Stereotypes of childbearing women: a look at some evidence. Midwifery 1990;6:1-8.

Green JM, Kitzinger JV, Coupland VA. Midwives' responsibilities, medical staffing structures and women's choice in childbirth. In: Robinson S, Thompson A, eds. Midwives, Research and Childbirth. Vol 3. Routledge, Chapman and Hall, London (in press).

Green JM. "Who is unhappy after childbirth?": Antenatal and intrapartum correlates from a prospective study. Journal of Reproductive and Infant Psychology 1990;8:175-83.

113. THE ROLE OF THE MIDWIFE IN RELATION TO WOMENS' EARLY EXPERIENCES OF BREASTFEEDING

January 1990 - September 1991

J Billingsley, MA Student, D Stears, Senior Lecturer. **Contact:** J Billingsley, Beverley Road, Canterbury, Kent CT2 7EN.

For full details see under Educational Studies (Record No. 113).

114. SOCIAL SUPPORT AND PREGNANCY OUTCOME

September 1985 - December 1991

Ann Oakley, Director, Social Science Research Unit, Sandra Stone, Project Administrator, Rosemary Marsden, Research Midwife, Carole Galen-Bamfield, Research Midwife, Sandra Buckle, Research Midwife, Rosemary Smith, Research Midwife, Lynda Rajan, Research Coordinator, Penrose Robertson, Computer Programmer. **Contact:** Ann Oakley, Social Science Research Unit, Institute of Education, University of London, 59 Gordon Square, London WC1H ONT. Tel: 071 636 1500 Ex 778

Funded as integral or additional part of a job by employer and by funding agency(ies): Department of Health, Institute of Education, Iolanthe Trust.

Abstract: (Not updated since 1991) The study was a randomized controlled trial of a social support intervention provided by research midwives to women at risk of low birthweight (LBW) delivery.

Women in four centres with a history of at least one previous LBW delivery were recruited and randomly allocated to be offered the social support intervention in addition to their normal antenatal care, or to receive normal antenatal care only. Five hundred and thirty-four women were invited to take part, and 509 agreed. Women allocated to the intervention group were mostly very positive about the intervention, which consisted of a 'minimum package' of three home visits, two brief contacts between these times, and provision of a twenty-four hour phone number. In fact, birthweight was not significantly different between intervention and control groups, but there were a number of significant health benefits to intervention group women and their babies.

Keywords: ANTENATAL CARE, HIGH RISK PREGNANCY, LOW BIRTHWEIGHT, SOCIAL SUPPORT

Oakley A. Social support in pregnancy: the 'soft' way to increase birthweight? Social Science and Medicine 1985;21:1259-68.

Oakley A. Is social support good for the health of mothers and babies? Journal of Reproductive and Infant Psychology 1988;6:3-21.

Oakley A. Smoking in pregnancy: smokescreen or risk factor? Sociology of Health and Illness 1989;11:311-35.

Oakley A, Rajan L, Grant A. Social support and pregnancy outcome: report of a randomised controlled trial. British Journal of Obstetrics and Gynaecology 1990;97:155-62.

Oakley A. Who's afraid of the randomised controlled trial? Some dilemmas of the scientific method and 'good' research practice. Women and Health 1989;15:25-59.

Oakley A, Rajan L. Social class and social support: the same or different? Sociology (details not confirmed).

Oakley A, Rajan L. Obstetric technology maternal emotional wellbeing: a further research note. Journal of Reproductive and Infant Psychology (details not confirmed).

Oakley A, Rajan L. Using medical care: the views of high risk mothers. Health Services Research 1991;5:651-69.

Oakley A, Rajan L, Robertson P. A comparison of different sources of information on pregnancy and childbirth. Journal of Biosocial Science. (details not confirmed)

Rajan L, Oakley A. Infant feeding practices in mothers at risk of low birthweight delivery. Midwifery 1990;6:18-27.

Rajan L, Oakley A. Low birthweight babies: the mother's point of view. Midwifery 1990;6:73-85.

Marsden R. Pregnancy home visiting study. Midwives Chronicle March 1989;102:86-7.

Buckle S. Meaningful relationships. Nursing Times 1988;102:41.

Oakley A. Who's afraid of the randomised controlled trial? Some dilemmas of the scientific method and 'good' research practice. In: Roberts H., ed. Women's Health Counts 1990;167-94.

Oakley A, Rajan L. The social support and pregnancy outcome study. In: Berendes H W, Kessel W and Yaffe S , eds. Prevention of Low Birthweight (details not confirmed).

115. REPORT ON THE KIDLINGTON TEAM MIDWIFERY SCHEME
April - November 1989

Pamela Watson, Not presently working, Alison Kitson, Head Research & Evaluation, Lesley Page, Director of Midwifery. **Contact:** Alison Kitson, Institute of Nursing, Radcliffe Infirmary, Oxford OX2 6HE. Tel: 0865 816667

For full details see under Management Studies (Record No. 115).

116. A STUDY OF THE ROLE AND RESPONSIBILITIES OF THE MIDWIFE
January 1978 - December 1983

Sarah Robinson, Senior Research Fellow, Josephine Golden, Research Associate, Susan Bradley, Research Associate, Keith Jacka, Statistician. **Contact:** Sarah Robinson, Nursing Research Unit, Kings College, London University, Cornwall House Annexe, Waterloo Road, London SE1 8TX. Tel: 071 872 3063/3057
For full details see under Management Studies (Record No. 116).

117. BOWEL CARE IN THE PUERPERIUM
October 1988 - November 1989

P F Samuel, Midwifery Sister. **Contact:** P F Samuel, Westminster Road, Poole, Dorset BH13 6JQ.

Formed part of a course. Funded by employer: Dorset Institute of Higher Education.

Abstract: The aim of this study was to find what, if any, treatment was most effective and acceptable to women to restore their normal bowel function after childbirth.

One hundred women following normal delivery were allocated consecutively to one of five groups, one control and four different treatments. The treatments used were Senokot, glycerine suppositories, high-fibre diets, Lactulose, and Fybogel Orange. Details of parity, pre-labour bowel preparation, length of labour, drugs used during labour, type of delivery and the presence or not of haemorrhoids and perineal sutures were all noted. The length of time from delivery to first defecation was recorded in hours. The outcomes were assessed with a questionnaire using mainly visual analogue scales. Staff perception of the study was ascertained using a questionnaire and each group was costed for financial implications.

The results showed that women were anxious about having their bowels open for the first time after childbirth. Their anxiety rose as time elapsed. Primigravidae were more anxious than multigravidae and the presence of perineal sutures increased anxiety levels. Results for the five treatment groups were not statistically significant. From the staff questionnaire, it was ascertained that midwives need to be more aware of mothers' anxieties concerning constipation in the puerperium. The costs of Lactulose and Fybogel Orange outweighed any small advantage they may have had in achieving earlier defecation. There was a statistically significant rise in anxiety in relation to the time to first defecation. The presence of perineal sutures also increased anxiety.

These findings show that if women had their bowels open sooner after childbirth and if they were given more education concerning their perineal sutures, their anxieties could be lessened.

Keywords: BOWEL FUNCTION, CONSTIPATION, LAXATIVES, POSTNATAL CARE, PUERPERIUM, SUTURES

118. INFANT FEEDING SURVEY
September 1990 - November 1991

Patricia Morris Thompson, Senior Midwife, Obstetrics & Gynaecology, Linda Green, Community Midwife, Pauline Cozer, Student Midwife, Lorraine Winthorpe, Parentcraft Co-ordinator, Josie Blanchard, Midwifery Tutor, Margaret Stockwell, Clinical Midwifery Manager, Maureen Keeting, Clinical Midwife Specialist. **Contact:** Patricia Morris Thompson, Leicester Royal Infirmary, Leicester LE1 5WW. Tel: 0533 541414 Ex 6416

Funded as integral or additional part of a job. 2-6 hours/week of own time spent.

Abstract: (Not updated since 1991) The purpose of the research project is to identify what factors influence choice of infant feeding and what factors influence failure to achieve the feeding method chosen.

A randomly selected group of 700 women will be included in the survey. A specially designed questionnaire which has been tested will be given to each woman at booking and the four sections will be filled in at booking, thirty-six weeks of pregnancy and two days and six weeks postnatally. There will be a quantitative analysis and recommendations will include an action plan to target groups with further education, health promotion and support in order to enable larger numbers of mothers to breastfeed successfully.

Keywords: ARTIFICIAL FEEDING, BREASTFEEDING (FAILURE), INFANT FEEDING, INFANT FEEDING (DECISIONS)

119. NEWLY QUALIFIED MIDWIVES: A STUDY OF THEIR CAREER INTENTIONS AND VIEWS OF THEIR TRAINING
January 1979 - December 1984

Sarah Robinson, Senior Research Fellow, Josephine Golden, Research Associate, Keith Jacka, Statistician. **Contact:** Sarah Robinson, Nursing Research Unit, Kings College, London University, Cornwall House Annexe, Waterloo Road, London SE1 8TX. Tel: 071 872 3063/3057
For full details see under Educational Studies (Record No. 119).

120. A STUDY OF THE CAREER PATTERNS OF MIDWIVES
January 1986 - December 1992

Sarah Robinson, Senior Research Fellow, Heather Owen, Research Associate, Keith Jacka, Statistician. **Contact:** Sarah Robinson, Nursing Research Unit, Kings College, London University, Cornwall House Annexe, Waterloo Road, London SE1 8TX. Tel: 071 872 3063/3057
For full details see under Educational Studies (Record No. 120).

121. EFFECTS OF SALT AND SAVLON BATH CONCENTRATE POST PARTUM

February - August 1985

Jennifer Sleep, Research Co-ordinator, Adrian Grant, Epidemiologist. **Contact:** Jennifer Sleep, Berkshire College of Nursing & Midwifery, Royal Berkshire Hospital, Craven Road, Reading, Berkshire RG1 5AN. Tel: 0734 877651

Funded as integral or additional part of a job by funding agency(ies): Oxford Regional Health Authority. 2-6 hours/week of own time spent.

Abstract: A wide range of remedies are currently recommended for the relief of perineal pain following childbirth. This study aimed to clarify the usefulness or otherwise of the routine addition of salt and Savlon concentrate during bathing in the immediate postpartum period, and comparing the results when no bath additives were used.

Eighteen hundred women recruited within twenty-four hours of vaginal delivery were randomly allocated to one of three ten-day bathing policies. Six hundred mothers were asked to add measured amounts of salt, 600 to add Savlon bath concentrate and 600 not to add anything to the bathwater. All analyses were based on the comparison between all women allocated to one or other of the bathing policies regardless of subsequent compliance because this comparison is free of selection bias. Outcome frequencies were compared using the chi-square test.

Overall, 90% of the women said that they followed their trial instructions. The response rate to the tenth-day questionnaire was 95%; 1,609 women returned their three-month questionnaire (89%). There were no statistically significant differences between the three groups in terms of perineal pain or the symptomatic relief afforded by the allocated policies at either ten days or three months postpartum. Overall, 93% reported that bathing had eased their discomfort during their first ten days after delivery. The pattern of wound healing was also similar in the three groups. These findings provide no support for the use of these particular additives in postpartum care; they are also more costly than bathing in plain water.

Keywords: BATH ADDITIVES, PAIN RELIEF (PERINEUM), PERINEAL CARE, PERINEAL HEALING, PERINEAL PAIN, SALT, SAVLON

Sleep J, Grant A. Effects of salt and savlon bath concentrate postpartum. Nursing Times 1988;84:55-7.

Grant A, Sleep J. Relief of perineal pain and discomfort after childbirth. In: Chalmers I, Enkin M, Kierse MJNC, eds. Effective Care in Pregnancy and Childbirth. Oxford: Oxford University Press 1989:1347-58.

Sleep J. Perineal management and care: A series of five randomised controlled trials. In: Robinson S, Thomson A M, eds. Midwives, Research and Childbirth. Vol. 2. London: Chapman Hall 1991:199-251.

Sleep J. Postnatal perineal care. In: Alexander J, Roche S, Levy V, eds. Midwifery Practice Series. Vol 3. Basingstoke: Macmillan Education Ltd. 1990:1-17.

Sleep J. An introduction to experimental method. Nursing Standard 1990;41:34-6.

122. RELIEF OF PERINEAL PAIN FOLLOWING CHILDBIRTH: A SURVEY OF MIDWIFERY PRACTICE

June - July 1987

Jennifer Sleep, Research Co-ordinator, Adrian Grant, Epidemiologist. **Contact:** Jennifer Sleep, Berkshire College of Nursing & Midwifery, Royal Berkshire Hospital, Craven Road, Reading, Berkshire RG1 5AN. Tel: 0734 877651

Funded as integral or additional part of a job by funding agency(ies): Oxford Regional Health Authority. 2-6 hours/week of own time spent.

Abstract: There is anecdotal evidence of a wide variation in what midwives prescribe for perineal pain following childbirth. A telephone survey was undertaken to find out what midwives actually recommend and to see whether practices vary between different units.

A random sample of fifty English maternity units was selected; this included thirty-six consultant and fourteen general practitioner units where births occurred during 1986. Using a structured interview technique, the senior midwife on duty at the time was asked to rank order the remedies most commonly recommended on her unit. Overall, the first-line management for perineal pain was oral analgesia (78% of units) although some units offered topical applications of ice, hydrocortisone and promoxine foam (Epifoam) or witch hazel. Paracetamol was the oral analgesic of choice for mild perineal pain but there was wide variation in the choice of preparations for more severe pain. The most widely recommended group of drugs (36%) each had a codeine constituent. Only three units reported ever using non-steroidal, anti-antiflammatory agents such as ibuprofen and mefanamic acid. The most popular topical treatment was ice (84%), followed by Epifoam (60%), witch hazel (12%) and lignocaine spray/gel (8%). Consultant units were more likely to offer electrical therapies such as ultrasound, heat and pulsed electromagnetic energy.

Given the wide range of oral analgesics currently available on the market, it was surprising to note the widespread use of codeine derivatives which have a tendency to cause constipation. These preparations would not seem the ideal choice for perineal pain, especially when several potentially useful alternatives could be prescribed, principally the non-steroidal anti-inflammatory drugs (NSAIDS). There is little available evidence of the long-term benefit of using ice, especially when packs are difficult to position accurately on the perineum. Few units used local anaesthetics despite evidence that they are both effective and inexpensive. The popularity of Epifoam would appear ill-considered, given concerns about its effect on wound healing in the long-term as well as its cost.

Keywords: MIDWIFERY PRACTICE, PAIN RELIEF (PERINEUM), PERINEAL CARE, PERINEAL HEALING, PERINEAL PAIN, POSTNATAL CARE

Sleep J, Grant A. Pelvic floor exercises in postnatal care. Midwifery 1987;3:158-64.

Grant A, Sleep J. Relief of perineal pain and discomfort after childbirth. In: Chalmers I, Enkin M, Kierse MJNC, eds. Effective Care in Pregnancy and Childbirth. Oxford: Oxford University Press 1989:1347-58.

Sleep J. Perineal management and care: A series of five randomised controlled trials. In: Robinson S, Thomson AM, eds. Midwives, Research and Childbirth. Vol 2. London: Chapman Hall 1991:199-251.

Sleep J. Postnatal perineal care. In: Alexander J, Roche S, Levy V, eds. Midwifery Practice Series. Vol 3. Basingstoke: Macmillan Education Ltd. 1990:1-17.

123. ULTRASOUND AND PULSED ELECTROMAGNETIC ENERGY TREATMENT FOR PERINEAL TRAUMA. A RANDOMISED PLACEBO-CONTROLLED TRIAL
February - December 1987

Jennifer Sleep, Research Co-ordinator, Adrian Grant, Epidemiologist, Jeannie McIntosh, Obstetric Physiotherapist, Hazel Ashurst, Computing Co-ordinator. **Contact:** Jennifer Sleep, Berkshire College of Nursing & Midwifery, Royal Berkshire Hospital, Craven Road, Reading, Berkshire RG1 5AN. Tel: 0734 877651

Funded as integral or additional part of a job by funding agency(ies): Oxford Regional Health Authority. 2-6 hours/week of own time spent.

Abstract: Ultrasound and pulsed electromagnetic energy therapies are increasingly used for perineal trauma sustained during childbirth. This study was designed to compare these electrical modalities with double-blind, placebo treatments begun within twenty-four hours of delivery for moderate or severe perineal trauma. Two main hypotheses were tested: 1) that ultrasound or pulsed electromagnetic energy therapy or both would reduce the frequency and severity of perineal pain on the tenth day after delivery; and 2) that active treatment would reduce the time to resumption of sexual intercourse and increase the frequency of pain-free intercourse three months after delivery.

A sample size of 400 women was pre-specified. A single pooled placebo group of the same size as the two actively treated groups was generated. Chi-square and t-tests with one-way analysis of variance were used where appropriate. Four hundred and fourteen women who had required instrumental assistance with delivery or who had sustained severe perineal trauma were recruited. All women received the allocated treatment which was double blind for each machine. Three treatments were given during a forty-eight-hour period. Pre- and post-therapy assessments were carried out by each mother and by the midwife researcher. The frequency and severity of perineal pain was assessed by the mother on the tenth day after delivery. Overall, more than 90% thought that treatment made their problem better.

There were no clear differences between the groups in outcome either immediately after treatment, or ten days or three months postpartum, other than more pain associated with pulsed electromagnetic energy treatment at ten days. Bruising looked more extensive after ultrasound therapy but then seemed to resolve more quickly. Neither therapy had an effect on perineal oedema or haemorrhoids. The place of these new therapies in postnatal care should be clarified by further controlled trials before they become part of routine care.

Keywords: DYSPAREUNIA, ELECTRICAL THERAPY, PERINEAL CARE, PERINEAL HEALING, PERINEAL PAIN, PERINEAL TRAUMA, POSTNATAL CARE, PULSED ELECTROMAGNETIC ENERGY, ULTRASOUND

Grant A, Sleep J, McIntosh J, Ashurst H. Ultrasound and pulsed electromagnetic energy treatment for perineal trauma. A randomised placebo-controlled trial. British Journal of Obstetrics and Gynaecology 1989;96:434-9.

Grant A. Sleep J. Relief of perineal pain and discomfort after childbirth. In: Chalmers I, Enkin M, Kierse MJNC,eds. Effective Care in Pregnancy and Childbirth. Oxford: Oxford University Press 1989:1347-58.

Sleep J. Perineal management and care: A series of five randomised controlled trials. In: Robinson S, Thomson AM, eds. Midwives, Research and Childbirth. Vol 2. London: Chapman Hall 1991:199-251.

Sleep J. Postnatal perineal care. In: Alexander J, Roche S, Levy V, eds. Midwifery Practice Series. Vol 3. Basingstoke: Macmillan Education Ltd. 1990:1-17.

124. DYSPAREUNIA ASSOCIATED WITH THE USE OF GLYCEROL-IMPREGNATED CATGUT TO REPAIR PERINEAL TRAUMA. REPORT OF A THREE YEAR FOLLOW UP STUDY
July 1985 - January 1986

Jennifer Sleep, Research Co-ordinator, Adrian Grant, Epidemiologist. **Contact:** Jennifer Sleep, Berkshire College of Nursing & Midwifery, Royal Berkshire Hospital, Craven Road, Reading, Berkshire RG1 5AN. Tel: 0734 877651

Funded as integral or additional part of a job by funding agency(ies): Oxford Regional Health Authority. 2-6 hours/week of own time spent.

Abstract: This study was designed to compare the use of chromic softgut with untreated chromic catgut for perineal repair following normal vaginal deliveries in respect of both short- and longer-term maternal morbidity.

Of 1000 consecutive women who had normal deliveries, 737 were judged to require perineal repair and were randomly allocated to be repaired through all the tissue layers with either glycerol-impregnated chromic catgut (softgut) or untreated chromic catgut. When assessed on the tenth postnatal day, women who had been sutured with softgut were 10% more likely to report perineal pain (p=0.015). There were no statistically significant differences between the groups with regard to healing by secondary intention or perineal breakdown.

The timing of resumption of sexual intercourse did not differ between the groups: 89% had resumed by three months postpartum; however, women who had been repaired with softgut were 33% more likely to suffer from dyspareunia at this time (p<0.025). Stratification by technique used to repair the perineal skin revealed that the differences between the materials in pain, dyspareunia and suture removal were more marked in the women who were repaired with interrupted sutures than in those repaired with continuous sub-cuticular stitches. The high rates of both short-term and long-term morbidity associated with the use of softgut appear to preclude the use of softgut for perineal repair. Furthermore, they demonstrate how important the choice of suture material may be for large numbers of women as they recover from traumatic vaginal delivery.

Keywords: CHROMIC CATGUT, DYSPAREUNIA, GLYCEROL-IMPREGNATED CATGUT, PERINEAL HEALING, PERINEAL PAIN, PERINEAL REPAIR, SUTURE MATERIALS

Grant A, Sleep J, Ashurst H, Spencer JAD. Dyspareunia associated with the use of glycerol-impregnated catgut to repair perineal trauma. Report of a 3 year follow up study. British Journal of Obstetrics and Gynaecology 1989;96:741-3.

Grant A, Sleep J. Relief of perineal pain and discomfort after childbirth. In: Chalmers I, Enkin M, Kierse MJNC, eds. Effective Care in Pregnancy and Childbirth. Oxford: Oxford University Press 1989:1347-58.

Sleep J, Perineal management and care: A series of five randomised controlled trials. In: Robinson S, Thomson AM, eds. Midwives, Research and Childbirth Vol 2. London: Chapman Hall 1991:199-251.

Sleep J. Postnatal perineal care. In: Alexander J, Roche S, Levy V, eds. Midwifery Practice Series. Vol 3. Basingstoke: Macmillan Education Ltd. 1990:1-17.

125. A RANDOMISED COMPARISON OF GLYCEROL-IMPREGNATED CHROMIC CATGUT WITH UNTREATED CHROMIC CATGUT FOR REPAIR OF PERINEAL TRAUMA
April 1982 - May 1983

Jennifer Sleep, Research Co-ordinator, Adrian Grant, Epidemiologist, Jo Garcia, Social Scientist, Diana Elbourne, Social Statistician, John Spencer, Registrar, Iain Chalmers, Director, NPEU. **Contact:** Jennifer Sleep, Berkshire College of Nursing & Midwifery, Royal Berkshire Hospital, Craven Road, Reading, Berkshire RG1 5AN. Tel: 0734 877651

Funded as integral or additional part of a job by employer and by funding agency(ies): Oxford Regional Health Authority, Maws/RCM Research Scholarship. Over 20 hours/week of own time spent.

Abstract: The purpose of the study was to conduct a longer-term follow-up of women who participated in a randomized controlled trial which compared glycerol-impregnated chromic catgut (softgut; soft-catgut-Braun, David and Geck Ltd; Gosport, UK) with untreated chromic catgut used for all layers in the repair of perineal trauma following normal vaginal deliveries (Spencer et al 1986, Record No. 124).

After a three-year period, 737 women who participated in the original trial were contacted by postal questionnaire; 70% responded. The respondent trial groups were very similar to the original trial groups in respect of descriptive details. A slightly higher proportion of women who responded in the 'softgut' group had given birth subsequently (44% v 38%); almost all of these had been vaginal and spontaneous. Women who had originally been sutured using 'softgut' were more likely to receive an episiotomy during their first subsequent delivery (25% v 14% p = 0.05). Sexual intercourse was reported as painful 1.7 times more often by women repaired with glycerol-impregnated catgut (P<0.02) even when the analysis was limited to women who had no subsequent deliveries. The results of this study suggest that glycerol-impregnated chromic catgut causes persistent dyspareunia and it may also increase the likelihood of episiotomy during subsequent delivery. Judged on this trial there is no place for its use in the repair of perineal wounds.

Keywords: CHROMIC CATGUT, DYSPAREUNIA, GLYCEROL-IMPREGNATED CATGUT, PERINEAL HEALING, PERINEAL PAIN, PERINEAL REPAIR, SUTURE MATERIALS

Sleep J. Perineal management - A midwifery skill under threat. Midwife, Health Visitor & Community Nurse 1987;23:455-8.

Spencer JAD, Grant A, Elbourne D, Garcia J, Sleep J. A randomized comparison of glycerol-impregnated chromic catgut with untreated chromic catgut for the repair of perineal trauma. British Journal of Obstetrics and Gynaecology 1986;93:426-30.

Sleep J. Perineal care: A series of five randomised controlled trials. In: Robinson S, Thomson AM, eds. Midwives, Research and Childbirth. Vol 2. London: Chapman Hall 1991:199-251.

Sleep J. Postnatal perineal care. In: Alexander J, Roche S, Levy V, eds. Midwifery Practice Series. Vol 3. Basingstoke: Macmillan Education Ltd. 1990:1-17.

Grant A, Sleep J. Relief of perineal pain and discomfort after childbirth. In: Chalmers I, Enkin M, Kierse MJNC, eds. Effective Care in Pregnancy and Childbirth. Oxford: Oxford University Press 1989:1347-58.

131. OXYTOCIN INFUSION DURING SECOND STAGE OF LABOUR IN PRIMIPAROUS WOMEN USING EPIDURAL ANALGESIA: A RANDOMISED DOUBLE BLIND PLACEBO CONTROLLED TRIAL
May 1987 - April 1989

N J Saunders, Senior Lecturer, Lucy Gilbert, Registrar, Robert Fraser, Senior Lecturer, Jacqueline Hall, Registrar, Phillip Mutton, Registrar, Ann Jackson, Senior House Officer, Douglas Edmonds, Obstetrician. **Contact:** Helen Spiby, Maternity Unit, Northern General Hospital, Herries Road, Sheffield S5 7AU. Tel: 0742 434343 blp 162

Funded as integral or additional part of a job, and by funding agency(ies): Birthright.

Abstract: Epidural analgesia is a widely used method of pain relief for labour in Britain. It is, though, associated with an increased incidence of instrumental vaginal delivery, particularly for occipito-posterior position. A prospective double-blind randomized controlled trial of oxytocin infusion, administered from the onset of the second stage of labour, was undertaken in three hospitals. Two hundred and twenty-six primiparous women with a singleton fetus presenting by the vertex, who were over thirty-seven weeks of gestation, and who received epidural anaesthesia during the first stage of labour, were eligible for inclusion. Pharmacy departments in Sheffield and London were asked to prepare trial infusions of oxytocin. In Sheffield, infusions of low-dose oxytocin in sodium chloride 0.9% and sodium chloride 0.9% only were prepared on the basis of random number allocations. In London, coded phials of oxytocin or placebo, which the ward staff would add to the infusion fluid, were similarly prepared. In both centres, the key to the coding system was retained by the pharmacist. Outcomes were assessed using Student's t-test and confidence intervals for differences in means, and the chi-square test for differences in proportions.

Treatment with oxytocin reduced the length of second stage and increased the rate of spontaneous delivery. No reduction in the proportion of women requiring Keilland's rotational forceps or Ventouse for persistent occipito-posterior position was achieved. Neither were any adverse fetal or neonatal effects observed.

Keywords: EPIDURALS, FORCEPS, INSTRUMENTAL DELIVERY, LABOUR, OXYTOCIN, PAIN RELIEF (LABOUR), SECOND STAGE, SECOND STAGE (MANAGEMENT)

Saunders NJ, Spiby H, Gilbert L, Fraser RB, Hall JM, Mutton PM, Jackson A, Edmonds DK. Oxytocin infusion during second stage of labour in primiparous women using epidural analgesia: a randomised double blind placebo controlled trial. British Medical Journal 1989;299:1423-6.

133. ANTENATAL SURVEY TO DEFINE THE QUALITY OF CARE IN THE WINCHESTER HEALTH AUTHORITY
October - October 1989
G Fairclough, Midwife Teacher. **Contact:** G Fairclough, Monnow Gardens, West End, Southampton SO3 3QD.
For full details see under Management Studies (Record No. 133).

134. IS NATURAL CHILDBIRTH GOING OUT OF FASHION?
January - September 1987
E R Buckley, Midwifery Sister, Pamela Hawthorne, Director of Nursing Studies, Barbara Payman, Course Tutor. **Contact:** E R Buckley, Glenorchy Cresent, Heron Ridge, Nottingham.

Formed part of a course. Funded by employer: Nottingham Health Authority.

Abstract: In view of the recent trend towards natural and active childbirth, it was decided to carry out a study to discover what mothers' wishes were for their care in labour, whether they were fulfilled and what percentage wanted natural childbirth methods. It was also decided to discover whether mothers were satisfied with their care in labour, and what their satisfaction was related to. Information was collected by means of an interview schedule, and forty-five first-time mothers were interviewed within forty-eight hours of delivery. The results were analyzed using SPSSx. It was found that only a small percentage (4%) of women wanted natural childbirth methods for labour and delivery. The great majority of mothers' wishes for their care in labour were fulfilled, and 96% of women were satisfied or very satisfied with their care in labour. Satisfaction with care appeared to be related to their relationships with their attendants in labour, rather than other factors such as the efficiency of pain relief or physical surroundings. This supports findings from other studies.

The implications of the findings are that relationships with carers in labour are the most important factor influencing satisfaction with care in labour. Spending large amounts of money on birthing beds, chairs and physical surroundings, therefore, does not appear to be justified. Priority should be given to providing high quality mid-wifery care in labour to ensure high levels of satisfaction with care.

Keywords: ACTIVE BIRTH, CONSUMER SATISFACTION, EXPERIENCE (WOMEN'S), LABOUR, LABOUR (SATISFACTION), RELATIONSHIPS, STAFF ATTITUDES

135. INTERPROFESSIONAL COMMUNICATION: A STUDY OF COMMUNITY MIDWIVES AND HEALTH VISITORS IN GLOUCESTER HEALTH DISTRICT
August 1989 - April 1990
T J McGrath, Midwife Teacher. **Contact:** T J McGrath, Lawn Rd, Ashleworth, Gloucester GL19 4JL.
For full details see under Management Studies (Record No. 135).

136. STUDY OF UMBILICAL CORD SEPARATION
March - December 1985
Y Stone, Community Services Manager, Maternity. **Contact:** Y Stone, Waverley Way, Carshalton Beeches, Surrey SM5 3LQ.
For full details see under Management Studies (Record No. 136).

138. "THEY KNOW WHAT THEY'RE DOING!"
January - December 1982
S Drayton, Nursing Officer, Colin Rees, Research Officer. **Contact:** S Drayton, Fidlas Road, Llanishen, Cardiff CF4 5NA.

12-20 hours/week of own time spent. Funded by employer and by funding agency(ies): Maws/RCM Research Scholarship.

Abstract: The hypotheses for the first part of this study were that an enema: 1) results in a quicker labour; 2) reduces faecal contamination of the delivery area; and 3) reduces the incidence of infection in mothers and babies.

Over a ten-week period, 222 women agreed to take part in the study, and were randomly allocated to an 'enema' or 'no enema' group. The results showed a similarity in the length of labour for both groups. There was no statistical difference in the incidence of soiling between the two groups in the first stage of labour, with over 85% in each group remaining clean. In the second stage of labour, this was reduced to 78% in the enema group and 58% in the no enema group. However, the soiling in the no enema group was slight and easy to remove. We suggest this is both acceptable to most midwives and 'manageable'.

Despite the increase in soiling in the no enema group, there was no significant difference in the incidence of infection between the two groups.

In our view, these results do not support the continued use of enemas for delivery; instead, they point to the need to assess the state of the woman's bowel in early labour, and to develop individual care plans. One of the easiest options is to ask the woman to open her bowels herself. Each woman in the study was asked two questions, which took the form of an interview. The first question consisted of two parts: 1) how do those who receive an enema describe the experience, and how do those who do not have one feel about not having one; and 2) how do both groups feel about having an enema with a future delivery?

Those who received an enema thought it was 'not as bad as expected', with a higher proportion of primigravid women answering in this way. Half those who did not receive an enema were 'relieved/delighted'. The second biggest category were 'unconcerned'. When asked how they would feel about a future enema, just under half in each group said they would not mind one way or the other.

We suggest and offer evidence that the reason many women are willing to accept enemas is the traditional nature of the procedure. The use of routine has led to an implicit trust in the 'good sense' of the professional. It is felt that 'they know what they're doing'.

Keywords: BOWEL FUNCTION, ENEMAS, FIRST STAGE, HOSPITAL POLICY, LABOUR, LABOUR (CARE), MIDWIFERY PROCEDURES, ROUTINES

Drayton S, Rees C. 'They know what they're doing'. Nursing Mirror (Midwifery Forum) 1984;159:4-8.
Drayton S, Rees C. Is anyone out there still giving enemas? In: Robinson S, Thompson AM, eds. Midwives, Research and Childbirth. Vol 1. Chapman Hall. 1989:139-53.

140. EVALUATION OF TWO ENDOTRACHEAL SUCTION REGIMES IN BABIES VENTILATED FOR RESPIRATORY DISTRESS SYNDROME
February 1987 - April 1988

G Wilson, Neonatal Sister (G), G Hughes, Research Nurse, J Rennie, Neonatologist, C Morley, Paediatrician. **Contact:** G Wilson, Fulbourn, Cambridge CB1 5DW.

2-6 hours/week of own time spent.

Abstract: All ninety-seven low birthweight babies in one unit, who were ventilated for respiratory distress syndrome during a period of fourteen months, were randomized to this study using sealed envelopes. They were allocated to receive endotracheal suction at either six or twelve hourly intervals. The methods used to assess the outcomes included: 1) a questionnaire to all staff; 2) observation of current practice within the unit; and 3) observation of the babies prior to, five minutes and fifteen minutes after endotracheal aspiration.

The main outcome measures for each group were: median time on ventilator; range of time ventilated; ventilated for more than seventy-two hours; pneumothorax; oxygen therapy for more than thirty days; all grades of intraventricular haemorrhage; and neonatal death.

The results showed no significant differences in respiratory outcome between the groups, and suggest that it is safe to aspirate endotracheal tubes infrequently during the first seventy-two hours in uncomplicated respiratory distress syndrome. As a result of this study, the nursing practice of routine suction is no longer carried out within this unit. We recommend that endotracheal suction should not be performed as a routine procedure on babies requiring ventilation for respiratory distress syndrome. We also recommend that suction should be performed only where necessary, that is: following a deterioration in the baby's condition; a fall in oxygenation/ saturation; or because of the presence of secretions in the endotracheal tube or the sound of secretions on auscultations of the lungs. Further research could address the following questions: 1) whether it is advisable to instill normal saline 0.5ml prior to suction or perform a dry suction; and 2) is the instillation of saline a necessary procedure to aspirate mucus more easily, and does it have any advantages or disadvantages?

Keywords: CARE COMPARISONS, ENDOTRACHEAL SUCTION, LOW BIRTHWEIGHT, NEONATAL CARE, RESPIRATORY DISTRESS SYNDROME, ROUTINES, VENTILATION

Wilson G, Hughes G, Rennie J, Morley C. Evaluation of two endotracheal suction regimes in babies ventilated for respiratory distress syndrome. Early Human Development 1991;25:87-9.

Wilson G, Hughes G, Rennie J, Morley C. Comparing endotracheal suction regimes. Nursing Times 1991;87:44.

Wilson G, Hughes G, Rennie J, Morley C. Evaluation of two endotracheal suction regimes in babies ventilated for respiratory syndrome. Neonatal Network 1992;11:43-5.

Wilson G, Hughes G, Rennie J, Morley C. Suction in neonates: How often is enough? Nursing Standard 1992;7:17.

142. A RANDOMISED TRIAL IN THE POST-OPERATIVE MANAGEMENT OF PATIENTS UNDERGOING ELECTIVE CAESAREAN SECTIONS
November 1990 - May 1991

J Aiken, Staff Midwife, M Thompson, Staff Midwife, K Hodges, Staff Midwife, J Botfield, Staff Midwife, L Grolys, Staff Midwife, V Menon, Consultant Obstetrician. **Contact:** J Aiken, Hemingway Road, Meir Hay, Longton, Stoke on Trent ST3 1SL.

Funded as integral or additional part of a job by employer. 2-6 hours/week of own time spent.

Abstract: (Not updated since 1991). Planned elective Caesarean Sections are rarely associated with serious post-operative complications, and significant morbidity is rare. Patients at North Staffordshire Maternity Hospital who had undergone elective

Caesarean Section prior to this study were only allowed to resume eating a normal diet considerably later than patients we had been used to caring for. This delay was often a source of complaint. This study was undertaken to test the hypothesis that an early resumption of normal dietary intake, following an uncomplicated elective Caesarean Section, will not significantly increase morbidity or delay transfer of the patient to community care.

A subjective assessment of the mother's feelings towards her recovery was made. All patients undergoing elective Caesarean Section were considered eligible for entry to the trial. Allocation to either study or control group was undertaken by using a sequence generated by random numbers contained in sealed envelopes. Following randomisation of approximately eighty mothers, the trial was then extended to include emergency Caesarean Sections and randomization was carried out post-operatively. The different management regimes for early or late resumption of a normal diet were available on all postnatal wards. Prior to Caesarean Section, all mothers were given a personalised questionnaire which was used to obtain information about the duration of intravenous infusion, day of first bowel movement, change in daily abdominal girth measurements and length of inpatient stay. In addition, a subjective assessment was made of the time at which the patient felt 'reasonably well', and whether they were encouraged to recommence a normal diet at the time they considered most appropriate. We do not intend to stratify according to method of anaesthesia. Two hundred women were entered into the study. Mean times of occurrence for each of the three outcome variables with confidence intervals were calculated.

Keywords: CAESAREAN SECTION, DIET, HOSPITAL POLICY, MATERNAL MORBIDITY, POSTNATAL CARE, POSTOPERATIVE CARE

144. COMPARISON OF APGAR SCORES WITH AND WITHOUT MECONIUM STAINED LIQUOR
November 1989 - May 1990
K Graham, Staff Midwife. **Contact:** K Graham, Carneybaun Park, Portrush, Co Antrim, Northern Ireland BT56 8PH.

Formed part of a course.

Abstract: The purpose of this research was to ascertain whether in the absence of abnormal fetal heart rate patterns, meconium-stained liquor was a sign of fetal distress, as measured by the Apgar scores.

The research was a retrospective study of 190 women: forty-one in an experimental group (those with meconium staining); and 149 in a control group (those with clear liquor). The inclusion criteria were as follows: spontaneous labour, no syntocinon, normal delivery, gestational age between thirty-seven to forty-two weeks, one dose of systemic analgesia, and no maternal or fetal abnormalities. The variables used were: period of gestation, maternal age, parity, colour of liquor, length of labour, administration of analgesia, length of time prior to delivery, weight of baby, and Apgar scores at one and five minutes.

The results were analyzed using an SPSSx computer package, Mann-Whitney U-test and chi-square. Measured at one minute, the Apgar scores were statistically lower ($p<0.01$) for meconium-stained liquor; the results at five minutes were much the same.

This small, retrospective study has raised some interesting observations. In our sample, we found that meconium stained liquor was a sign of fetal distress in the absence of abnormal fetal heart rate patterns. Infants over forty weeks gestation also had lower one-minute Apgar scores - which may be due to placental insufficiency at term. Similarly, infants over 4030g had lower one-minute Apgar scores, which may be due to post-maturity. The length of labour was also influenced by maternal age, which could be attributed to the fact that an older woman is more likely to have had a previous pregnancy. Further work is needed to substantiate these observations. In the meantime, meconium-stained liquor should be treated as an indication of fetal distress.

Keywords: APGAR SCORES, FETAL DISTRESS, FETAL HEART RATE, FETAL MONITORING, LABOUR, LIQUOR (CLEAR), LIQUOR (MECONIUM STAINED), MECONIUM

145. MIDWIVES' AND MOTHERS' PERCEPTIONS OF THE TRANSITION TO PARENTHOOD
October 1986 - October 1991
T A Goodenough, Research student. **Contact:** T A Goodenough, Berkeley Rd, Bishopston, Bristol B67 8HG.

Formed part of a course. Over 20 hours/week of own time spent.

Abstract: (Not updated since 1991). This research grew out of a desire to see improved communication between mothers and midwives during the transition to parenthood. The term 'transition to parenthood' was taken to mean the period from late pregnancy up to the end of the first six postnatal weeks. Midwives' and mothers' perceptions of the mothers' experience were studied to compare concepts, attitudes and expectations that might affect communication between them.

Women who took part in the study were approached through National Health Service and National Childbirth Trust parentcraft classes. Fifty-two women completed the study. Midwives were approached through two teaching hospitals. Ninety-one midwives completed the study of whom thirty-three were qualified and fifty-eight were students. For analysis, and where appropriate, the midwives were subdivided into those with and without children. This was in order to highlight the differences in perceptions arising from previous firsthand experience of late pregnancy and early parenthood. The research was divided into two parts:
1. Study of the perceptions of mothers' experience of the transition to parenthood as seen by midwives and the mothers themselves. Data were collected using the following questionnaires: perceptions of mother's self; perceptions of mother's social support networks; perceptions of mother's health locus of control; perceptions of parentcraft education. The questionnaires were administered to the mothers at two visits - the first at thirty-six to thirty-eight weeks of pregnancy, the second at the end of the sixth

postnatal week. The midwives completed both antenatal and postnatal sections of the questionnaires at one session.

2. For mothers only, variables which represented some of the outcomes of the transition to parenthood were measured in the early postnatal weeks. This was in order to discover how mothers' concepts, attitudes and expectations may be related to outcomes, including: labour length, pain relief in labour, feeding practice, and the quality and nature of interactions of mother and baby. Additional data for this section were collected by giving the mothers the following questionnaires: expectations and perceptions of childbirth; expectations and perceptions of the neonate. The mothers also filled out diary data sheets. These were completed for one twenty-four-hour period each week for the first six postnatal weeks, and provided data concerning the baby's activities and interactions.

A short extension to the main study has now been added. This involved exploring the perceptions of a mother's self as held by young women with no firsthand experience of the transition to parenthood. Thirty-four young women completed the perceptions of self questionnaire, and the data generated will be used as a contrast and control to the perceptions of the mothers and midwives. Multivariate analysis is now complete and it is hoped to have the study written up by October 1991.

Keywords: ADAPTATION TO MOTHERHOOD, ADAPTATION TO PARENTHOOD, COMMUNICATION, EXPERIENCE (WOMEN'S), MIDWIVES, PERCEPTIONS OF PARENTHOOD (MIDWIVES'), PERCEPTIONS OF PARENTHOOD (WOMEN'S)

149. IDENTIFICATION AND ANALYSIS OF THE HEALTH EDUCATION NEEDS OF YOUNG PREGNANT WOMEN
October 1988 - October 1990
F M Telfer, Midwife Teacher. **Contact:** F M Telfer, Lincoln Circus, Nottingham NG7 1BG.

Formed part of a course. Over 20 hours/week of own time spent.

Abstract: The purpose of this study was to identify the health education needs of pregnant women who were a) twenty-five years of age or below and b) having their first baby. The study was conducted in the antenatal clinic of a hospital in the north west of England. Women attended the clinic nine to seventeen weeks after conception to register for delivery at the hospital.

A survey method was used with a questionnaire for completion by the respondent. This was followed by a semi-structured interview and a formal 'booking in' interview, which forms a part of the midwifery records. The questionnaire was designed specifically for this study, and reviewed by a statistician and the research supervisor; the semi-structured interview forms were derived from 'A Study of the Antenatal Booking Interview' (Methven, 1982). Both the questionnaire and the interview forms were modified as the result of a pilot study, which was conducted a month before the study began. The sample size was thirty women.

The data from the questionnaire were analyzed using SPSSx. The qualitative data were transcribed from tape recordings of the interviews, and quoted under the appropriate headings in the interview forms. The data were then reviewed for significance, together with the findings from the questionnaire, and compared to the objectives of the study as a whole. The women were found to be highly motivated in their desire to become successful mothers. Their receptiveness to health education was also found to be high. At the time of the interview, their knowledge of self-care in pregnancy derived almost entirely from their mothers, older sisters, friends and magazines.

The main finding was that means should be provided to assist and encourage a woman to make the earliest possible contact with a midwife, and preferably when the pregnancy is first known about. Such a mechanism would allow the woman to receive advice and health education in confidence. Recommendations are made as to how this might be accomplished. The use of literature is proposed, and especially where this could be enclosed with pregnancy testing kits. The need for parenting to receive greater attention in schools and in further education is also identified.

Keywords: ANTENATAL BOOKING INTERVIEW, ANTENATAL CARE, ANTENATAL EDUCATION, HEALTH EDUCATION, MIDWIFE'S ROLE, PRIMIPARAE

Telfer FM. Identification and analysis of the health education needs of young pregnant woman. Unpublished MSc. dissertation. University of Manchester 1990.

Telfer FM. Health education needs of young pregnant women. Research and the Midwife Conference Proceedings 1991:36-42.

151. TO SWAB OR NOT TO SWAB!
January - May 1990
A Berry, Sister, Neonatal Unit. **Contact:** A Berry, Euston Parade, Belfast BT6 9BX.

Formed part of a course. 6-12 hours/week of own time spent. Funded by employer: Eastern Health & Social Services Board.

Abstract: This was a small, retrospective study which included forty-eight infants in a neonatal intensive care unit. The study was designed to investigate whether or not the routine practice of swabbing the carrier sites of all infants admitted to the unit from peripheral hospitals was necessary. Of the forty-eight cases, sixteen laboratory results were not available in the case notes. This was probably due to one of two occurrences: either the laboratory reports were not put into the case notes, or the carrier site swabs were not taken. Of the remaining thirty-two cases, no treatment was ordered for those with a positive result. In conclusion, it is suggested that swabbing infants routinely may not be necessary and should only be performed if signs of sepsis are apparent or suspected. It may also be a needless disturbance to the sick or pre-term infant. Further work is needed to confirm this observation.

Keywords: CARRIER SITE SWABS, HOSPITAL POLICY, NEONATAL CARE, NEONATAL UNITS, ROUTINES

152. KETOSIS IN LABOUR: A STUDY OF LOW-RISK WOMEN WHO HAVE EATEN WITHIN FOUR HOURS PRIOR TO GOING INTO ESTABLISHED LABOUR

November 1989 - February 1990

V Wherry, Midwifery Sister and Family Planning Nurse, D Stables, Midwifery Tutor.
Contact: V Wherry, Gayleighs, Rayleigh, Essex SS6 9LX.

Funded as integral or additional part of a job. Own time spent.

Abstract: Following the appointment of an obstetric anaesthetist, all women were forbidden from taking food of any kind or fluids other than water, even in very early labour. This was felt to be an erosion of the midwives' role. It was also felt to compromise the women's likelihood of having labour without medical intervention. The hypotheses for this study were that women who have eaten within four hours prior to being in established labour would be: 1) less likely to require IVI for treatment of ketosis; 2) less likely to have their labours accelerated; and 3) less likely to have obstetric intervention at delivery.

The subjects included fifty primigravida and multigravida women. The criterion for entry into the study was women who had taken food or fluids within four hours prior to being in established labour. For the purposes of the study, established labour was deemed to be where there was cervical dilatation of 3 cms, effacement of the cervix and descent of the presenting part, accompanied by regular and effective contractions. The methodology used was a short questionnaire which was completed by the midwife while the woman was still in labour. Chi-square statistical analysis was used to analyze the data.

Two thirds of all the women had not eaten a full meal before admission to hospital, preferring high carbohydrate snacks. They appeared not to want to eat in the last 24 hours before delivery. The numbers were too small for confident statements of association but those women who delivered between midnight and midday were more likely to have IVI commenced than those who delivered between midday and midnight. Remaining details to be confirmed.

Keywords: CONFLICTING ADVICE, DIET (LABOUR), HOSPITAL POLICY, HYDRATION (LABOUR), KETOSIS, LABOUR

153. WOMEN-CENTRED CARE: A MIDWIFERY-BASED SCHEME WHICH PROVIDES WOMEN WITH INCREASED CHOICES AND CONTROL

April 1989 - October 1990

Charlette Middlemiss, Midwife Researcher, Paul A Atkinson, Supervisor. **Contact:** Charlette Middlemiss, Princess of Wales Hospital, Coity Road, Bridgend, Mid-Glamorgan, S Wales CS31 1RQ. Tel: 0656 662166 blp 2308

For full details see under Management Studies (Record No. 153).

154. THE EXPERIENCE OF ANTENATAL HOSPITALISATION
June 1987 - April 1990

Susan Kirk, Research Associate. **Contact:** Susan Kirk, Department of Nursing, University of Liverpool, The Whelan Building, PO Box 147, Liverpool L69 3BX. Tel: 051 794 5682

Formed part of a course. 2-6 hours/week of own time spent.

Abstract: In this study, a survey was used to investigate the experiences of women hospitalised in pregnancy. A convenience sample of fifty women was interviewed using a structured schedule. Each woman also completed the Antepartum Hospital Stressors Inventory (AHSI). The data from the structured schedule and the AHSI were analyzed using the SPSSx program.

A number of problems associated with hospital life were highlighted. The main problem identified was that of boredom, which may be related to the large increase in smoking that was found to occur following admission to hospital. Women with children at home expressed great concern, particularly with regard to the effect of the separation. A major cause of anxiety for all women would appear to be the health of their unborn baby. Many women also expressed feelings of guilt, low self-esteem and negative body image. It was found that the sample had received a low level of parentcraft education both prior to and during hospitalisation. A majority of the sample expressed a generally positive attitude towards information-giving from professionals, although in certain aspects a level of dissatisfaction was noted.

The recommendations from the research centre on providing individualised, family-centred care based upon a health model, relieving boredom, providing parentcraft education and planned information-giving, and considering options to hospitalisation.

Keywords: ANTENATAL CARE, ANTENATAL EDUCATION, EDUCATION FOR PARENTHOOD, EXPERIENCE (WOMEN'S), FAMILIES, HOSPITALISATION, PREGNANCY, SMOKING, STRESS (MATERNAL)

Kirk SA. The experience of antenatal hospitalisation. Research and the Midwife Conference Proceedings 1988.

Kirk SA. The experiences of women hospitalised in pregnancy. Nursing Times 1989;85:58.

Kirk SA. The experience of antenatal hospitalisation. Unpublished MSc. thesis, University of Manchester.

Kirk SA. The health needs of women hospitalised in pregnancy. In: Robinson S, Thomson AM, eds. Midwives, Research and Childbirth Vol 3. Chapman & Hall (in press).

155. FEEDING AND GROWTH PATTERNS OF INFANTS IN A NEONATAL UNIT

June 1989 - October 1994

S Lang, Research Midwife, C Lawrence, Senior Lecturer in Statistics. **Contact:** S Lang, St Leonards Avenue, Exeter, Devon EX2 4DL.

Funded as integral or additional part of a job and by funding agency(ies): The Jean Boxall Memorial Trust Fund. Over 20 hours/week of own time spent.

Aims of the study: 1. To identify factors which influence growth and feeding outcome of infants who are preterm, sick or otherwise compromised.
2. To identify any distinct feeding patterns in babies fed breast milk and those fed infant formula milk which may influence length of hospital stay.
3. To examine the role of neonatal staff in the eventual feeding method of the infant at discharge.

Ethics committee approval gained: Yes

Research design: Descriptive – Qualitative and Quantitative – Survey/Case Study

Data collection:
Techniques used:
1. Records of observations.
2. Case notes and Kardex review.
3. Interviews with parents.
4. Semi-structured interviews with members of medical/nursing staff.
5. Weekly discussion with Paediatric Unit Secretary.
6. Diaries of significant events in the first year which could influence feeding outcome (eg infection, drug therapy).

Time data were collected:
Prospectively from admission of an infant to the neonatal unit - to discharge.
Follow up data were collected at the 6 week OP appointment and at any further appointments - following discharge of an infant.
Data were also sent from the Paediatric Unit if any of the infants in the study were re-admitted to hospital during their first year.

Testing of any tools used:
Pilot study with 152 babies

Topics covered:
i) Admission and discharge details, family social history for each baby.
ii) Details of daily feeding regimes for each baby from admission to discharge including method of feeding, type of diet, frequency of feeds, expected and actual fluid intakes.
iii) Interim data which could affect infants' nutritional and growth patterns and eventual method of feeding ie periods of infection, phototherapy etc.

iv) Sequential growth measurements for each baby

v) Staff training and knowledge of lactation

Setting for data collection:

Neonatal unit

Details about sample studied:

Planned size of sample:

600 infants

Rationale for planned size:

To include full range of gestations, weights and clinical conditions

Entry criteria:

All infants admitted to the neonatal unit over a 15 month period.

Sample selection:

Consecutive admissions

Actual sample size:

600

Response rate:

100%

Follow up:

Yes

Response rate:

60% overall

Stage follow up carried out:

At the 6 week out patient clinic and thereafter at any clinic appointment. Follow up of any infant admitted to the Paediatric Unit during its first year.

Problems:

Families moving from the area or on holiday. Poor response from other units, after transfer of the infant.

Intervention, Outcome and Analysis:

Analysis:

Paradox 3

SPSSX via SWURCC and Minitab

Statistical tests:

a) Survival analysis

b) Chi-square

c) Multi variate analysis

d) Principle component analysis, growth modelling, allometry and logistic regression

Results: There were five main results:

1. On a neonatal unit successful breastfeeding at discharge was influenced by the method of feeding used during the transition period between gastric tube feeding and the establishment of breastfeeding. Using bottles during this period significantly reduced the incidence of successful breastfeeding, particularly for pre-term infants, whereas cup feeding significantly increased the establishment of breastfeeding.

2. Infants discharged breastfeeding had shorter periods of hospitilisation than infants discharged forumla feeding, when matched for gestation, clinical condition and birth weights. However there were social class differences with shorter hospital stay and increased breastfeeding rates in SC I, II and III compared to SC IV and V.

3. Breast milk expressed by pump was frequently in excess of the infant's requirements. Supplementation was commonly given. However, by making use of the fat rich hindmilk, growth (ie weight, HC and length) was satisfactorily maintained, and reduced the need for the amount of supplementation.

4. Infants of mothers who intended to breastfeed, tended to be heavier at birth than infants of a mother who intended to artificially feed. But at discharge the trend was for breastfed infants to be lighter than formula fed infants.

5. The staff of a neonatal unit have a wide variety of backgrounds. Knowledge of, and skills in lactation are equally variable. This can have an effect on the advice and help a mother intending to breastfeed is given and can influence the eventual feeding outcome.

Recommendations for further research: i) The effects of a skill based training workshop for neonatal staff in the needs of the breastfeeding mother and infant.

ii) A randomised controlled study of cup feeding to assess its effect on maturation of the suck, swallow and breathing reflexes; earlier establishment at the breast or bottle; and suitability as a method of feeding at discharge of preterm infants still requiring the occasional supplement.

Keywords: ARTIFICIAL FEEDING, BREASTFEEDING, BREASTMILK, HOSPITALISATION (DURATION), INFANT FEEDING, INFANT FORMULAE, NEONATAL CARE, NEONATAL UNITS, OUTCOMES (NEONATAL)

Lang S. Cup feeding: An alternative method. Midwives Chronicle 1994;107:70-175.

158. SURVEY OF DISTRICT MIDWIFERY POLICIES - ANTENATAL AND POSTNATAL CARE
October 1990 - October 1991
Jo Garcia, Social Scientist, Mary J Renfrew, Director, Midwifery Research Programme, Pam Hughes, Project Secretary, Hazel Ashurst, Computer Co-ordinator. **Contact:** Jo Garcia, National Perinatal Epidemiology Unit, Radcliffe Infirmary, Oxford OX2 6HE. Tel: 0865 224170
For full details see under Management Studies (Record No. 158).

159. THE NPEU POSTNATAL CARE PROJECT
February 1990 - December 1993

Jo Garcia, Social Scientist, Sally Marchant, Research Midwife, Pam Hughes, Secretary. **Contact:** Jo Garcia, National Perinatal Epidemiology Unit, Radcliffe Infirmary, Oxford OX2 6HE. Tel: 0865 224170

For full details see under Management Studies (Record No. 159).

162. SURVEY OF INFANT FEEDING PRACTICES
November 1987 - May 1988

Mary J Renfrew, Midwife Researcher. **Contact:** Mary J Renfrew, National Perinatal Epidemiology Unit, Radcliffe Infirmary, Oxford OX2 6HE. Tel: 0865 224876

Funded as integral or additional part of a job by employer: Oxford Health Authority.

Abstract: The purpose of the study was to investigate infant feeding practices, with special reference to breastfeeding in the Oxford area. A six-part survey was carried out. The methods used were: 1) collation of routinely collected data on infant feeding; 2) chart audit of 399 consecutive deliveries to establish initiation, discontinuation and supplementation rates among breastfeeding mothers; 3) a questionnaire to a sample of one in four staff (response rate of 53%) to examine knowledge about and attitudes to infant feeding; 4) direct observation of care given on delivery suite and postnatal wards (total of nine periods of observation ranging in length from three-and-a-half hours to thirty minutes); 5) interviews with special care baby unit staff to establish infant feeding practice and problems; 6) diaries completed by women regarding their experience of infant feeding in hospital.

The results showed that staff were generally knowledgeable about and committed to breastfeeding. Problems identified included an 8% discontinuation rate before discharge home, and the fact that only 27% of breastfed babies were fully breastfed in hospital; the remainder received additional fluids. Mothers did not routinely receive skilled care at the first feed, and the clinical skill of those most closely involved with helping mothers to breastfeed was not always of the highest quality. Recommendations arising from the report relate to the practice of all those caring for women after birth: midwives, paediatricians, obstetricians, nursery nurses, auxiliary nurses and special care unit nurses. More integration of care between the staff is required.

Keywords: BREASTFEEDING, BREASTFEEDING (DURATION), BREASTFEEDING (INCIDENCE), BREASTFEEDING (SUPPORT), MIDWIFERY SKILLS, POSTNATAL CARE, STAFF ATTITUDES

Renfrew MJ. Survey of Infant Feeding Practice in the Oxford District 1987-1988. Report submitted to the Director of Midwifery Services, John Radcliffe Hospital, Oxford 1988.

165. A STUDY TO DETERMINE IF DIRECT CARE REDUCES WITH INCREASING GRADE OF MIDWIFE

October 1990 - March 1991

M M Heggie, Midwifery Lecturer. **Contact:** M M Heggie, Gleneldon Rd, Streatham, London SW16 2BZ.

For full details see under Management Studies (Record No. 165).

167. AROMATHERAPY IN LABOUR

June - December 1990

C Blamey, Staff Midwife, E Burns, Clinical Specialist/Lecturer Practitioner, H Ashurst, Computing Co-ordinator, C Sapsford, Aromatherapist, R Cecil, Aromatherapist, M J Renfrew, Midwife Researcher. **Contact:** C Blamey, Nine Acres Close, Charlbury, Oxford OX7 3RB.

Funded as integral or additional part of a job by John Radcliffe Hospital. 2 hours/week of own time spent.

Aims of the study: To assess the effectiveness of essential oils in labour.

Ethics committee approval gained: No

Research design: Descriptive – Qualitative and Quantitative – Ethnography
    Data collection:
        Techniques used:
            Records of observation
        Time data were collected:
            During labour or after delivery
            Prior to transfer out of delivery suite
        Testing of any tools used:
            Evaluation sheet piloted
        Topics covered:
            Which oils were used
            When, how and why they were used
            Analgesia
            Labour outcome
            Perceptions of effectiveness - mothers' and midwives'
            Adverse effects
        Setting for data collection:
            Hospital delivery suite

    Details about sample studied:
        Planned size of sample:
            All women using aromatherapy in 6 months
        Rationale for planned size:
            Total population

Entry criteria:
  Inclusion: Women in established labour
  Exclusion: Multiple allergies
Sample selection:
  Random
Actual sample size:
  585
Response rate:
  100

Intervention, Outcome and Analysis:
  Analysis:
    SPSS

Results: 585 women participated: 384 primigravidae, 201 multigravidae. 880 uses of oils were given. Overall 62.5% women found oil(s) "effective" while 11.6% women found them "ineffective". The remaining 24.9% were ambivalent or declined to record an opinion.

Keywords: AROMATHERAPY, COMPLEMENTARY THERAPIES, ESSENTIAL OILS, LA-BOUR

168. THE CONTRIBUTION OF THE NEONATAL MIDWIFE TO THE VERY LOW BIRTHWEIGHT BABY AND HIS/HER PARENTS
January 1986 - January 1992
V Fletcher, Midwife, Fetal Assessment Unit/Day Care. **Contact:** V Fletcher, Randolph Road, Broomhill, Glasgow G11 7LG.

6-12 hours/week of own time spent.

Aims of the study: To describe the nursing content of the management of the very low birthweight baby (<1500g) and his/her parents with particular reference to the promotion of mothering skills. Specifically to a) describe the care plan, its orientation and implementation, b) examine the nature and content of nursing care, c) describe the assessment of parental needs - methods used and time allocated and d) describe the continuity of nursing care into the community.

Ethics committee approval gained: Yes

Research design: Descriptive – Qualitative – Case Study

  Data collection:
    Techniques used:
      Demographic records
      Semi-structured interviews
      Questionnaires
      Rating scales

Time data were collected:
    1 week post delivery to 6 weeks post discharge
Testing of any tools used:
    Questionnaires pre-tested with parents and staff
Topics covered:
    Physical involvement (touch and handling)
    Care giving involvement
    Parentcraft provision
    Breastfeeding outcomes
    Anxiety
    Affection - development of affectionate ties with infants
    Preparation for discharge
    Continuity of care into the community
    Community support
    Relationship with staff during infants' hospitalisation
Setting for data collection:
    Hospital and community

Details about sample studied:
Planned size of sample:
    24
Rationale for planned size:
    Constraints of the method
Entry criteria:
    Infants weighing 1500g or less
    No congenital anomalies
Sample selection:
    Consecutive admissions over 18 months
Actual sample size:
    20
Response rate:
    83% initially
    67% at follow up stages

Intervention, Outcome and Analysis:
Analysis:
    Identification of themes

Results: Neonatal midwives attempted to individualise the care of families but mothers were anxious and their behaviours were a reflection of their willingness to conform to staff expectation rather than a genuine desire for physical contact with the infant. A suggestion is made that mothers should be reassured that they are not expected to establish a relationship with their baby before they feel ready to do so. Additional written information was perceived by the mothers to be desirable and they would have liked more counselling.

Mothers who were particularly vulnerable to problems included those who had had a previous adverse outcome of pregnancy, and those lacking social support. Serious medical complications in the baby was an important contributing factor in a mothers' unwillingness to become involved in mothering tasks.

Transition from hospital to home presented problems and community HVs and GPs were perceived as inappropriate people to consult about everyday problems of child care: they were seen to lack interest and knowledge. The study suggests paediatric liaison midwives, known to the women, were more appropriate people to visit the family after discharge.

Keywords: ADAPTATION TO MOTHERHOOD, ADAPTATION TO PARENTHOOD, EXPERIENCE (WOMEN'S), INDIVIDUALISED CARE, MIDWIVES (NEONATAL), NEONATAL CARE, NURSES (NEONATAL), RELATIONSHIPS, VERY LOW BIRTHWEIGHT

169. INFANT FEEDING SURVEY AT A BRITISH MILITARY HOSPITAL, RINTELN, BRITISH ARMY OF THE RHINE
October 1990 - March 1991
D Noble, Nursing Officer, Midwifery. **Contact:** D Noble, Dunston, Gateshead, Tyne and Wear NE11 9QR.

Funded as integral or additional part of a job by employer. 2-6 hours/week of own time spent.

Aims of the study: To discover whether the percentage of successful breastfeeding mother was poorer at a British Military Hospital than in the national United Kingdom.

Ethics committee approval gained: No

Research design: Descriptive – Qualitative and Quantitative – Survey

> **Data collection:**
> > **Techniques used:**
> > > Questionnaires
> > **Time data were collected:**
> > > Over 6 months
> > **Testing of any tools used:**
> > > Questionnaire piloted
> > **Topics covered:**
> > > Demographic information
> > > Family influence
> > > Attitudes to breastfeeding
> > > Influencing factors
> > **Setting for data collection:**
> > > Military hospital, Rinteln

> **Details about sample studied:**
> > **Planned size of sample:**
> > > All patients delivered during a six month trial period

Rationale for planned size:
Total population
Entry criteria:
Women delivering in a British Military hospital
Sample selection:
Inclusive
Actual sample size:
556
Response rate:
22%

Intervention, Outcome and Analysis:
Analysis:
Content analysis

Results: Percentages of breastfeeding mothers at the British Military Hospital were not less than those in the civilian United Kingdom. Attitudes did not appear to be biased. More effort could be made to influence women to breastfeed who have pre-conceived ideas inclining them to bottle feed.
High motivation and enthusiasm is required from midwives.
Exposure to the topic should begin prior to childbearing.
The ongoing Gulf War appeared to cause family disruption and might have influenced feeding practice in this study period.

Keywords: ANTENATAL EDUCATION, BREASTFEEDING, BREASTFEEDING (DURA-TION), BREASTFEEDING (SUPPORT), MIDWIVES

170. INDUCTION OF LABOUR: A COMPARISON OF A SINGLE PROSTAGLANDIN E2 VAGINAL TABLET WITH AMNIOTOMY AND INTRAVENOUS OXYTOCIN
June 1981 - June 1982
A A Calder, Professor of Obstetrics, James H Kennedy, Lecturer, Peter Stewart, Senior Registrar, David H Barlow, Registrar, Edith M Hillan, Research Sister. **Contact:** Edith M Hillan, Department of Nursing Studies, University of Glasgow, Glasgow G12 8QQ. Tel: 041 339 8855 Ex 4053

Funded as integral or additional part of a job by employer: Greater Glasgow Health Board, University of Glasgow.

Aims of the study: To compare the efficacy and acceptability of a single vaginal tablet of Prostaglandin E2 with amniotomy and intravenous oxytocin for induction of labour.

Ethics committee approval gained: Yes

Research design: Experimental – Qualitative and Quantitative – Randomized Controlled Trial

Data collection:
    Techniques used:
        Case note review.
        Questionnaires.
    Time data were collected:
        Questionnaires - 48 hours after delivery.
        Other data - during and following delivery.
    Testing of any tools used:
        Pilot study carried out.
    Topics covered:
        Satisfaction of mothers.
        Amount of analgesia required.
        Blood loss at delivery.
        Incidence of neonatal jaundice.
    Setting for data collection:
        Hospital

Details about sample studied:
    Planned size of sample:
        100
    Rationale for planned size:
        Advice of statistician.
    Entry criteria:
        Parity 1 or 2.
        Singleton pregnancy.
        Cephalic presentation at 38-42 weeks gestation.
    Sample selection:
        First 100 women who met above criteria and gave informed consent.
    Actual sample size:
        100
    Response rate:
        100% - questionnaires.

Intervention, Outcome and Analysis:
    Interventions used:
        Group 1: Forewater amniotomy and simultaneous intravenous oxytocin controlled by a Cardiff infusion system (maximum dosage 32m - units/minute).
        Group 2: Vaginal tablet of 3mg prostaglandin E2 in a lactic acid base placed in the posterior fornix. Membranes were ruptured 6 hours later or sooner if there was regular uterine activity and cervical dilation had reached 4cm.
    Main outcomes measured:
        Satisfaction of mothers
        Blood loss
        Analgesia requirements
        Neonatal jaundice

Analysis:

SPSSX

Results: Four of the women in Group 2 (PGE2) required additional intravenous oxytocin to achieve delivery. The prostaglandin group had a longer mean overall induction-delivery interval but a shorter amniotomy-delivery interval than the women in the amniotomy/oxytocin group. Women treated with PGE2 expressed a higher level of satisfaction with their method of induction, required less analgesia, had a lower blood loss at delivery and their babies had a lower incidence of neonatal jaundice.

It was concluded that in women with a favourable cervix, labour could be reliably induced with a single vaginal tablet of PGE2 followed by amniotomy. The reduced requirement of analgesia suggests that the gradual onset of contractions produced by PGE2 was better tolerated. Further advantages were reduced blood loss and less neonatal jaundice. For the women, the main advantages were freedom of movement and the gradual onset of uterine activity.

Keywords: LABOUR (INDUCTION), PROSTAGLANDIN E2, RANDOMIZED CONTROLLED TRIAL

Hillan EM. Starting Labour. Unpublished MSc thesis. University of Strathclyde 1983.
Hillan EM. Advances in care. Nursing Mirror 1984;159:i-vii.
Kennedy JH, Stewart P, Barlow DH, Hillan E, Calder AA. Induction of labour: a comparison of a single prostaglandin E2 vaginal tablet with amniotomy and intravenous oxytocin. British Journal of Obstetrics and Gynaecology 1982;89:704-7.

171. A COMPARATIVE ASSESSMENT OF AN AUTOMATED BLOOD MICROPROCESSOR FOR FETAL BLOOD PH MEASUREMENTS IN THE LABOUR WARD

June 1982 - June 1983

Peter Stewart, Consultant Obstetrician, Edith M Hillan, Research Sister. **Contact:** Edith M Hillan, Department of Nursing Studies, University of Glasgow, Glasgow G12 8QQ. Tel: 041 339 8855 Ex 4053

Funded as integral or additional part of a job by employer: Greater Glasgow Health Board.

Aims of the study: To compare a new fully automated, self-calibrating blood pH analyser with a standard reference instrument for the measurement of pH of fetal scalp and umbilical cord blood samples.

Ethics committee approval gained: Yes

Research design: Descriptive – Quantitative – Comparative assessment

Data collection:
> **Techniques used:**
>> Analysis of recordings
>
> **Time data were collected:**
>> Immediately following delivery
>
> **Testing of any tools used:**
>> Pilot study carried out
>
> **Topics covered:**
>> pH
>
> **Setting for data collection:**
>> Hospital

Details about sample studied:
> **Planned size of sample:**
>> 106
>
> **Rationale for planned size:**
>> Advice of statistician
>
> **Entry criteria:**
>> Details not confirmed
>
> **Sample selection:**
>> Convenience
>
> **Actual sample size:**
>> 106
>
> **Response rate:**
>> 100%

Intervention, Outcome and Analysis:
> **Analysis:**
>> Paired t-test

Results: The range of the 106 samples as measured by the reference instrument was 7.07-7.54 pH units and the range of the differences between the two methods of analysis using the same blood sample was 0-0.075 pH units. The mean of the signed differences was -0.004 (SD 0.025) and a paired t-test of these differences gave a t-value of -1.640 (df 105) which was not statistically significant. The number of differences greater than 0.04 pH units was 14 (13%). In three of these cases the reading from the reference instrument was higher than the reading from the 220 instrument; in the other 11 samples the 220 instrument gave a higher reading. Overall the 220 instrument gave more high readings (54) than low readings.

The 220 pH system was found to obviate the need for trained technicians and the blood sample size of 10-15 μl was easier to obtain from the fetal scalp than the 50 μl size required by the reference instrument. The 220 system proved easy to operate and was reasonably reliable. The results suggest that multiple samples should be taken to reduce the chance of isolated errors. The major disadvantage of the 220 system was that cartridges for each sample cost £6.50 which means it may not be economical where multiple estimations are required and where trained technicians are readily available.

Keywords: AUTOMATED BLOOD MICROPROCESSOR, FETAL BLOOD PH, LABOUR WARD, PH ANALYSIS

Stewart P, Hillan E, Calder AA, Nicol SM. A comparative assessment of an automated blood microprocessor for fetal blood pH measurements in the labour ward. British Journal of Obstetrics and Gynaecology 1983;90:522-4.

172. THE UNRIPE CERVIX: MANAGEMENT WITH VAGINAL OR EXTRA-AMNIOTIC PROSTAGLANDIN E2
June 1982 - June 1983

A A Calder, Professor of Obstetrics, Peter Stewart, Senior Registrar, James H Kennedy, Lecturer, Edith M Hillan, Research Sister. **Contact:** Edith M Hillan, Department of Nursing Studies, University of Glasgow, Glasgow G12 8QQ. Tel: 041 339 8855 Ex 4053

Funded as integral or additional part of a job by employer: Greater Glasgow Health Board, University of Glasgow.

Aims of the study: To compare the efficacy of vaginal prostaglandin E2 tablets with the more conventional extra amniotic route in women with an unripe cervix admitted for induction of labour.

Ethics committee approval gained: Yes

Research design: Experimental – Qualitative and Quantitative – Randomized Controlled Trial

> **Data collection:**
> > **Techniques used:**
> > > Questionnaires to women.
> > > Case note review.
> > **Time data were collected:**
> > > Questionnaire - 48 hours after delivery.
> > > Other data - during and following labour.
> > **Testing of any tools used:**
> > > Pilot study carried out.
> > **Topics covered:**
> > > Feelings about method of induction.
> > > Progress in labour.
> > > Duration of labour.
> > > Mode of delivery.
> > > Condition of baby at birth.
> > **Setting for data collection:**
> > > Hospital

Details about sample studied:
> **Planned size of sample:**
>> 62
>
> **Rationale for planned size:**
>> Convenience
>
> **Entry criteria:**
>> Primigravidae with unripe cervix.
>
> **Sample selection:**
>> Convenience
>
> **Actual sample size:**
>> 62
>
> **Response rate:**
>> 100%

Intervention, Outcome and Analysis:
> **Interventions used:**
>> Group 1: Vaginal tablet of 3mg prostaglandin E2 repeated if necessary after 18 and 24 hours, Amniotomy performed after labour established.
>>
>> Group 2: 450 mg PGE2 in tylose gel into the amniotic space. 18 hours later amniotomy and IV oxytocin.
>
> **Main outcomes measured:**
>> Discomfort.
>> Degree of embarassment.
>> Onset of labour.
>> Duration of labour.
>> Mode of delivery.
>> Condition of baby at birth.
>
> **Follow up:**
>> Not applicable.
>
> **Analysis:**
>> SPSSX

Results: The treatment regime in Group 2 (extra amniotic PGE2) produced a more reliable cervical ripening effect and rapid onset of labour than that of Group 1 (tablets). Only 4 women, however, in Group 1 failed to labour after treatment with 3 vaginal tablets. There were no differences between the two groups in the duration of labour, mode of delivery or condition of the baby at birth. The regime of vaginal PGE2 tablets did not significantly reduce the need for oxytocin but women in Group 1 did appreciate the avoidance of an IV infusion early in labour, thus enabling them to be ambulant. Most women found amniotomy and IV infusion unpleasant. The alternative regime using vaginal tablets and deferred amniotomy is simple, less invasive and was found to be highly acceptable in terms of discomfort and embarrassment in the assessment of the women themselves.

Keywords: CERVICAL RIPENING, PROSTAGLANDIN E2, RANDOMIZED CONTROLLED TRIAL, UNRIPE CERVIX

Hillan EM. Starting labour. Unpublished MSc. thesis; University of Strathclyde 1983.

Hillan EM. Advances in care. Nursing Mirror 1984;159:i-vii.

Stewart P, Kennedy JH, Hillan E, Calder AA. The unripe cervix: management with vaginal or extra-amniotic prostaglandin E2. Journal of Obstetrics and Gynaecology 1983;4:90-3.

173. A RANDOMISED STUDY TO ASSESS THE BENEFITS AND HAZARDS OF DELIVERY IN A BIRTHING CHAIR
June 1983 - June 1984

A A Calder, Professor of Obstetrics, Edith M Hillan, Research Sister, Peter Stewart, Senior Registrar. **Contact:** Edith M Hillan, Department of Nursing Studies, University of Glasgow, Glasgow G12 8QQ. Tel: 041 339 8855 Ex 4053

Funded as integral or additional part of a job and by funding agency: Greater Glasgow Health Board.

Aims of the study: To assess the benefits and hazards associated with delivery in a birthing chair. The specific objectives were to assess whether the sitting position affected:

1) the duration of the second stage or particularly the duration of active pushing;

2) the incidence of instrumental delivery;

3) the incidence of episiotomy or other perineal damage;

4) the condition of the infant at birth;

Ethics committee approval gained: Yes

Research design: Experimental – Quantitative – Randomized Controlled Trial

Data collection:
> **Techniques used:**
>> Observation.
>> Case note review.
>
> **Time data were collected:**
>> During labour and delivery.
>
> **Testing of any tools used:**
>> Pilot study carried out.
>
> **Topics covered:**
>> Details of labour and delivery.
>> Condition of the baby at birth.
>
> **Setting for data collection:**
>> Hospital (university teaching).

Details about sample studied:
> **Planned size of sample:**
>> 500

Rationale for planned size:
Advice of statistician.

Entry criteria:
Singleton pregnancy.
Cephalic presentation.
37-42 weeks gestation.

Sample selection:
Randomly allocated towards end of first stage of labour.

Actual sample size:
500

Response rate:
100%

Intervention, Outcome and Analysis:

Interventions used:
Group 1: delivery in birthing chair.
Group 2: delivery in conventional dorsal recumbent position in bed.

Main outcomes measured:
Duration of labour.
Perineal damage.
Blood loss.
Condition of baby at birth.
Mode of delivery.
Active pushing time.

Analysis:
SPSSx

Results: There was no significant difference in the duration of second stage between those women delivering in a chair and those in bed. However, when the duration of active pushing was examined both primigravidae and multigravidae delivered in the chair had significantly shorter mean pushing time. A significantly greater proportion of primigravidae delivered in the birthing chair achieved a spontaneous delivery and this was especially marked in the group of women delivered with epidural analgesia. There was no significant difference in the mode of delivery between the two groups of multigravidae. Multigravidae delivered in the birthing chair had a significantly higher mean blood loss at delivery and also appeared to have a higher incidence of primary postpartum haemorrhage (blood loss >500 mls) although these results did not reach statistical significance. Perineal damage was significantly reduced for all women delivered in the birthing chair and this remained significant amongst primigravidae even when forceps deliveries were excluded. The mean birth weight and condition of the infants at birth was similar regardless of the place of delivery.

Delivery in the birthing chair appeared to help overcome the difficulty of delivering spontaneously while under epidural block. Several women were noticed to develop marked perineal and vulval oedema during delivery in the chair although no other deleterious effects were noted and spontaneous resolution occured in all cases.

Keywords: BIRTH CHAIR, BLOOD LOSS, DELIVERY, EPISIOTOMY, INSTRUMENTAL DELIVERY, RANDOMIZED CONTROLLED TRIAL, SECOND STAGE (DURATION)

Hillan EM. Posture for labour and delivery. Midwifery 1985;1:19-23.

Hillan EM. A randomised study to assess the benefits of delivery in a birthing chair. In: Proceedings of the 20th Congress of the International Confederation of Midwives. Sydney 1984:216-23.

Stewart P, Hillan E, Calder AA. A randomised trial to evaluate the use of birth chair for delivery. Lancet 1983;1:1296-8.

Hillan EM. The birthing chair trial. Research and the Midwife Conference, Manchester 1983:22-37.

174. CAESAREAN SECTION VERSUS VAGINAL DELIVERY: A COMPARISON OF OUTCOMES

June 1985 - June 1989

Edith M Hillan, University Lecturer, Malcolm MacNaughton, Professor of Obstetrics, Gillian M McIlwaine, Senior Epidemiologist. **Contact:** Edith M Hillan, Department of Nursing Studies, University of Glasgow, Glasgow G12 8QQ. Tel: 041 339 8855 Ex 4053

Funded by Scottish Office Home & Health Department.

Aims of the study: To compare a group of primigravidae delivered by emergency Caesarean Section with a comparable group of women delivered vaginally to assess the effect of the delivery method on:

1. the immediate, short term and long term morbidity experienced by the women.
2. women's views of the labour and delivery experience.
3. the resumption of sexual activity and the attitude of the women to future pregnancies.

Ethics committee approval gained: Yes

Research design: Descriptive – Qualitative and Quantitative – Survey

Data collection:
    Techniques used:
        1. Case note review.
        2. Hospital review.
        3. Postal questionnaire.
        4. Home interview.
    Time data were collected:
        1. Retrospectively.
        2. 3rd or 4th postnatal day.
        3. 3 months after delivery.
        4. 6 months after delivery.

Testing of any tools used:

All instruments were piloted

Topics covered:

1. Maternal and infant characteristics; labour and delivery data including the indications for instrumental or Caesarean delivery; perineal damage; blood loss; type of anaesthesia; operative morbidity; post-operative morbidity; length of postnatal stay.

2. Antenatal experiences; time of first seeing, holding and feeding baby; postnatal pain, discomfort and problems; rating of labour and delivery experience; infant feeding - intended and actual.

3. Women's knowledge of reasons for instrumental/operative delivery; maternal health since delivery; morbidity; drug therapy; infant health; infant feeding practices.

4. Women's health since delivery; infant health and feeding practices; retrospective rating of labour and delivery experience; resumption of sexual intercourse; sexual difficulties; plans for future pregnancies.

Setting for data collection:

Hospital and community

Details about sample studied:

Planned size of sample:

50 primigravidae delivered by emergency Caesarean Section (study group).

50 primigravidae delivered vaginally (control group).

Rationale for planned size:

Convenience

Entry criteria:

Primigravidae with no major antenatal complications; height > 155cm; 37-42 weeks gestation.

Study group - delivered by emergency Caesarean Section during the course of labour.

Control group - delivered vaginally.

Sample selection:

Control group - next primigravida who met the criteria for entry after a subject had entered the study group.

Actual sample size:

Study group - 50

Control group - 50

Response rate:

1,2 - 100%

3 - 91%

4 - 88%

Intervention, Outcome and Analysis:
Analysis:
SPSSx

Results:

Aim 1: Women delivered by Caesarean Section had longer labours, developed more complications during the course of labour and required an increased number of obstetric interventions compared with women delivered vaginally. The blood loss at delivery was also greater and 18% of women in the study group required blood transfusion compared with only 2% in the control group.

The patterns of recorded morbidity were different in the two groups of women due to the different delivery methods. Most of the morbidity in the control group was related to perineal trauma sustained at delivery, whereas in the study group a wide variety of morbidity was documented, much of which was infectious. It was apparent that many of the problems the women complained of in the postnatal period were not recorded in either the medical or midwifery notes.

Three months after delivery 51% of the study group stated that they felt back to normal and 40% felt less healthy than before the pregnancy compared with 70% and 28% in the control group. Six months after delivery 38% of the women delivered by Section still did not feel back to normal health and a further 12% were still taking medication for problems experienced since delivery. In the group delivered vaginally, 30% still did not feel they were back to normal and a further 2 women said they were just back to normal having completed courses of antidepressant therapy. The problems still being complained of included tiredness, depression, backache and wound pain. In the majority of these cases multiple complaints were made.

Aim 2: When the women were interviewed on the 3rd or 4th postnatal day, 60% of the study group said the labour was worse than anticipated and 24% said it was better. The corresponding figures for the control group were 44% and 32% respectively. In 64% of the study group the partner was present in theatre for delivery compared with 80% of partners in the group delivered vaginally. Women delivered vaginally saw, held and fed their infants sooner than those delivered by Caesarean Section. Women in the study group were more likely to complain that they did not get enough rest in the postnatal ward and that it was more difficult for them to cope with the demands of looking after the baby because of the pain and other discomforts they were experiencing. A higher proportion of the study group (48% v 18%) also said they would like more information about the events during the intrapartum period before discharge from hospital.

At the end of the interview the women were also asked if they felt the hospital could have done anything to make things better for them in the antenatal and postnatal periods. Areas for improvements were:

1. failure of communication between women and the staff; occured in all areas from antenatal care to the postnatal wards.
2. lack of realistic preparation for labour, delivery and parenthood.
3. lack of support and conflicting advice from midwives, especially in the postnatal ward.

Aim 3

Women delivered by Caesarean Section resumed intercourse sooner than those delivered vaginally and had fewer sexual problems after the birth. By the time of the home interview 2 women delivered vaginally had still not resumed intercourse compared with none of the women delivered by section.

Six months after the birth, women in the study group were more likely to attribute a reluctance to have another pregnancy due to the inexperience on this occasion than those who delivered vaginally (9 compared with 1).

Recommendations for further research: Large-scale systematic studies to determine the morbidity associated with different delivery methods considering not only the immediate, but also the short and long term effects.

Keywords: CAESAREAN SECTION, CAESAREAN SECTION INDICATORS, DELIVERY, INFANT CHARACTERISTICS, LABOUR, MATERNAL CHARACTERISTICS, MATERNAL MORBIDITY, SEXUAL PROBLEMS, WOMEN'S VIEWS

Hillan EM. Caesarean Section versus vaginal delivery: a comparison of outcomes. Journal of Psychosomatic Obstetrics and Gynaecology 1989;10:144.

Hillan EM. Outcomes of Caesarean delivery. Unpublished PhD thesis. University of Glasgow 1990.

Hillan EM. Decision making in Caesarean Section. Theoretical Surgery 1990;3:155.

Hillan EM. An overview of recent trends in Caesarean Section. Nursing Standard 1990;25:24-7.

Hillan EM. Caesarean Section: historical background. Scottish Medical Journal 1991;5:150-4.

Hillan EM. Decison making in Caesarean Section. Journal of Medical Decision Making 1991;1:69.

Hillan EM. Caesarean Section: maternal risks. Nursing Standard 1991;48:26-9.

Hillan EM. Caesarean Section: perinatal risks. Nursing Standard 1991;48:37-9.

Hillan EM. Caesarean Section: psychosocial morbidity. Nursing Standard 1991;50:30-3.

Hillan EM. Research and audit: women's views of Caesarean Section. In: Roberts H (ed). Women's Health Matters. London: Routledge. 1992:157-75.

Hillan EM. Short-term morbidity associated with Caesarean Section. Birth 1992;4:190-4.

Hillan EM. Monitoring the effects of Caesarean Section. Nursing Times 1992;24:50-1.

Hillan EM. Short term morbidity associated with Caesarean Section. Journal of Clinical Nursing 1992;2:107-8.

Hillan EM. Caesarean Section: psychosocial morbidity. Midwives Information and Resource Service Midwifery Digest 1992;2:182-5.

Hillan EM. Caesarean Section: perinatal risks. Midwives Information and Resource Service Midwifery Digest 1992;3:313-5.

Hillan EM. Issues in the delivery of midwifery care. Journal of Advanced Nursing 1992;1:274-8.

Hillan EM. Maternal-infant attachment following Caesarean delivery. Journal of Clinical Nursing 1992;1:33-7.

Hillan EM. Caesareans - a cause for concern? Johnson and Johnson Digest Number 3, 1994 (in press).

175. OUTCOMES OF CAESAREAN DELIVERY
June 1985 - June 1989
Edith M Hillan, University Lecturer, Malcolm MacNaughton, Professor of Obstetrics, Gillian M McIlwaine, Senior Epidemiologist. **Contact:** Edith M Hillan, Department of Nursing Studies, University of Glasgow, Glasgow G12 8QQ. Tel: 041 339 8855 Ex 4053

Funded by Scottish Office Home & Health Department.

Aims of the study: 1. To describe the current practice with regard to Caesarean Section in a large university teaching hospital and to determine the indications for the performance of the operation.

2. To determine the operative and post-operative morbidity associated with Caesarean Section and to compare the morbidity by the timing of the operation: elective versus emergency Caesarean Section; sub-groups of women delivered by emergency Caesarean Section; women delivered during the first stage of labour versus those delivered during the course of the second stage.

3. To describe the short-term effects of Caesarean delivery for the mother and her baby including: the health of women after discharge from hospital and to describe the reported morbidity; women's knowledge of the reasons for the performance of the caesarean section; the health of infants since discharge from hospital; infant feeding practices.

Ethics committee approval gained: Yes

Research design: Descriptive – Qualitative and Quantitative – Survey

> **Data collection:**
> > **Techniques used:**
> > > 1,2 - Case note review
> > > 3 - Postal questionnaire
> > **Time data were collected:**
> > > 1,2 - Retrospectively
> > > 3 - 3 months after delivery
> > **Testing of any tools used:**
> > > Pilot study
> > **Topics covered:**
> > > Maternal and infant characteristics.
> > > Indications for Caesarean delivery.
> > > Status of surgeon.
> > > Type of anaesthesia.
> > > Operative morbidity.
> > > Post-operative morbidity.
> > **Setting for data collection:**
> > > Hospital and community.

Details about sample studied:
  Planned size of sample:
    All women delivered by Caesarean Section during a one year period in a university teaching hospital (n=619).
  Rationale for planned size:
    All women delivered by Caesarean Section during a one year period in a university teaching hospital (n=619).
  Entry criteria:
    1,2 - women having a Caesarean Section.
    3 - women who experienced a perinatal loss or where the neonatal outcome was uncertain were excluded (n=31).
  Sample selection:
    Consecutive Caesarean Sections.
  Actual sample size:
    1,2 - n=619
    3 - n=588
  Response rate:
    1,2 - 100%
    3 - 76%

  Intervention, Outcome and Analysis:
    Analysis:
      SPSSx

Results: Aims 1 and 2
Elective surgery was performed in 220 (36%) of cases and in the remaining 399 (64%) the operation was carried out as an emergency procedure. In over 65% of the cases more than one indication for the performance of the Caesarean Section was recorded in the case record and these were not necessarily ordered in terms of priority. Ultimately four main indications - dystocia, breech presentation, previous Caesarean delivery and fetal distress - were found to be responsible for over 87% of the operations performed.

Twelve (2%) women in the study population had incisions other than low transverse. A further 41 women (6.8%) had extensions or tears of the original uterine incision and in 16 cases the extension involved both uterine angles, the upper uterine segment, cervix or vagina. Emergency Caesarean Section was associated with more extensions of the uterine incision, an increased incidence of bladder trauma, a greater mean blood loss, increased incidence of blood loss >500mls and subsequently an increased requirement for intra-operative blood transfusion when compared with elective delivery, and this was particularly marked where a period of labour had occurred before delivery. The highest incidence of operative complications was found in women delivered after the onset of the second stage of labour.

Only 9.5% of the women had no recorded morbidity in the postnatal period. Infectious morbidity which might be directly attributable to the mode of delivery occurred in 21.7% of cases during the hospital stay and 26.7% of the women received antibiotic therapy. The most commonly encountered categories of infectious morbidity were urinary tract infection (11%), wound infection (7%), intra-uterine infection (4%) and chest infection (4%) and these were more frequently associated with emergency caesarean section.

Aim 3: 13% of those who replied either did not know or gave completely wrong explanations for the performance of the Caesarean Section and a further 14% were only partially right in the comprehension.

Three months after the birth, 35% of the women still did not feel back to normal and 28% felt less healthy than before the pregnancy. The most common complaints following delivery were wound pain, wound leakage, tiredness, backache, constipation, wind, depression and sleeping difficulties. In some women these had persisted since the delivery.

Although 43% of the respondents indicated that they had planned to breast feed before delivery, only 35% actually attempted to do so. One month after delivery only 19% were still breast feeding and by 3 months 9% were totally breast feeding and a further 2% were combining breast and bottle feeding.

Recommendations for further research: Large-scale systematic studies to determine the morbidity associated with different delivery methods.

Keywords: CAESAREAN SECTION, CAESAREAN SECTION INDICATORS, DELIVERY, INFANT CHARACTERISTICS, LABOUR, MATERNAL CHARACTERISTICS, MATERNAL MORBIDITY, SEXUAL PROBLEMS, WOMEN'S VIEWS

Hillan EM. Caesarean Section versus vaginal delivery: a comparison of outcomes. Journal of Psychosomatic Obstetrics and Gynaecology 1989;10:144.

Hillan EM. Outcomes of Caesarean delivery. Unpublished PhD thesis. University of Glasgow 1990.

Hillan EM. Decision making in Caesarean Section. Theoretical Surgery 1990;3:155.

Hillan EM. An overview of recent trends in Caesarean Section. Nursing Standard 1990;35:24-7.

Hillan EM. Caesarean Section: historical background. Scottish Medical Journal 1991;5:150-4.

Hillan EM. Decision making in Caesarean Section. Journal of Medical Decision Making 1991;1:69.

Hillan EM. Caesarean Section: maternal risks. Nursing Standard 1991;48:26-9.

Hillan EM. Caesarean Section: perinatal risks. Nursing Standard 1991;49:37-9.

Hillan EM. Caesarean Section: psychosocial morbidity. Nursing Standard 1991;50:30-3.

Hillan EM. Research and audit: women's views of Caesarean Section. In: Roberts H (ed). Women's Health Matters. London: Routledge. 1992:157-75.

Hillan EM. Short-term morbidity associated with Caesarean Section. Birth 1992;4:190-4.

Hillan EM. Monitoring the effects of Caesarean Section. Nursing Times 1992;24:50-1.

Hillan EM. Short-term morbidity associated with Caesarean Section. Journal of Clinical Nursing 1992;2:107-8.

Hillan EM. Caesarean Section: psychosocial morbidity. Midwives Information and Resource Service Midwifery Digest 1992;2:182-5.

Hillan EM. Caesarean Section: perinatal risks. Midwives Information and Resource Service Midwifery Digest 1992;3:313-5.

Hillan EM. Issues in the delivery of midwifery care. Journal of Advanced Nursing 1992;1:274-8.

Hillan EM. Maternal-infant attachment following Caesarean delivery. Journal of Clinical Nursing 1992;1:33-7.

Hillan EM. Caesareans - a cause for concern? Johnson and Johnson Digest Number 3, 1994 (in press).

183. MIDWIVES' PERSONAL EXPERIENCE OF BREASTFEEDING
September 1988 - September 1989

Sally C McMulkin, Senior Midwife Tutor, Rosaleen Malone, Midwife Teacher. **Contact:** Sally C McMulkin, c/o National Board for Nursing,, Midwifery and Health Visitors, c/o Directorate of Estate Services, Stoney Road, Dundonald Belfast BT16 OUS. Tel: 0232 523877

2 hours/week of own time spent. Funded by National Board for Nursing, Midwifery & Health Visiting.

Aims of the study: To determine whether midwives' professional knowledge and experience enhanced their personal experience of breastfeeding.

Ethics committee approval gained: No.

Research design: Descriptive – Qualitative and Quantitative – Survey

> **Data collection:**
> > **Techniques used:**
> > > Questionnaire.
> > **Time data were collected:**
> > > During statutory Refresher Courses and in-service study days during the period September 1988 to September 1989.
> > **Testing of any tools used:**
> > > Questionnaire piloted.
> > **Topics covered:**
> > > Breastfeeding.
> > > Professional knowledge.
> > **Setting for data collection:**
> > > Hospital and community.
>
> **Details about sample studied:**
> > **Planned size of sample:**
> > > 214
> > **Rationale for planned size:**
> > > Available number presenting.
> > **Entry criteria:**
> > > Midwives who had personally breastfed a baby.

Sample selection:
Convenience
Actual sample size:
210
Response rate:
100%

Intervention, Outcome and Analysis:
Analysis:
SPSSx
Chi-square
Pearson
Continuity correction
Likelihood ratio
Mantel-Haenszel
Fishers Exact Test 1 tailed and 2 tailed

Results: Data obtained supported the positive correlation of theory to practice translated into the personal experience of the practising midwife. Midwives who wish to feed their own babies require as much support and reassurance as any newly delivered mother. There is evidence that the most supportive person for those midwives who successfully breastfed was the midwife practising in hospital.

Recommendations for further research: Replication study with much larger sample. It would be interesting to undertake a separate study to ascertain midwives' knowledge of the physiology of lactation and its application in practice in comparison to research data in this area from the United States.

Keywords: BREASTFEEDING, BREASTFEEDING (PERSONAL EXPERIENCE), BREASTFEEDING (STAFF KNOWLEDGE), BREASTFEEDING (SUPPORT), EXPERIENCE (MIDWIVES'), MIDWIFERY PROCEDURES (INFLUENCES)

McMulkin S, Malone R. Midwives' personal experience of breastfeeding. Proceedings of 23rd International Confederation of Midwives 1993:1271-84.

184. IRON SUPPLEMENTATION DURING PREGNANCY
September 1989 - May 1990
P Graham, Community Midwife, Z McNeill, Community Midwife, A Allen, Community Midwife, P Lewis, Community Midwife, H Bell, Community Midwife, M McGroggan, Community Midwife. **Contact:** P Graham, Leighinmohr Avenue, Ballymena, Co Antrim, Northern Ireland BT42 2AR.

Formed part of a course. Funded by employer: Northern Health and Social Services Board.

Aims of the study: To explore the need for routine iron supplementation in pregnancy, treatment compliance, and factors which influence compliance.

Ethics committee approval gained: No

Research design: Descriptive – Qualitative and Quantitative – Simple Descriptive Study

> **Data collection:**
> > **Techniques used:**
> > > Semi-structured interview.
> > > Case note review.
> > **Time data were collected:**
> > > September 1989 to December 1990.
> > **Testing of any tools used:**
> > > Piloted with 5 community midwives.
> > **Topics covered:**
> > > Treatment compliance.
> > > Factors which influence compliance.
> > > Haemoglobin levels.
> > > Side effects of iron supplementation.
> > **Setting for data collection:**
> > > Community.

> **Details about sample studied:**
> > **Planned size of sample:**
> > > Maximum obtainable during study period.
> > **Rationale for planned size:**
> > > Total population.
> > **Entry criteria:**
> > > Mothers who delivered live, full term infants.
> > > No medical complications up to and including third postnatal day.
> > **Sample selection:**
> > > Random.
> > **Actual sample size:**
> > > 110 mothers (retrospective study).
> > **Response rate:**
> > > 100%.

> **Intervention, Outcome and Analysis:**
> > **Analysis:**
> > > Chi-square test.
> > > SPSSx

Results: A greater compliance rate and toleration were found in those women who were prescribed iron for a specific reason than in those who were routinely advised to supplement their intake. Recommendations were made that antenatal policy should be modified to determine actual need for iron therapy rather than recommending iron for all pregnant women.

Recommendations for further research: Development of more accurate predictors of anaemia.

Keywords: COMPLIANCE, IRON, IRON SUPPLEMENTS, PREGNANCY, ROUTINES

185. TO EXAMINE THE USE OF CHLORHEXIDINE ACETATE AS A SWABBING LOTION ON LABOURING WOMEN
April 1992 - March 1994
Sheelagh Calkin, Research Midwife. **Contact:** Sheelagh Calkin, Labour Ward, Crawley Hospital, West Green Drive, Crawley, W Sussex RH11 7DH. Tel: 0293 527866 Blp 134

Funded as integral part of job by employer: Crawley Hospital, and by LORS, South West Thames Regional Health Authority.

Aims of the study: To investigate whether women in labour need to be swabbed with an antiseptic solution.

Ethics committee approval gained: Yes

Research design: Experimental – Quantitative – Randomized Controlled Trial

Data collection:
Techniques used:
Bacteriological swabbing - vagina and ear.
Questionnaires.
Records of observations.
Time data were collected:
Bacteriological swabs - 3rd postnatal day.
Questionnaires - within 10 days.
Testing of any tools used:
Pilot study February - April 1992.
Topics covered:
Bacterial colonisation.
Comfort of mother.
Details of labour.
Perineal healing.
Setting for data collection:
Hospital Community Mostly urban

Details about sample studied:
Planned size of sample:
3000 women.
Rationale for planned size:
Low perinatal infection rate.
Entry criteria:
Exclusion:
Women booked for an elective Caesarean Section.
Inability to read English.
Prolonged rupture of membranes.
Preterm labour.

Sample selection:
> Interviewed at 36 weeks to obtain consent.
> Randomly allocated to one of two groups - chlorhexidine acetate or tap water.

Actual sample size:
> Recruitment ongoing.

Intervention, Outcome and Analysis:
Interventions used:
> Women were swabbed with chlorhexidine acetate or tap water.

Main outcomes measured:
> Bacteriological assays.
> Comfort of women.
> Perineal healing.

Analysis:
> Not yet decided.

Keywords: CHLORHEXIDINE, LABOUR, POSTNATAL INFECTION, SWABBING, TAP WATER, VAGINAL EXAMINATIONS

186. A STUDY OF THE CURRENT PRACTICE OF USING THE NON-STRESS CARDIOTOCOGRAPH
December 1990 - March 1991

Helen Rowe, Midwifery Sister/Research development. **Contact:** Helen Rowe, Warrington Hospital NHS Trust, Lovely Lane, Warrington WA5 1QG. Tel: 0925 35911 Ex 2344

Funded as integral or additional part of a job by employer.

Aims of the study: To raise research awareness at a local level.
To determine the clinical value of the non-stress cardiotocograph.

Ethics committee approval gained: No

Research design: Descriptive – Qualitative and Quantitative – Simple Descriptive Study

Data collection:
Techniques used:
> Demographic data recorded on special proforma.

Time data were collected:
> December 1990 to March 1991.

Testing of any tools used:
> Not necessary.

Topics covered:
> Demographic data.
> Indication for CTG.
> Duration and outcome of (labour) CTG.

Setting for data collection:
Maternity unit (consultant).

Details about sample studied:
Planned size of sample:
All women during the planned time period who had CTGs performed.
Rationale for planned size:
Convenience.
Entry criteria:
All antenatal women who had a CTG.
Sample selection:
Convenience.
Actual sample size:
517 women having a total of 1236 CTGs.

Interventions, Outcomes and Analysis:
Analysis:
Manual using index cards. Simple descriptive statistics only.

Results: Indications for CTG were pregnancy induced hypertension/pre-eclampsia 19.6%, decreased fetal movements 16.3%, intra uterine growth retardation 15.7%, early labour 11.0%, spontaneous rupture of membranes 6.3% and miscellaneous reasons 25.4%. A small number of women with intra uterine growth retardation received serial CTGs. There was a dramatic fall in routine CTGs over the study period from 9.7% in the first month to 2.1% in final month, with a mean of 5.7%.

It was concluded that many CTGs were performed for unclear reasons and to be seen to be doing something. In some cases midwives are conducting CTGs against their own clinical judgement. Recommendations are made to engage in discussion with medical colleagues around this topic.

A high number (16.3%) of CTGs were performed for decreased fetal movements - this was considered an unacceptably high rate. Following discussions with medical colleagues the routine use of fetal activity charts was discontinued in line with current research evidence. Targeting of special groups is now undertaken.

Recommendations for further research: A repeat study would be beneficial to assess whether this change has affected the antenatal CTG rate for decreased fetal movements, as well as investigating trends in rates of routine CTGs.

Keywords: CARDIOTOCOGRAPHY, CLINICAL JUDGEMENT, MIDWIFE'S ROLE, NON-STRESS TESTS, PREGNANCY

187. ARMY WIVES IN NORTHERN IRELAND AND THEIR SOURCES OF HELP AND SUPPORT POSTNATALLY
September 1991 - April 1992
D Daly, Staff Midwife. **Contact:** D Daly, Movilla Road, Downpatrick, Co. Down BT30 6JW.

Formed part of a course. 6-12 hours/week of own time spent.

Aims of the study: To describe the attitudes and feelings of a group of wives of military personnel towards motherhood. To explore their perceptions of help and support in the postnatal period.

Ethics committee approval gained: Yes

Research design: Descriptive – Qualitative – Ethnography/Phenomenology

    Data collection:
        Techniques used:
            Semi-structured interviews.
            Case note review.
        Time data were collected:
            Day 2 and day 14 following delivery.
        Testing of any tools used:
            None.
        Topics covered:
            Perceptions of sources of help and support postnatally.
            Impact of army life.
            Perceptions of husband's role.
        Setting for data collection:
            Hospital and community.

    Details about sample studied:
        Planned size of sample:
            5 women.
        Rationale for planned size:
            Availability of respondents. Time factor.
        Entry criteria:
            Wives of army personnel.
        Sample selection:
            Convenience.
         Actual sample size:
            3 women.
        Response rate:
            100%

Interventions, Outcomes and Analysis:
   Analysis:
      Content analysis.

Results: Army life was perceived as having a clearly defined social structure with the army first priority in the husband's life. The mothers all described a feeling of uncertainty relating to their husband's ability to be with them during labour and the necessity for contingency plans to be made. There was a feeling of awkwardness in hospital when they mixed with non-military wives. All experienced tiredness postnatally related to their need to cope alone and the repetitive tasks following transfer home.

All the women perceived their husbands as helpful in the home and with the baby. The nature of help was varied but the most important element was having him around. During his absence, arrangements were made with mothers and mothers-in-law. Friendships were regarded as superficial.

When problems arose professionals were the main source of help. Concerns frequently related to security although services in hospital were perceived as flexible. It is recommended that military wives may require additional support particularly where husbands are away from home.

Recommendations for further research: A study conducted over a longer period of time with a larger group of women in order to elicit perceptions of support and help when midwifery care had ceased for some time.

Keywords: ADAPTATION TO MOTHERHOOD, ARMY WIVES, EXPERIENCE (WOMEN'S), LABOUR, POSTNATAL SUPPORT, PREGNANCY, PUERPERIUM, SOCIAL SUPPORT

188. MIDWIFE MANAGED DELIVERY UNIT: A CLINICAL, SOCIAL AND ECONOMIC EVALUATION
December 1991 - December 1993
Fiona M Cruickshank, Research Sister, Labour Ward, Gordon D Lang, Consultant Obstetrician, Joan M Milne, Clinical Midwifery Manager, Dana Blyth, Research Assistant, Moira Turner, Project Assistant, Vanora Hundley, Research Fellow, Charis Glazener, Wellcome Research Fellow. **Contact:** Vanora Hundley, Aberdeen Maternity Hospital, Cornhill Road, Aberdeen AB9 2ZA. Tel: 0224 681818 Ex 53875

Funded as integral or additional part of a job and by funding agency: Scottish Office Home and Health Department.

Aims of the study: To evaluate whether there are differences between delivering in a midwife managed unit and a consultant supervised labour ward which have implications for the future planning of obstetric services.

Ethics committee approval gained: Yes

Research design: Experimental – Qualitative and Quantitative – Randomized Controlled Trial

Data collection:
    Techniques used:
        Questionnaires.
        Interviews.
        Case note review.
    Time data were collected:
        Mothers' questionnaires (on discharge from hospital).
        Interviews (postnatally).
        Midwives' questionnaires (following delivery).
    Testing of any tools used:
        Questionnaires piloted.
    Topics covered:
        Women's satisfaction.
        Demographic, delivery and obstetric data.
        Staff satisfaction.
        Costing.
    Setting for data collection:
        Hospital.

Details about sample studied:
    Planned size of sample:
        2700
    Rationale for planned size:
        Based on statistical advice and power calculations.
    Entry criteria:
        Inclusion:
        Women booking for antenatal care at Aberdeen Maternity Hospital.
        Assessed as low risk on set criteria.
        Exclusion:
        1. Pre-existing maternal disease eg, hypertension, severe renal disease, epilepsy, diabetes mellitus, thyroid disease and rhesus Iso immunisation.
        2. Past adverse obstetric history - eg previous Caesarian Section, intrauterine growth retardation (<5th centile), eclampsia or severe pre-eclampsia, primary post partum haemorrhage or previous poor obstetric outcome.
        3. Primigravidae <150cms tall.
        4. Pregnancies resulting from in vitro fertilisation.
        5. Maternal age over 35 years.
    Sample selection:
        Randomly allocated to midwives unit or labour ward.
    Actual sample size:
        3451 eligible, 2844 agreed to participate.

Response rate:
95% of 2844

Interventions, Outcomes and Analysis:
Interventions used:
Random allocation to midwives unit or labour ward.
Main outcomes measured:
Maternal satisfaction.
Staff satisfaction.
Obstetric and neonatal outcomes - maternal and perinatal morbidity/mortality.
Comparison of relative costs of care.
Analysis:
SPSS

Keywords: CONSULTANTS, CONSUMER SATISFACTION, EXPERIENCE (WOMEN'S), LABOUR, MATERNAL OUTCOMES, MIDWIFE MANAGED DELIVERY UNIT, MIDWIFERY MANAGED CARE, OUTCOMES (PERINATAL)

189. A SURVEY OF SYSTEMS OF MIDWIFERY CARE IN SCOTLAND
November 1990 - October 1991
Tricia Murphy-Black, Research Fellow. **Contact:** Tricia Murphy-Black, Research and Development Adviser, Simpson Memorial Maternity Pavilion, Lauriston Place, Edinburgh EH3 9EF. Tel: 031 229 2477 Ex 4357
For full details see under Management Studies (Record No. 189).

190. MIDWIVES' OCCUPATIONAL EXPOSURE TO NITROUS OXIDE
April 1992 - May 1992
C Newton, Midwife. **Contact:** C Newton, May Lodge Drive, Rufford Abbey Park, Newark NG21 9DE.

Funded as integral or additional part of a job by employer. 2-6 hours/week of own time spent.

Aims of the study: To investigate the levels of nitrous oxide to which midwives are occupationally exposed.

Ethics committee approval gained: Yes

Research design: Descriptive – Qualitative and Quantitative – Action Research

Data collection:
Techniques used:
Records of nitrous oxide exposure.
Diffusers.

Time data were collected:
> During midwives' working hours on labour ward, while attending women using nitrous oxide over a 7 hour period.

Topics covered:
> Levels of occupational exposure to nitrous oxide.

Setting for data collection:
> Labour ward in hospital.

Details about sample studied:
> **Planned size of sample:**
>> 15
>
> **Rationale for planned size:**
>> Financial and time restrictions.
>
> **Entry criteria:**
>> All midwives working on labour ward during the data collection period.
>
> **Sample selection:**
>> Inclusive.
>
> **Actual sample size:**
>> 15
>
> **Response rate:**
>> 100%

Interventions, Outcomes and Analysis:
> **Analysis:**
>> Diffusers sent from Nottingham to Burnley for analysis.

Results: It was demonstrated that whilst working on labour suite midwives are at times exposed to unacceptable levels of nitrous oxide.

Recommendations for further research: Further research is urgently needed to evaluate the effects of such exposure.

Keywords: MIDWIVES, NITROUS OXIDE, OCCUPATIONAL HEALTH

Newton C. Hazards of N_2O exposure. Nursing Times 1992;88:50.

192. PSYCHOSOCIAL FACTORS INFLUENCING TEENAGE SEXUAL ACTIVITY AND USE OF CONTRACEPTION
June - December 1992
Vivien Woodward, Midwife Teacher. **Contact:** Vivien Woodward, Midwifery Education Department, Rosie Maternity Hospital, Robinson Way, Cambridge CB2 2SW. Tel: 0223 217692

Formed part of a course. 12-20 hours/week of own time spent. Funded by employer.

Aims of the study: To compare teenagers who become unintentionally pregnant and

teenagers who have never been pregnant but who are attending a family planning clinic for contraception on:-
1. family or partner stability.
2. communication with a parent or stable sexual partner about sexual matters.
3. levels of self esteem.

Ethics committee approval gained: Yes

Research design: Descriptive – Qualitative and Quantitative – Case Study/Comparison of two groups.

Data collection:
Techniques used:
Anonymous self-completed questionnaires.
Rosenbergs self-esteem scale.
Time data were collected:
During clinic session.
Testing of any tools used:
Small pilot study (5 subjects) from each group.
Topics covered:
Teenagers' living arrangements.
Details of school, employment and academic achievements.
Self-esteem.
Communication with others about sex related issues.
Details of menarche, sexual history, use of contraception and associated problems.
Contact with family doctor/Family Planning Clinic.
Setting for data collection:
Community based Family Planning Clinic.
Antenatal and gynaecology clinics in a hospital.

Details about sample studied:
Planned size of sample:
3 groups of 30 (90 in total)
Rationale for planned size:
Time factor.
Appropriate for planned statistical analysis.
Entry criteria:
Exclusion:
Over 19 years of age.
Married at time of conception.
Planned pregnancy.
Previous unplanned pregnancy (FP clinic only).
Sample selection:
Convenience and opportunistic.
Actual sample size:
77 questionnaires issued.

Response rate:
92%
Antenatal clinic - 30
Family planning clinic - 31
Gynaecology clinic - 10

Interventions, Outcomes and Analysis:
Analysis:
SPSS.
Frequencies.
Mann Whitney U test (2 tailed) using 0.05 level of significance.
Chi-square test (Yates continuity correction with small numbers).
Pearson coefficient of correlation.

Results: The two groups were matched for age, ethnic group and academic achievement. Self-esteem scores were similarly matched preventing further analysis.

Teenagers attending the antenatal clinic (ANC) had longer term relationships with their boyfriends (P=0.02) and were more likely to be cohabiting (P=0.0008) than teenagers in Family Planning Clinics (FPC) who were more likely to be living with parents. Levels of unemployment were significantly higher in the ANC group (P=0.00001). Few significant differences between the groups emerged in relation to communication with either parents or a stable partner generally. However, teenagers attending ANC sought information about sexual matters more from mothers than the FPC group (P=0.03) who preferred books (P=0.02). ANC teenagers preferred to discuss personal feelings with boyfriends (P=0.05) and the FPC teenagers discussed personal rules and values with peers (P=0.04).

Recommendations for further research: Investigation into the perception that teenagers have of their relationship with parents and its effect on teenage pregnancy rates.

How teenagers' perception of women's role in society, either traditional or "modern" is influenced by their main source of information and possible effects on contraceptive behaviour and attitudes towards pregnancy.

Keywords: ADOLESCENTS, CONTRACEPTION, PREGNANCY, SELF ESTEEM, SEXUAL ACTIVITY

193. CONFLICTING ADVICE ON BREASTFEEDING. WHAT ARE WE SAYING NOW?
December 1988 - September 1989
S J Tarry, Midwifery Sister, E Collins, Midwifery Sister, S Green, Staff Midwife, J Harvey, Staff Midwife, A Jarman, Staff Midwife. **Contact:** S J Tarry, Quarry Park Road, Exeter EX2 5PB.

6-12 hours/week of own time spent. Funded by employer and by funding agency(ies): Staff Enterprise Fund, Elizabeth Clark Trust.

Aims of the study: To determine whether conflicting advice is given to breastfeeding mothers and to investigate the need for updating of current guidelines and policies.

Ethics committee approval gained: Yes

Research design: Descriptive – Qualitative – Ethnography

Data collection:
> **Techniques used:**
>> Structured questionnaire.
>> Analysis of records.
>> Diaries.
>
> **Time data were collected:**
>> Questionnaires - March 1989.
>> Diaries - during first ten days of breastfeeding.
>
> **Testing of any tools used:**
>> 10% pilot study of questionnaire.
>
> **Topics covered:**
>> Breastfeeding.
>> Advice - conflicting.
>> Weight of baby.
>> Additional fluids.
>
> **Setting for data collection:**
>> Consultant unit and 4 satellite GP units and community.

Details about sample studied:
> **Planned size of sample:**
>> 175 midwives, student midwives and nursery nurses.
>> 10 women.
>
> **Rationale for planned size:**
>> Staff: All those working in Exeter Health Authority.
>> Mothers: 10 women asked to complete diaries to give additional information.
>> Feed charts - all charts for 1 month.
>
> **Entry criteria:**
>> Questionnaires - all staff.
>> Diaries - women from a parentcraft class being run by one of the research team.
>> - intending to breastfeed
>> - first time mothers
>> Feed charts - all those kept in Exeter Maternity Unit for month of January 1989.
>
> **Sample selection:**
>> Staff - inclusive.
>> Diaries - willing participants.
>> Feed charts - all kept for 1 month.
>
> **Actual sample size:**
>> 175 questionnaires.
>> 10 diaries.

Response rate:
Questionnaires - 68%
Diaries - 60%
Interventions, Outcomes and Analysis:
Analysis:
Simple statistics.

Results: Additional fluids - 29% of staff thought that artifical feeds should be used when mothers had "milk insufficiency". According to the feed charts in January 1989, 48% of babies received complementary feeds of water, dextrose or formula feeds though nearly half of these were on one occasion only.

Baby's weight - Fluctuations of 150-180g daily were considered important by the majority of the staff. Where there was loss of just over 10% of birth weight by day 3, 10% of respondents would give top ups of formula feed.

Initial feed - 67% of staff indicated that the initial breastfeed should take place immediately after delivery or within the first hour. The remainder would allow up to 12 hours post delivery. 94% thought the timing of the first feed important.

Recommendations for further research: Further work is needed to clarify the issues raised by this research.

Keywords: BREASTFEEDING, BREASTFEEDING (ATTITUDES OF STAFF), BREASTFEEDING (INFORMATION), BREASTFEEDING (STAFF KNOWLEDGE), BREASTFEEDING (SUPPORT), CONFLICTING ADVICE (FEEDING), PUERPERIUM

195. CHARACTERISATION OF LONG-TERM POSTPARTUM HEALTH PROBLEMS
May 1992 - December 1993
E G Knox, Professor of Epidemiology (Retired), Christine MacArthur, Senior Research Fellow, Margo Lewis, Consultant Anaesthetist, Debra Bick, Research Midwife. **Contact:** Debra Bick, Department of Public Health and Epidemiology, Medical School, University of Birmingham, Edgbaston, Birmingham B15 2TT. Tel: 021 414 6772

Funded as integral part of a job by funding agency: Department of Health.

Aims of the study: To ascertain the nature and severity of long-term health problems ocurring after childbirth.

Ethics committee approval gained: Yes

Research design: Descriptive – Qualitative and Quantitative – Survey

Data collection:
Techniques used:
1. Postal questionnaire - whole group.
2. Midwife interview - all symptomatic women and 20% sample of non-symptomatic.
3. Obstetric case note review.

Time data were collected:
Postal questionnaire - 6-7 months postpartum.
Interview - 8-12 months postpartum.

Testing of any tools used:
Pilot study carried out in June 1992. 52 women were sent a questionnaire, 34 responded (65.4%) and 10 women were interviewed.

Topics covered:
Long term health problems - symptoms and severity. Quality of life - including potential symptom triggers.
Social and obstetric factors.
Opinions on postnatal care.

Setting for data collection:
Community.

Details about sample studied:
Planned size of sample:
1500 women.

Rationale for planned size:
Large enough to give data on less common symptoms and to take account of inter-related factors.

Entry criteria:
Inclusion: Women who delivered at Birmingham Maternity Hospital.
Exclusion: Perinatal deaths.
Asian women.

Sample selection:
All women delivering at the Birmingham Maternity Hospital.

Actual sample size:
1,606

Response rate:
79.6%

Interventions, Outcomes and Analysis:
Analysis:
Multi-variate discriminant analysis.
Multi-way tabulation.
Content analysis.

Results: Not yet available.

Keywords: EPIDURALS, LONG TERM OUTCOME, POSTNATAL HEALTH, PUERPERIUM

196. THE FIRST MONTH OF MOTHERHOOD
March - September 1991
L Cowan, Team Midwife. **Contact:** L Cowan, Church Street, Watlington, Oxfordshire OX9 5QR.

Formed part of a course.

Aims of the study: To explore the experience of the postnatal period for primiparous women in the East End of Glasgow.

Ethics committee approval gained: Yes

Research design: Descriptive – Qualitative – Ethnography

Data collection:
Techniques used:
Review of routine data.
Questionnaire to mothers.
Semi-structured interviews.
Time data were collected:
Questionnaires - 9th postnatal day.
Interviews - on or around the 28th postnatal day.
Testing of any tools used:
Interview guide tested on friends with babies and in two pilot interviews.
Topics covered:
Change in the mother - physical, emotional and social.
Social support.
Maternity services.
Setting for data collection:
Community - urban.

Details about sample studied:
Planned size of sample:
20 for qualitative interviews
Rationale for planned size:
To allow comparison with other comparable studies.
Time factor.
Entry criteria:
Candidates for a larger study being conducted concurrently.
Primiparous women.
Vaginal delivery.
Baby not in SCBU for more than 24 hours.
Sample selection:
Convenience.
Actual sample size:
29 women.

Response rate:
69%

Interventions, Outcomes and Analysis:
   Analysis:
      Content analysis.
      Categorisation of themes.
      Simple frequencies.

Results: Perineal pain was the most frequently mentioned physical change and was sometimes severe. It was linked to episiotomy and forceps delivery. Emotional change was dominated by anxiety and the "baby blues" although improved mood was also reported. Social changes were generally positive and many reported improved relationships with partners and mothers. The quality of relationships was not influenced by marriage as distinct from co-habitation. Excellent lay support was widely available. Maternity services were generally well regarded but confusion existed regarding the function of different health professionals. Continuity of care was appreciated by women but was often poor from midwives. Care tended to conform to the "medical" model.

Recommendations include improved preparation towards realistic expectations of the postpartum period. Improvement in continuity of care and a move towards a natural model incorporating principles from stress and coping theory is advocated.

Recommendations for further research: More exploration of the "normal" experience of early motherhood.

Keywords: ADAPTATION TO MOTHERHOOD, CONSUMER SATISFACTION, EXPERIENCE (WOMEN'S), MATERNITY SERVICES, PERINEAL PAIN, POSTNATAL SUPPORT, PUERPERIUM

197. NON-ASIAN PREGNANCY HOME VISITING PROJECT
January 1992 - December 1993
Judy Dance, Research Nurse, Carol Hoare, Linkworker, Sharon Fuery, Linkworker, Rosemary Osborne, Clerical Assistant. **Contact:** Judy Dance, Room 06 : Community Offices, Yardley Green Unit, East Birmingham Hospital, Yardley Green Road, Birmingham B9 5PX. Tel: 021 766 6611 Ex 2306

Funded as integral or additional part of a job by employer.

Aims of the study: To test the hypothesis that women who receive additional health education and social support from a linkworker will have better pregnancy outcomes than women who receive routine antenatal care.

Ethics committee approval gained: Yes

Research design: Experimental – Quantitative – Randomized Controlled Trial

Data collection:
    Techniques used:
        Interviews.
        Questionnaires.
        Case note review.
    Time data were collected:
        Antenatally at 'booking clinic' in hospital.
        Postnatally 6/52.
    Testing of any tools used:
        Questionnaires and interview schedules tested on 10 people.
    Topics covered:
        Obstetric outcomes
        Problems
        Support
        Analgesia
        Delivery
        Type of feeding
        Source and type of information received
        Smoking
        Postnatal examination.
    Setting for data collection:
        Hospital 'booking clinic'.
        Participants' homes.

Details about sample studied:
    Planned size of sample:
        400 women - 200 experimental, 200 controls
    Rationale for planned size:
        Statistical calculation.
    Entry criteria:
        1. Non-Asian primigravidae.
        2. Non-Asian pregnant women with a previous history of a low birthweight baby or perinatal death not associated with:
        i) a multiple birth,
        ii) an elective Caesarean Section,
        iii) a gross congenital abnormality.
        3. All recruited women booking not later than 24 weeks gestation.
    Sample selection:
        Random.
    Actual sample size:
        Recruitment ongoing.

Interventions, Outcomes and Analysis:
    Interventions used:
        In addition to routine antenatal care, a minimum of 3 home visits from a Caucasian linkworker whose role is to provide basic health education/information and social support.

Main outcomes measured:
> Pregnancy outcomes, birthweight/gestation, delivery, analgesia, problems (mother/infant), feeding, uptake of postnatal examination, knowledge obtained, mothers' opinions on care received and shortfalls.

Analysis:
> SPSSx

Keywords: ANTENATAL CARE, HOME CARE, LINKWORKERS, LOW BIRTHWEIGHT, PREGNANCY, SOCIAL SUPPORT

198. HEALTH BEHAVIOUR IN PREGNANCY: ROLES AND RESPONSIBILITIES IN ANTENATAL CARE

August 1990 - August 1993

Pamela Foley, Research Midwife. **Contact:** Pamela Foley, Antenatal Clinic, Maternity Unit, Bradford Royal Infirmary, Bradford, West Yorkshire BD9 6RJ. Tel: 0274 542200 Ex 4511

Funded as integral or additional part of a job partially by employer: Bradford NHS Hospitals Trust. Formed part of a course. 6-12 hours/week of own time spent.

Aims of the study: An investigation of altered health behaviour in pregnancy: influencing factors; roles and responsibilities of pregnant women and health professionals; and the ethical issues.

Ethics committee approval gained: Yes

Research design: Descriptive – Qualitative and Quantitative – Ethnography

Data collection:
> **Techniques used:**
>> Interviews.
>> Historical review of Bradford archives.
>
> **Time data were collected:**
>> 1990 - 1993.
>
> **Testing of any tools used:**
>> Details to be confirmed.
>
> **Topics covered:**
>> Health behaviour.
>> Influencing factors.
>> Roles and responsibilities of health professionals.
>> Ethical issues.
>
> **Setting for data collection:**
>> Hospital and community.

Details about sample studied:
   Planned size of sample:
      150 pregnant women.
      40 health professionals.
   Rationale for planned size:
      Time constraints.
   Entry criteria:
      Pregnant women at 36/37 weeks gestation.
      Health professionals working in antenatal care in Bradford.
   Sample selection:
      Random.
   Actual sample size:
      160 pregnant women.
      36 health professionals.
   Response rate:
      Details to be confirmed.

Interventions, Outcomes and Analysis:
   Analysis:
      SPSS - PC

Results: Not yet available.

Keywords: ANTENATAL CARE, ANTENATAL EDUCATION, HEALTH BEHAVIOUR, HEALTH BELIEFS, HEALTH PROMOTION, MIDWIFE'S ROLE, PREGNANCY

199. IPSWICH CHILDBIRTH STUDY
May 1992 - October 1994
C Mackrodt, Research Midwife, B S Gordon, Midwifery Clinical Specialist, E Fern, Head of Midwifery, S Ayers, Computer Programmer, A Grant, Epidemiologist. **Contact:** B S Gordon, Colchester Road, Ipswich, Suffolk IP4 3BT.

Funded as integral or additional part of a job and by funding agency: National Birthday Trust; Directorate of Public Health Medicine; Locally Organised Research Scheme.

Aims of the study: 1. To compare the differences in pain, comfort and healing between suturing the perineum using the standard 3 layer approach and using a 2 layer approach leaving the skin edges apposed and unsutured.
2. To compare pain, comfort and healing rates between perineal repairs using chromic catgut and polygalactin 210 (vicryl) for suturing.

Ethics committee approval gained: Yes

Research design: Experimental – Qualitative and Quantitative – Randomized Controlled Trial

Data collection:
    Techniques used:
        Questionnaires.
        Records of observations.
    Time data were collected:
        Postnatally:
        - 24-48 hours;
        - 10-14 days;
        - 2-3 months.
    Testing of any tools used:
        Tested on a small number of women.
    Topics covered:
        Pain.
        Healing.
        Comfort.
    Setting for data collection:
        Hospital and community.

Details about sample studied:
    Planned size of sample:
        1500 women.
    Rationale for planned size:
        Statistically calculated.
    Entry criteria:
        Inclusion: Normal deliveries.
        1st and 2nd degree tears or episiotomies.
        Exclusion: 3 degree tears.
        Lacerations which do not involve perineal skin.
    Sample selection:
        Randomised to trial groups.
    Actual sample size:
        Recruitment ongoing

Interventions, Outcomes and Analysis:
    Interventions used:
        1. One group to have 2 layer approach to perineal repair leaving skin edges apposed and unsutured.
        2. One group to have perineal repair using polygalactin 210 (vicryl) for suturing.
    Main outcomes measured:
        Pain.
        Healing.
        Comfort.
        Resumption of sexual intercourse and degree of dyspareunia.
        General well being.

NB. Tandem study for those women having 'simple' instrumental deliveries, started June 1993.
Sample size 200-300.
Separately randomised.

Keywords: PERINEAL HEALING, PERINEAL PAIN, PERINEAL REPAIR, PERINEUM, PUERPERIUM, SUTURES, SUTURING

200. ASSESSMENT OF ANALGESIC AND LAXATIVE USE ON TWO POSTNATAL WARDS AT PRINCESS MARY MATERNITY HOSPITAL, NEWCASTLE UPON TYNE

March - September 1992

T Lind, Clinical Director of Obstetrics and Gynaecology, Catherine M Hall. **Contact:** Catherine M Hall, Pharmacy Department, Royal Victoria Infirmary, Queen Victoria Road, Newcastle Upon Tyne NE1 4LP. Tel: 091 232 5131 x24488

Funded as integral or additional part of a job by employer: District Health Authority. Formed part of a course. 6-12 hours/week of own time spent.

Aims of the study: To investigate prescribing of analgesics and laxatives on two postnatal wards.

Ethics committee approval gained: Yes

Research design: Descriptive – Qualitative and Quantitative – Case Study

Data collection:
Techniques used:
Pain measured on verbal-descriptor scale and visual analogue scale.
Interview.
Questionnaires to mothers.
Records by pharmacists.
Questionnaires to pharmacists in other hospitals.
Time data were collected:
Mothers: twice daily for duration of stay in hospital.
Pharmacist in study hospital - throughout study period.
Other pharmacists - one-off enquiry.
Testing of any tools used:
No formal tests of questionnaires were done.
Topics covered:
Pain including treatment and side effects of treatment.
Prescribing by doctors and midwives - including on discharge.
Use of topical agents.
The cost of medications prescribed.
Setting for data collection:
Hospital

Details about sample studied:
Planned size of sample:
100-150
Rationale for planned size:
Large enough sample to produce meaningful results. Feasible given time constraints.
Entry criteria:
Primigravidae.

Any women following Caesarean Section.
Sample selection:
All patients who met the entry criteria between Monday and Friday.
Actual sample size:
156; 148 questioned, 8 refused.

271 questionnaires to other pharmacists; 192 replied.
Response rate:
95% mothers.

78% pharmacists.

Interventions, Outcomes and Analysis:
Analysis:
Simple frequencies and content analysis.

Results: The study investigated analgesic and laxative prescribing at Princess Mary Maternity Hospital (PMMH) and other maternity units in the UK. 37% of units had an analgesic policy and 32% had a laxative policy. Paracetamol was frequently prescribed in 95% of departments. Lactulose was the most widely used laxative (77% of units).

148 patients, on two wards at PMMH, were questioned after a first baby by vaginal delivery or any Caesarean Section to determine the degree of postpartum pain experienced. 89% of vaginal deliveries and 95% of Caesarean Sections had suffered pain since delivery. Pain was described as moderate in 23% of vaginal deliveries and 37% of Section patients.

Co-codaprin and paracetamol were the most frequently prescribed analgesics. The most frequently reported adverse effect was constipation. 26% of patients taking co-codaprin complained of constipation compared with 10% of patients taking paracetamol. 32 laxative prescriptions were written during the study - 23 for lactulose and 11 for senna. Senna was recommended as the drug of choice for relief of postpartum constipation.

Elsewhere in maternity hospitals a wide range of analgesics are prescribed most of which are on a prn basis. The majority of hospitals prescribe lactulose; less than half of the hospitals use senna. Despite the fact that research has shown that Epifoam is of little value, many hospitals still use it regularly. There is clearly a role for clinical pharmacists to work with medical and midwifery staff to review their analgesic and laxative prescribing.

Keywords: CAESAREAN SECTION, LAXATIVES, PAIN ASSESSMENT, PAIN RELIEF (PRESCRIBING), PRESCRIBING PATTERNS, PUERPERIUM

202. A RANDOMISED TRIAL OF AMNIHOOK VERSUS AMNICOT FOR AMNIOTOMY IN LABOUR

January - June 1991

M Harris, Staff midwife, E Cooper, Labour Ward Sister. **Contact:** M Harris, Compass Drive, Plympton, Plymouth, Devon PL7 5DX.

Funded as integral or additional part of a job.

Aims of the study: To compare the efficacy, maternal acceptability and incidence of scalp trauma of amnicot and amnihook for ARM.

Ethics committee approval gained: Yes

Research design: Experimental – Quantitative – Randomized Controlled Trial

Data collection:
Techniques used:
Records of observations - scalp trauma.
Visual analogue scales.
Verbal analogue.
Time data were collected:
At time of ARM.
Scalp trauma: 24 hours after delivery.
Testing of any tools used:
Pilot study of 10 women.
Topics covered:
Obstetric data.
Operator ease.
Discomfort in women.
State of infant scalp.
Setting for data collection:
Hospital

Details about sample studied:
Planned size of sample:
100
Rationale for planned size:
Feasibility.
Entry criteria:
In established labour.
Cervix 3cms or more dilated.
Sample selection:
Convenience.
Actual sample size:
50 women in each group - it took 6 months to recruit 100 women. There were no refusals. (The midwives selected those they considered "suitable" thus this sample may represent cooperative, communicative women).

147

Response rate:
100%

Interventions, Outcomes and Analysis:
Interventions used:
Amnihook or amnicot used to rupture membranes in labour.
Main outcomes measured:
Ease of use of instrument by operator.
Maternal discomfort.
Scalp trauma.
Analysis:
Chi-square.
T-tests.
Mann-Whitney U test.
Confidence intervals using C/A package.

Results: There was a trend towards less patient discomfort in the amnicot group (NSS). Damage to the fetal scalp was significantly less in the amnicot group. When the cervix was posterior the amnicot was easier to use but small scratches to the fetal scalp were more likely. Where the cervix was anterior there was less discomfort and fewer scratches in the amnicot group.

Recommendations for further research: Further larger studies with adequate design and numbers are required using operators of varying experience to assess if findings can be extended into clinical practice.

Keywords: AMNICOT, AMNIHOOK, ARTIFICIAL RUPTURE OF THE MEMBRANES, EXPERIENCE (WOMEN'S), LABOUR

203. DOES ARTIFICIAL RUPTURE OF THE MEMBRANES IN SPONTANEOUS LABOUR AT TERM BENEFIT MOTHER AND/OR BABY?

October 1990 - March 1991

M Chesney, Midwife Teacher. **Contact:** M Chesney, Newhouse Close, Wardle, Rochdale, Lancs OL12 9LW.

Funded as integral or additional part of a job. Formed part of a course. 12-20 hours/ week of own time spent.

Aims of the study:
1. To examine the effects of artificial rupture of membranes (ARM).
2. To compare the effects of ARM with those of spontaneous rupture of membranes (SRM).
3. To determine whether there are benefits to mother and/or baby from ARM.

Ethics committee approval gained: No

Research design: Descriptive – Quantitative – Comparative Study from Case Notes

Data collection:
Techniques used:
Case note review.
Time data were collected:
1990-1991
Topics covered:
Length of labour.
Rupturing of membranes.
Hospital/community delivery.
Apgar scores.
Setting for data collection:
Hospital and community deliveries.

Details about sample studied:
Planned size of sample:
100 hospital and 100 home births.
Rationale for planned size:
Consecutive deliveries during data collection period.
Entry criteria:
Normal delivery.
No epidural.
No augmentation.
Not induced ie. no syntocinon.
Sample selection:
Convenience
Actual sample size:
100 normal deliveries in hospital.
100 normal deliveries in home.
Response rate:
100%

Interventions, Outcomes and Analysis:
Analysis:
Statistical package on computer.

Results: Mothers delivered in hospital who had an ARM had a mean length of labour of 8 hours 6 minutes. For those whose membranes ruptured spontaneously the mean was 8 hours. For those delivered at home the means were 6 hours 4 minutes and 5 hours 6 minutes respectively.

Fourteen babies born in hospital had an Apgar score of 7 or less one minute after birth. There were no differences in the SRM and ARM groups. Only one baby had an Apgar score of 7 or less in the home delivery group. It was concluded that the length of labour and condition of the baby at birth were not improved by carrying out an ARM.

Recommendations for further research: A large RCT is needed to test these findings.

Keywords: ARTIFICIAL RUPTURE OF THE MEMBRANES, EXPERIENCE (WOMEN'S), LABOUR, LABOUR (DURATION), OUTCOMES (MATERNAL), OUTCOMES (NEONATAL)

204. COMMUNITY MIDWIVES' VIEWS AND EXPERIENCES OF HOME BIRTH

November 1991 - October 1992

E Floyd, Midwifery Lecturer Practioner. **Contact:** E Floyd, Copt Hewick, Ripon, N Yorks HG4 5BY.

Formed part of a course. 6-12 hours/week of own time spent. Funded by employer and by Iolanthe Trust.

Aims of the study: To quantify and explore community midwives' experience of home births in order to identify factors which influence positive or negative feeling.

Ethics committee approval gained: No

Research design: Descriptive – Qualitative and Quantitative – Survey/Ethnography

Data collection:
> **Techniques used:**
>> Self-completion questionnaires.
>> In depth interviews with a stratified sub sample of the questionnaire subjects.
>> Critical incident technique.
> **Time data were collected:**
>> February to May 1992.
> **Testing of any tools used:**
>> Pilot study of questionnaire November 1991.
>> Pilot study of interview schedule December 1991.
> **Topics covered:**
>> a) Questionnaire:
>> demographic and career details,
>> length of time practising,
>> number of home deliveries,
>> experience of and willingness to book women for home birth.
>> b) Interview:
>> experience of home birth,
>> beliefs,
>> education and training experience.
> **Setting for data collection:**
>> 3 adjacent Health Authorities in West London.

Details about sample studied:
> **Planned size of sample:**
>> 56 community midwives.
>
> **Rationale for planned size:**
>> All community midwives in 3 health authorities.
>
> **Entry criteria:**
>> All full time community midwives practising in February 1992.
>
> **Sample selection:**
>> All in a geographical area.
>
> **Actual sample size:**
>> 56
>
> **Response rate:**
>> 78%

Interventions, Outcomes and Analysis:
> **Analysis:**
>> a) Quantitative data from questionnaire analysed by descriptive statistics and Chi-square testing.
>>
>> b) Qualitative data from one open question on questionnaire and interview transcripts analysed using manifest and latent content analysis techniques.

Results: The mean number of home births undertaken by this group of 44 midwives in the previous year (1991) was 2 although 14 (32%) had not undertaken any. The total number undertaken in these midwives' careers ranged from 0-131 and the average (median) number was only 6. 4 (9%) reported they had never undertaken a home birth.

Although 33 (77%) stated they were happy booking low risk women, half never offered women the choice. These factors were unrelated to the midwives' total home birth experience, their age, training or own motherhood. The qualitative data showed that half of the midwives were strongly positive about home birth and only 6 (15%) were strongly negative. Midwives' views were found to be influenced by the quality of their past home birth experiences, their perception of their role as midwives and of the role of women as well as by the support they perceived from colleagues, managers and doctors.

Recommendations for further research: Replication of study in other areas with a higher or very low home birth rate.
Women's experiences of home birth, their beliefs and expectations about place of birth to explore how women make choices.

Keywords: COMMUNITY MIDWIVES, EXPERIENCE (MIDWIVES'), HOME BIRTHS, MIDWIFE'S ROLE

205. BIRTH OUTCOMES IN BRADFORD PAKISTANIS: INFLUENCE OF SOCIOECONOMIC AND CULTURAL FACTORS AND IMPLICATIONS FOR HEALTH SERVICES
December 1991 - December 1993

Iain Smith, Project Manager, Health Care Needs Assessment, Sue Proctor, Research Midwife, Waqar Ahmad, Lecturer, Asian Studies, Alison Macfarlane, Medical Statistician, Gulshan Karbani, Genetic Counsellor (Leeds General Infirmary). **Contact:** Sue Proctor, Clinical Epidemiology Research Unit, New Mill, Victoria Road, Saltaire BD18 3LD. Tel: 0274 366128/366026

Funded as integral or additional part of a job and by locally organised research scheme.

Aims of the study: To establish the influence of consanguinity in relation to other personal and social factors on birth outcomes in Bradford Pakistani families.

Ethics committee approval gained: Yes

Research design: Descriptive – Qualitative and Quantitative – Case Control Cohort Study

> **Data collection:**
>> **Techniques used:**
>>> Case note review.
>>> Interviews.
>> **Time data were collected:**
>>> Interviews - Summer 1992 to 1993, during pregnancy.
>>> Case note review - November 1991 to August 1993, after delivery.
>> **Testing of any tools used:**
>>> Tested interview schedules on 5 women.
>> **Topics covered:**
>>> Interviews:
>>> demographic data,
>>> diet,
>>> access to services,
>>> history of consanguinity.
>>> Case note review:
>>> obstetric history,
>>> delivery details,
>>> anthropometric measures.
>> **Setting for data collection:**
>>> Case notes - in hospital.
>>> Interviews - conducted in community.

> **Details about sample studied:**
>> **Planned size of sample:**
>>> Case note review - about 4000 women.
>>> Interviews - 80-100

Rationale for planned size:

Statistician's advice.

Case notes - determined by number of deliveries to Pakistani women in Bradford over 2 year period.

Entry criteria:

Case notes:

- every Pakistani born/ethnic origin woman who is a Bradford resident at time of delivery.

- every third delivery to UK born/ethnic origin caucasian woman in each hospital's register.

Interviews:

- booked for care at Bradford Royal Infirmary.

- every Pakistani born/ethnic origin woman who is a Bradford resident at time of delivery.

- every third UK born/ethnic origin caucasian woman who is a Bradford resident at time of delivery.

Sample selection:

Interviews - first 5 women approached (from booking clinic appointments list) - every week.

Actual sample size:

Case notes to date - 4049 (complete database)

Interviews to date - 75

Interventions, Outcomes and Analysis:

Analysis:

SPSSx

SPSS PC

Keywords: CONSANGUINITY, ETHNIC GROUPS, MUSLIMS, OUTCOMES (NEONATAL), PAKISTANIS, PERINATAL MORTALITY

Proctor SR, Smith IJ. A reconsideration of the factors affecting birth outcome in Pakistani Muslim families in Britain. Midwifery 1992;8:76-81.

206. A RANDOMISED CONTROLLED TRIAL COMPARING VICRYL WITH BLACK SILK IN PERINEAL SKIN SUTURING FOLLOWING CHILDBIRTH

March - October 1992

Mark Roberts, Registrar, Christine Lumsdon, Clinical Midwife Manager, Doris Johnson, Clinical Midwife Specialist, Lesley Richardson, Midwifery Sister, Sally Coleman, Senior Staff Midwife. **Contact:** Doris Johnson, Maternity Unit, Leazes Wing, Royal Victoria Infirmary, Newcastle Upon Tyne NE1 4LP. Tel: 091 273 8811 Ex 22307

Funded as integral or additional part of a job by employer, and by Ethicon UK Ltd. 2 hours/week of own time spent.

Aims of the study: To test the hypothesis: subcuticular polyglactin 910 (vicryl) is associated with less short term pain and no greater long term morbidity than interrupted black silk, when used to repair perineal trauma following childbirth.

Ethics committee approval gained: Yes

Research design: Experimental – Quantitative – Randomized Controlled Trial

Data collection:

Techniques used:

Questionnaires

Time data were collected:

1. Immediately after repair of the perineum.
2. On day 5 postpartum.
3. 3 months postpartum.

Testing of any tools used:

This is pilot study.

Topics covered:

Demographic data,
gestation,
birthweight,
type of delivery,
grade of person suturing,
nature of perineal trauma,
details of repair,
pain.
Disability - problems with sexual intercourse, breast feeding, sitting, bowels and perineum.

Setting for data collection:

Hospital and community.

Details about sample studied:

Planned size of sample:

100 women (50 experimental, 50 control)

Rationale for planned size:

To enable long term follow up.

Entry criteria:

Inclusion:

Must have given consent for follow up.
All second degree perineal tears and episiotomies.
Must live in Newcastle.

Exclusion:

First and third degree tears or episiotomies.
Complicated repairs.
Operator unwillingness to use either method of repair.

Sample selection:

Random allocation at point of perineal repair.

Actual sample size:
100 women (50 experimental, 50 control)
Response rate:
91% at 5 days.
92% at 3 months.

Interventions, Outcomes and Analysis:
Interventions used:
Group A have perineal skin repaired with black silk W2524T (no 2/o) using interrupted "mattress" technique.
Group B have perineal skin repaired with 3/o coated vicryl (polyglactin 910) on a cutting needle.
Main outcomes measured:
Pain.
Disability - problems with sexual intercourse, sitting, bowels, breast feeding.
Complications with perineal healing.
Cosmetic result.
Analysis:
Computer Software: Excel for Windows (spread sheets), Minitab (data analysis). Statistical analysis - Chi-squared test.

Results: Confidential

Keywords: PERINEAL HEALING, PERINEUM, PUERPERIUM, SILK, SUTURE MATERIALS, SUTURING, VICRYL

208. MIDWIVES' PERCEPTIONS OF THEIR RELATIONSHIP WITH CLIENTS
April 1989 - October 1990
B H McCrea, Lecturer, Valerie Crute, Lecturer. **Contact:** B H McCrea, Department of Nursing & Health Visiting, University of Ulster, Cromore Road, Co Londonderry BT52 1SA. Tel: 0265 44141 Ex 4362

Funded as integral or additional part of a job by employer: Faculty Research Committee. 2-6 hours/week of own time spent.

Aims of the study: To examine midwives' understanding of the factors which affect the development of a therapeutic relationship with clients.

Ethics committee approval gained: Yes

Research design: Descriptive – Qualitative – Ethnography

Data collection:
Techniques used:
In depth interviews.

Time data were collected:
July to September 1989.
Testing of any tools used:
Pilot study of interview schedule with 5 practising midwives.
Topics covered:
Nature of clients.
Therapeutic and nontherapeutic relationships.
Needs and interests.
Conflicts.
Dilemmas and their resolutions.
Setting for data collection:
One maternity unit in a teaching hospital in urban area.

Details about sample studied:
Planned size of sample:
No set number of midwives were required.
Rationale for planned size:
Voluntary response was a key factor in the design.
Entry criteria:
Practising midwives.
Ward Sister/Staff midwife grades.
Volunteers.
Sample selection:
Volunteers recruited.
Actual sample size:
80 invited, 16 responded.
Response rate:
20%

Interventions, Outcomes and Analysis:
Analysis:
Content analysis. Dilemma analysis.

Results: A complex picture emerged of the factors which affect midwives' relationships with their clients. Four main issues were identified: the nature and value of the midwives' role; recognition of authority and autonomy in this role; emotional involvement with clients; and maintenance of personal integrity. When midwives were successful in managing these issues the relationship became therapeutic for the client. Mismanagement of these issues resulted in dilemmas which inhibited development of meaningful relationships. A recommendation was made for educational and organisational change and the provision of support services to facilitate effective management of the factors which affected interaction.

Keywords: CONFLICT, MIDWIFE-MOTHER RELATIONSHIP, NON-THERAPEUTIC RELATIONSHIP, THERAPEUTIC RELATIONSHIP

McCrea BH, Crute V. Midwife/client relationship: Midwives' perspectives. Midwifery 1991;7:183-92.
McCrea BH. Valuing the midwife's role in the midwife/client relationship. Journal of Clinical Nursing 1993;2:47-52.

209. EVALUATION OF A NEW PARENTHOOD PROGRAMME AVAILABLE FOR PRIMIGRAVIDAE
January 1993 - June 1994

Norma Aikman, Sister in Charge, Tricia Murphy-Black, Research Fellow. **Contact:** Norma Aikman, Parenthood Department, Simpson Memorial Maternity Pavilion, Lauriston Place, Edinburgh EH3 9EF. Tel: 031 229 2477 Ex 4411

2-6 hours/week of own time spent. Funded by employer: Health Board.

Aims of the study: To identify the outcome of changes to a parenthood programme. This programme involves active involvement of the clients in determining the content and the increased variety in teaching/learning methods used.

Ethics committee approval gained: Yes

Research design: Descriptive – Qualitative and Quantitative – Survey

Data collection:
Techniques used:
Self-completion questionnaires.
Time data were collected:
On completion of the Parenthood programme (pre-natal group 1) and within 48 hours of delivery (post-natal group 2).
Testing of any tools used:
Pre-testing and pilot study was undertaken with 30 primigravid women, 15 pre-natal and 15 post-natal, in November 1992.
Topics covered:
Parenthood programme for primigravidae.
Setting for data collection: Hospital, urban.

Details about sample studied:
Planned size of sample:
500 (200 pre-natal, 300 postnatal).
Rationale for planned size:
To ensure that less motivated clients who did not complete the Parenthood programme are included in the sample.
Entry criteria:
Exclusion:
Within the post-natal group mothers of a sick baby or stillbirth. Medically unfit women.
Sample selection:
Convenience sample.
Actual sample size:
Recruitment ongoing.

Keywords: CONSUMER LED EDUCATION, CONSUMER SATISFACTION, EDUCATION FOR PARENTHOOD, MIDWIFERY EDUCATION (CURRICULUM), PRIMIGRAVIDAE

210. THE PROVISION OF CARE AT A MIDWIVES' ANTENATAL CLINIC

January 1982 - January 1984

Ann Thomson, Senior Lecturer. **Contact:** Ann Thomson, School of Nursing Studies, University of Manchester, Coupland III Building, Coupland Street, Manchester M13 9PL. Tel: 061 275 5342

Funded as integral or additional part of a job by employer: University of Manchester. 6-12 hours/week of own time spent.

Aims of the study: 1. To describe the characteristics of women referred to a teaching midwives' antenatal clinic (TMC).
2. To assess whether those who attended the TMC came within the groups identified as being at low obstetric risk. If not, were they noted as being at high risk and was appropriate care targetted to them?
3. Was continuity of care provided?
4. Were problems which occurred in labour, the puerperium and the perinatal period identified antenatally.

Ethics committee approval gained: Yes

Research design: Descriptive – Quantitative – Survey

Data collection:
Techniques used:
Extracted from medical records.
Time data were collected:
June 1983 to January 1984.
Testing of any tools used:
Data collection sheet piloted.
Topics covered:
Attendance at teaching midwives' antenatal clinic. Obstetric risk.
Continuity of care.
Intra- and post-natal outcomes.
Demographic details.
Setting for data collection:
District General Hospital in North of England.

Details about sample studied:
Planned size of sample:
All women referred to TMC in 1 calendar year.
Rationale for planned size:
Inclusive population.
Entry criteria:
Women who had been referred by an obstetrician to the TMC during 1982.
Sample selection:
Referrals.

Actual sample size:
142

Interventions, Outcomes and Analysis:
Analysis:
SPSSx computer programme.
Chi-square.

Results: The teaching midwives were providing care for a group of relatively young women. A high proportion were primiparous and came from the lower SE groups. There was no indication in the records that these women were at potentially high obstetric risk. Consequently no additional care was specifically targetted to them. Continuity of care was not achieved and it is recommended that greater effort be made in this area. As in other studies there was an under-detection and over-diagnosis of IUGR. There was a high referral rate to the obstetrician. It is recommended that women should be booked initially by midwives and subsequently referred to obstetricians as necessary.

Recommendations for further research: Further evaluation of midwife-provided antenatal care.
Further studies on the detection of IUGR.

Keywords: ANTENATAL CARE, ANTENATAL CLINICS, CONTINUITY OF CARE, MIDWIFE'S CARE, MIDWIFERY MANAGED CARE, MIDWIVES' CLINIC, PREGNANCY, RISK ASSESSMENT

Thomson A M. Providing care at a midwives' antenatal clinic. In: Robinson S, Thomson A M, eds. Midwives, Research and Childbirth 1991;2. London: Chapman & Hall.

211. AN INVESTIGATION OF THE EFFECTS OF ADMISSION TO HOSPITAL ON PREGNANT WOMEN'S SMOKING BEHAVIOUR
January 1991 - September 1992
Ann Thomson, Senior Lecturer. **Contact:** Ann Thomson, School of Nursing Studies, University of Manchester, Coupland III Building, Coupland Street, Manchester M13 9PL. Tel: 061 275 5342

Funded as integral or additional part of a job by employer: University of Manchester. 6-12 hours/week of own time spent.

Aims of the study: To investigate the effect of admission to hospital on pregnant women's smoking behaviour.

Ethics committee approval gained: Yes

Research design: Descriptive – Quantitative – Survey

Data collection:
Techniques used:
Interview using structured schedule.
Time data were collected:
After the 20th week of gestation up to before labour had started.
Testing of any tools used:
Questionnaire developed and tested by Bachelor of Nursing Students.
Topics covered:
Number of cigarettes smoked before pregnancy, during pregnancy prior to admission to hospital and since admission to hospital; factors affecting change in smoking behaviour in hospital and in general; reason for admission to hospital; demographic information.
Setting for data collection:
Hospital.

Details about sample studied:
Planned size of sample:
As many as available during data collection period.
Rationale for planned size:
Time factor.
Entry criteria:
Smoked 1 cigarette a day on admission or at the time of interview.
Gestation 20 weeks and over.
'In patient' for at least 48 hours.
Fully mobile (ie not on bed rest).
Not in labour.
Sample selection:
Convenience.
Actual sample size:
41
Response rate:
100%

Interventions, Outcomes and Analysis:
Analysis:
Amdhal computer SPSSx. Wilcoxon signed ranks test.

Results: The women appeared to be aware of the dangers of smoking in pregnancy in that they reported a significant decrease in the number of cigarettes smoked in pregnancy when compared with the number smoked pre-pregnancy ($Z = -2.6359$, $p = 0.0084$). However, following admission to hospital the number of cigarettes smoked increased, although the difference did not quite reach statistical significance ($Z = -1.7876$, $p = 0.0738$). The major reason given by the women for this increase was 'boredom'.

Recommendations for further research: After instituting procedures which have been shown to reduce the need for admission to hospital in pregnancy there is a need to investigate ways in which boredom can be reduced for these women who have to be admitted to hospital in pregnancy.

Keywords: ADMISSIONS, ANTENATAL CARE, PREGNANCY, SMOKING, TERATOGENS, TOBACCO

Thomson AM. If you are pregnant and smoke admission to hospital may damage your baby's health. Journal of Clinical Nursing 1993;2:111-19.

Thomson AM. The effect of admission to hospital on pregnant women's smoking behaviour. In: Proceedings of 1993 ICM Triennial Congress, Vancouver 1993:1899-1916.

213. A CRITICAL STUDY OF THE ROLE, IMPACT AND IMPLICATIONS OF MIDWIVES' PARTICIPATION IN CHILD PROTECTION CONFERENCES

February - September 1993

E J Clarke, Midwifery Tutor. **Contact:** E J Clarke, Canterbury Close, Off Glasshouse Lane, Kenilworth CV8 2PU.

Formed part of a course. 12-20 hours/week of own time spent.

Aims of the study: To investigate midwives' involvement in child protection (CP) case conferences.

Objectives:

a) To identify which midwives working in the community have been involved in CP case conferences in the last 12 months in Solihull and Birmingham Heartlands Hospitals.

b) To investigate the frequency of attendance.

c) To classify the type of case conference attended eg. pre-birth.

d) To identify a core sample for qualitative study of their experiences of C.P. case conferences.

Ethics committee approval gained: Yes

Research design: Descriptive – Qualitative and Quantitative – Survey

> **Data collection:**
> > **Techniques used:**
> > > Questionnaire - all midwives working in the community.
> > > Interview - core sample.
> > **Time data were collected:**
> > > Questionnaire - March/April 1993.
> > > Interviews - August/September 1993.

Testing of any tools used:
>Piloted questionnaires and interviews with 5 midwives.

Topics covered:
>Experience and support.
>Midwives' attitude, knowledge and training.

Setting for data collection:
>Community.

Details about sample studied:

Planned size of sample:
>All midwives working in the community in Solihull Health Authority and Birmingham Heartlands NHS Trust.

Rationale for planned size:
>Questionnaire to all midwives. Individual interviews with those who have participated in CP conferences.

Entry criteria:
>For interviews: experience of participation in conferences.

Sample selection:
>Supervisor of midwives identified all staff currently working in the community.

Actual sample size:
>51

Response rate:
>76.5% - questionnaires.
>Results of questionnaires identified that 53.8% of midwives working in the community had experience of attending child protection case conferences.
>52.4% - gave consent to be interviewed about their experiences.

Interventions, Outcomes and Analysis:

Analysis:
>Simple frequencies.
>Content analysis.

Results: Examination of the 39 returned questionnaires revealed that 21 midwives (53.8%) had experience of attending child protection case conferences, 18 midwives had not. Eleven of the 21 (52.4%) consented to be interviewed about their experiences.

Recommendation for practice as a result of the research:

1. Multi disciplinary training in child protection is essential.

2. No midwife should be expected to attend a CP case conference for the first time alone.

3. All midwives should receive adequate instruction in child protection procedures.

4. Welfare services should consider sharing the responsibility for organisation of training with other disciplines. Priority should be given to multi-disciplinary training as opposed to inter-disciplinary training.

5. A multi-disciplinary training co-ordinator should be appointed.

6. Midwives should be invited to all pre-birth case conferences.

Recommendations for further research: 1. Larger studies to include all midwives in a given area. This would enable a rate of attendance at case conferences by midwives to be established.

2. A further study to interview midwives from other areas of the country to establish if experiences are similar to Birmingham midwives.

Keywords: CASE CONFERENCES, CHILD ABUSE, CHILD PROTECTION CASE CONFERENCES, MIDWIFE'S ROLE

214. WOMEN'S EXPERIENCE OF MATERNITY CARE IN MID SURREY
April 1990 - February 1991
R Coppen, Midwifery Lecturer, P Kolodij, Computer Student Postgraduate, A Coppen, Consultant Psychiatrist, P Wilson, Quality Assurance Manager. **Contact:** R Coppen, Furlong House, Tattenham Crescent, Epsom Downs, Surrey KT18 5NY.

Formed part of a course. Funded as integral or additional part of a job by employer: Community Health Council. Over 20 hours/week of own time spent.

Aims of the study: To obtain women's views of maternity care in mid Surrey and to determine areas for improvement.

Ethics committee approval gained: No

Research design: Descriptive – Qualitative and Quantitative – Survey

   Data collection:
      Techniques used:
         Questionnaires.
      Time data were collected:
         Day of discharge postnatally (minimum 2 days, maximum 10 days).
      Testing of any tools used:
         Questionnaires were based on selection of questions produced by the Social Survey Division OPCS (Mason 1989).
      Topics covered:
         Antenatal, intrapartum and postnatal care (including care in the community).
      Setting for data collection:
         Hospital based - maternity unit.

   Details about sample studied:
      Planned size of sample:
         300 women
      Rationale for planned size:
         1. Manageable number for the researcher.
         2. Funds (limited).
         3. Sample size enough to fulfil aims of the study.

Entry criteria:
> *Inclusion:* - Mothers admitted to the maternity unit over the period 1 April to 3 June 1990.
> *Exclusion:* - homebirths.

Sample selection:
> Random.

Actual sample size:
> 300

Response rate:
> 67%

Interventions, Outcomes and Analysis:
Analysis:
> SPSSx

Results: Most deliveries were normal and conducted by midwives. 44% were primiparous, 55% multiparous. The Caesarean Section rate was 19% and the forceps delivery rate 10%. 44% of labours were accelerated. Epidural anaesthesia was the most effective form of pain relief, but was used in only 17% of cases. Pethidine injections were perceived as least effective pain relief in labour but were given to 39% of the women. 33% had episiotomies and 52% perineal tears. 77% were monitored at some stage in their labours with the majority comfortable with the process. Most women delivered in the propped up position supported by pillows but one fifth wanted to adopt alternate positions. Postnatally 70% breastfed the baby, 14% bottle fed, with the remaining 16% adopting both methods.

Overall 80% of the mothers were very satisfied with the care they had received. As many as 90% felt they had had enough explanation, help and advice about feeding the baby, but a quarter would have liked more help with handling, settling and looking after the baby in the longer term. A third were worried or confused by conflicting advice.

Areas identified for improvement were greater attention to individualised care, better pain relief and less intervention in labour. Postnatally, a third of women were unhappy with the state of the wards and lack of facilities and a third did not like the visiting hours. Some complained about the quantity and quality of the food served to them. Following their discharge home, a third expressed concerns over their own health and recovery.

Keywords: ANTENATAL CARE, COMMUNITY CARE, CONSUMER SATISFACTION, EXPERIENCE (WOMEN'S), LABOUR, MATERNITY SERVICES, POSTNATAL CARE

Coppen R. Maternity services excel in Epsom General Hospital. NCT Newsletter, Autumn 1991:15.
Unpublished report to Director of Nursing/Midwifery Services Epsom Health Care Trust and to all Clinical areas in Epsom General Hospital Maternity Unit.

216. SEMI-STRUCTURED POST-NATAL GROUPS AND WOMENS' EXPERIENCE OF CHILDBIRTH
January 1991 - June 1993
J A Gillen, Independent midwife. **Contact:** J A Gillen, Kingston Road, Didsbury, Manchester M20 8RZ.

6-12 hours/week of own time spent.

Aims of the study: To explore:
1. the historical roots which led to the medical profession's dominant approach in defining experience of childbirth.
2. the feelings of women in relation to their experience of pregnancy and childbirth.
3. the appropriateness of group work as a means for women to share and understand their experience.

Ethics committee approval gained: No

Research design: Descriptive – Qualitative – Historical/Group Discussion

   Data collection:
   Techniques used:
         Tape recording.
         Questionnaires.
   Time data were collected:
         Between 6 weeks and 3 months postnatally.
   Testing of any tools used:
         Questionnaire piloted.
   Topics covered:
         Experiences of pregnancy and childbirth.
   Setting for data collection:
         Home of researcher.

   Details about sample studied:
   Planned size of sample:
         24 (6-8 women in each group, 4 groups).
   Rationale for planned size:
         Availability of women; requirements for focus group studies.
   Entry criteria:
         Belonging to pre-existing antenatal group.
   Sample selection:
         Taken from pre-existing NCT antenatal groups.
   Actual sample size:
         24
   Response rate:
         100%

Interventions, Outcomes and Analysis:
    Analysis:
        Content analysis.

Results: 1. The women found it difficult to describe their birth experience as it related to them rather than their care-takers.
2. They had a need to have the events of labour explained to them.
3. The group participants found a great deal of support from each other in coming to terms with both their birth experience and their new role as mother.
4. They needed "permission" to acknowledge what is/was important to them in pregnancy and labour.
5. Women could only acknowledge their own sense of powerlessness in childbirth through the experience of others.
6. Focused postnatal groups seem to be very important to help women come to terms with labour.
7. Historical review of the literature demonstrated that medical intervention in childbirth has taken place and affected women's experiences.

Keywords: EXPERIENCE (WOMEN'S), POSTNATAL SUPPORT, SUPPORT GROUPS

217. THE PLACE OF BIRTH: ARE WOMEN GIVEN A CHOICE?
October 1992 - May 1993
L Lathan, Community Midwife. **Contact:** L Lathan, Farthing Drive, Letchworth, Herts SG6 2TR.

Formed part of a course. 2-6 hours/week of own time spent.

Aims of the study: 1. To identify the information women need when making a choice in the place of birth.
2. To determine if alterations or improvements in present midwifery practice are needed.

Ethics committee approval gained: Yes

Research design: Descriptive – Qualitative and Quantitative – Survey

    Data collection:
        Techniques used:
            Questionnaires
        Time data were collected:
            Within two weeks of the birth.
        Testing of any tools used:
            Pilot study - 5 subjects.
        Topics covered:
            Place of birth.
            The information women want.
            Sources of information.
            Factors which influence their choice.

Setting for data collection:
Hospital and community.

Details about sample studied:
Planned size of sample:
40
Rationale for planned size:
Limit of defined geographical area.
Entry criteria:
Primigravida.
Normal vaginal delivery.
A live baby.
A planned hospital or home birth.
Postnatal period of less than 2 weeks.
In a defined geographical area.
For home births - the geographical area was extended to district and multiparae were included.
Sample selection:
Convenience.
Actual sample size:
41
Response rate:
98%

Interventions, Outcomes and Analysis:
Analysis:
Content analysis. Computer - Minitab for stats.

Results: Women found it easy to ask for information about their choices in birth place, and most found the information adequate. The majority looked to their midwife as their main source of information.

More than half would not discuss their choice with a professional, because either they were certain in their choice, assumed they had no choice or only discussed their choice with family or friends. All the mothers thought they should have a choice, but not all considered the eventual place of birth had been their choice. Retrospectively all mothers felt the place of birth had been right for them.

Seeing hospital as the safest place was the main factor in women's choice of hospital as the birth place. Seeing home as a personal relaxed place was the main factor in women's choice of home birth.

Recommendations for further research:
1. Larger study for statistically significant data.
2. Replication study involving only multips to make data comparable between hospital and home births.
3. Repeat study following introduction of Health Authority leaflet on choices in child birth.
4. Professionals' views on offering choices in birth place.

Keywords: CHOICE, CONSUMER SATISFACTION, INFORMED CHOICE, PLACE OF BIRTH

219. IDENTIFYING THE KEY FEATURES OF CONTINUITY OF CARE IN MIDWIFERY
February - October 1992

Tricia Murphy-Black, Research and Development Adviser. **Contact:** Tricia Murphy-Black, Research and Development Adviser, Simpson Memorial Maternity Pavilion, Lauriston Place, Edinburgh EH3 9EF. Tel: 031 229 2477 Ex 4357

Funded as integral or additional part of a job by Scottish Office Home & Health Department.

Aims of the study: To determine the key features of continuity of care identified by midwives and mothers.

Ethics committee approval gained: No

Research design: Descriptive – Qualitative and Quantitative – Group Interviews

Data collection:
    Techniques used:
        Group interviews.
    Time data were collected:
        Between 3 days and 8 months postnatally.
    Testing of any tools used:
        None.
    Topics covered:
        Continuity of care.
        Organisation.
        Politics.
    Setting for data collection:
        Four hospitals and community units; two rural and two urban.

Details about sample studied:
    Planned size of sample:
        4 groups of midwives, 4 groups of mothers.

Rationale for planned size:
Two groups each from units with team midwifery and units without team midwifery.

Entry criteria:
Expert midwives from one Unit who were:
practising in any department apart from special care baby unit,
of any grade,
on day or night duty,
full or part time.
Each team of midwives to be represented.

Sample selection:
Convenience sample (of mothers) and by expertise (for midwives).

Actual sample size:
37 midwives and 19 mothers.

Response rate:
Unknown.

Interventions, Outcomes and Analysis:
Analysis:
Content analysis of transcribed interview data.
Cross tabulation of quantitative data.

Results: The midwives identified key features of continuity of care in midwifery in two areas - carers and caring. Flexibility was a crucial factor.

In terms of the carers, the organisation, locally based care, midwives' clinic and caseloads were all important features of the structure. Relationships and social visits were key elements of the process.

In terms of the caring, key features in the structure were policy, documentation and assessment; and in the process were individualised care and partnership.

Maternal views of the key features of continuity of care in midwifery included social visits and shift to shift communication in the process of care. Outcomes in terms of having a known midwife in labour, continuity of carer, choice and control, support, a midwife as advocate, consistent advice and expectations met, were all important factors.

Recommendations for further research: Identification of the influence of continuity of care on maternal and neonatal outcomes.

Keywords: CONSUMER OPINION, CONSUMER SATISFACTION, CONTINUITY OF CARE, EXPERIENCE (WOMEN'S), MIDWIFE'S CARE

Murphy-Black T. Identifying the key features of continuity of care in midwifery. Nursing Research Unit Report, Department of Nursing Studies, University of Edinburgh 1993.

220. ROUTINE POSTNATAL HAEMOGLOBIN ESTIMATIONS
March - June 1992
N Perry, Midwife, Postnatal Ward. **Contact:** N Perry, Beacon Square, Clifton Village, Rotherham, South Yorkshire S66 7RZ.

Funded as integral or additional part of a job by employer: Doncaster Royal Infirmary & Montagu NHS Trust. 2-6 hours/week of own time spent.

Aims of the study: Taking into account physiological changes that occur in blood volume during pregnancy and the puerperium, are routine postnatal haemoglobin estimations necessary and cost effective? Is a protocol needed to identify those at risk of developing postnatal anaemia.

Ethics committee approval gained: No

Research design: Descriptive – Quantitative – Retrospective case note review

> **Data collection:**
> > **Techniques used:**
> > > Case note review.
> > **Time data were collected:**
> > > Retrospectively.
> > **Topics covered:**
> > > Postnatal haemoglobin estimations.
> > **Setting for data collection:**
> > > Hospital.

> **Details about sample studied:**
> > **Planned size of sample:**
> > > 350
> > **Rationale for planned size:**
> > > All deliveries in a selected month.
> > **Entry criteria:**
> > > All women who delivered in January and who had a haemoglobin estimation performed whilst in hospital.
> > **Sample selection:**
> > > Random selection of a month in which all notes and postnatal details would be available.
> > **Actual sample size:**
> > > 324

> **Interventions, Outcomes and Analysis:**
> > **Analysis:**
> > > Manual.

Results: A protocol was identified (after discussion with managers) early in the study to determine those at risk of developing postnatal anaemia. Using this protocol all case notes were checked looking at antenatal and postnatal haemoglobin levels and estimated blood loss at delivery. The study showed that less than 43% of postnatal haemoglobins were necessary (by using protocol). It also showed that 5.25% of haemoglobins of 8.0g/dl-10g/dl would have been missed. Further investigation (on the basis that a 500ml blood loss drops the haemoglobin by 1g) when looking at pre-delivery and first postnatal haemoglobin results, showed that many estimated blood losses at delivery were underestimated and greater care was needed.

In the light of these results, it was agreed by managers and medical personnel that postnatal haemoglobins were not cost effective or necessary.

Keywords: ANAEMIA, BLOOD LOSS ESTIMATION, COST-BENEFIT ANALYSIS, HAE-MOGLOBIN LEVELS, POSTNATAL CARE

221. ANTENATAL WOMEN TO CARRY THEIR OWN OBSTETRIC RECORD: AN EVALUATION OF A NEWLY INTRODUCED PROGRAMME
February - December 1993
Helen Rowe, Practice Development/Research Midwife, Marie Collier, Staff Midwife.
Contact: Helen Rowe, Warrington Hospital NHS Trust, Lovely Lane, Warrington WA5 1QG. Tel: 0925 35911 Ex 2344

Funded as integral or additional part of a job.

Aims of the study: To assess whether the introduction of a system of women carrying their own obstetric record is as administratively effective as the current system of centrally held records.

Ethics committee approval gained: No

Research design: Descriptive – Qualitative and Quantitative – Evaluation/descriptive comparison.

> **Data collection:**
> **Techniques used:**
> Specifically designed checklist.
> **Time data were collected:**
> Checks carried out at 24,30,36 weeks and post delivery.
> **Testing of any tools used:**
> No.
> **Topics covered:**
> Availability of notes - reasons for non availability.
> Filing of special routine test results, scan and LVS results. Legibility of record entries and condition of records.
> **Setting for data collection:**
> Consultant led maternity unit - in mainly urban area but including outlying rural areas. Data collected in both hospital and community settings.

Details about sample studied:
    Planned size of sample:
        192 (96 women carrying own notes [one consultant], 96 women
        hospital held notes [three consultants]).
    Rationale for planned size:
        10% of consultants' last year antenatal bookings.
    Entry criteria:
        Exclusion: any women who miscarried.
    Sample selection:
        Convenience.
    Actual sample size:
        186
    Response rate:
        97%

Interventions, Outcomes and Analysis:
    Analysis:
        Descriptive statistics.
        Chi-square test.

Results: Not yet available.

Keywords: ANTENATAL CARE, CLIENT HELD NOTES/RECORDS, MEDICAL RECORDS

222. A RANDOMIZED CONTROLLED TRIAL OF AEROBIC AND PELVIC FLOOR EXERCISES IN PREGNANCY
December 1991 - April 1994
G Lee, Research Midwife, M McNabb, Senior Lecturer, S Challenger, Service Evaluation Officer. **Contact:** G Lee, Kirkstall Road, London SW2 4HF.

Funded as integral or additional part of a job and by funding agency(ies): Primary Care Development Fund of South East Thames Regional Health Authority, Special Trustees of St Thomas's Hospital and Maws Award. Over 20 hours/week of own time spent.

Aims of the study: To test the hypothesis that performing regular aerobic exercise during pregnancy will result in
a) a shorter duration of spontaneous labour
b) a lower mean pulse rate during labour
c) a lower perceived pain level during labour
d) a lower incidence of stress incontinence three months following delivery
e) birth weight differences between the study and control group.

Ethics committee approval gained: Yes

Research design: Experimental – Qualitative and Quantitative – Randomized Controlled Trial

Data collection:

Techniques used:

Randomized controlled trial.

Time data were collected:

At recruitment, delivery and 3 months postnatally.

Testing of any tools used:

Small pilot on people who attended parentcraft reunion.

Topics covered:

Length of labour.

Pulse rate.

Perceived pain.

Stress incontinence postnatally.

Baby's birth weight.

Setting for data collection:

Hospital

Details about sample studied:

Planned size of sample:

360 (180 in each group)

Rationale for planned size:

To obtain statistically significant results.

Entry criteria:

Primigravidae.

Prepared to participate in a planned programme of aerobic exercise. Non-smokers.

No medical problems.

Sample selection:

Random

Actual sample size:

370

Response rate:

67%

Interventions, Outcomes and Analysis:

Interventions used:

Aerobic exercise for 60 minutes, 3 times a week at 60-70% of age related maximal heart rate.

Main outcomes measured:

Length of labour.

Perceived pain during labour.

Incidence of stress incontinence at 12 weeks postpartum.

Baby's birth weight.

Analysis:

Mann-Whitney U test.

Results: Not yet available.

Keywords: AEROBIC EXERCISE, PELVIC FLOOR, PELVIC FLOOR EXERCISES, PREGNANCY, STRESS INCONTINENCE, URINARY INCONTINENCE

223. WHO'S ACCOUNTABLE? WHO'S TO BLAME? LITIGATION IN PERINATAL CARE
February 1991 - April 1992
A Symon, Research Midwife. **Contact:** A Symon, Douglas Street, Stirling, Scotland FK8 1NT.

Formed part of a course.

Aims of the study: 1. To explore the incidence of perinatal litigation.
2. To gauge the response of a small group of midwives to a perceived rise in litigation.
3. To assess the possibilities for legal reform.

Ethics committee approval gained: No

Research design: Descriptive – Qualitative – Survey

Data collection:
   Techniques used:
      1. Literature review to assess incidence of litigation.
      2. Semi-structured interviews.
   Time data were collected:
      At respondents' convenience.
   Testing of any tools used:
      Draft schedule tested with one G grade midwife.
   Topics covered:
      Litigation.
      Levels of supervision.
      Levels and timing of documentation.
      Use of Apgar scores.
      Midwife-obstetrician relationships.
   Setting for data collection:
      Hospital

Details about sample studied:
   Planned size of sample:
      20
   Rationale for planned size:
      Availability and within time constraints.
   Entry criteria:
      Registered midwives/qualified obstetric specialists.
   Sample selection:
      Convenience.
   Actual sample size:
      16 midwives, 2 obstetricians approached.
   Response rate:
      100%

Interventions, Outcomes and Analysis:
    Analysis:
        Content analysis.

Results: 1. The incidence of medical negligence litigation is increasing sharply, due in large part to a rising incidence within perinatal care. Cerebral palsy is a major cited factor.
2. Those midwives surveyed were aware of the threat of litigation, but this was not a pressing factor in the working day. Most midwives were unaware of the workings of the law concerning negligence.
3. A conclusion drawn from contact with consumer groups is that support for the introduction of no-fault compensation has grown, and is now supported by the British Medical Association and the Royal College of Midwives.
The Government however has chosen not to reform the law concerning alleged negligence.
Consumer groups have expressed the fear that no-fault compensation may reduce accountability.

Recommendations for further research: 1. Conduct a comprehensive survey of the incidence and nature of perinatal litigation.
2. Explore in depth the response of midwives and obstetricians to the perceived threat of litigation.
3. Examine the role of relevant consumer groups.
(all in planning).

Keywords: ACCOUNTABILITY, DELIVERY, EXPERIENCE (MIDWIVES'), LABOUR, LITIGATION, MATERNITY SERVICES, NEGLIGENCE, PERINATAL CARE

225. THE MIDWIFERY DEVELOPMENT UNIT (MDU); A RANDOMIZED CONTROLLED TRIAL
July 1992 - July 1995

Deborah Turnbull, Project Manager, Mary McGinley, Head of Midwifery Services, Barbara Maclennan, Area Nurse, Midwifery, Ian Greer, Professor of Obstetrics and Gynaecology, Gillian M McIlwaine, Consultant Public Health Women's Health. **Contact:** Deborah Turnbull, Midwifery Development Unit, Glasgow Royal Maternity Hospital, Rottenrow, Glasgow G4 ONA. Tel: 041 552 3400

Funded as integral or additional part of a job and by funding agency(ies): Scottish Office.

Aims of the study: A comparison of midwifery led care in the Midwifery Development Unit (MDU) and the existing pattern of shared care between midwives, obstetricians and general practitioners.

It is hypothesized that Midwifery Development Unit care offers women:
    a) a lower rate of intervention,
    b) with the same (or more favourable) outcomes,
    c) same complication rates,

d) greater continuity of care and carer,

e) and greater satisfaction with care.

Ethics committee approval gained: Yes

Research design: Descriptive/Experimental – Qualitative and Quantitative – Survey/ Randomized Controlled Trial/Action Research

Data collection:

Techniques used:

1. Women: self-report questionnaires and interviews; case note review; observation.

2. Midwives: self-report questionnaires, interviews.

Time data were collected:

Women: questionnaires and interviews -34/35 weeks; 7 weeks postnatally; 7 months postnatally; case note review - retrospective.

Observation - antenatal, intrapartum and postnatal.

Testing of any tools used:

All tools have been designed and tested with local women, with the exception of the Edinburgh Postnatal Depression Scale.

Topics covered:

Satisfaction (midwives' and women's).

Postnatal depression.

Continuity of care.

Setting for data collection:

The Glasgow Royal Maternity Hospital.

Details about sample studied:

Planned size of sample:

2300 (1150 experimental women and 1150 control women).

Rationale for planned size:

This sample size has 99% power to detect, at the 0.05 level, a 5% difference between the experimental and control groups, if the characteristics occur in at most 10% of the women overall.

Entry criteria:

Women must live in the geographical catchment area served by the community midwives at Glasgow Royal Maternity Hospital and be experiencing a normal healthy pregnancy. Clinical exclusion criteria have been designed by senior clinical midwives in consultation with obstetricians. There were over 30 criteria that fall into the following groups: booking, social, physical, genetic, medical, obstetric, gynaecological, psychological and other.

Sample selection:

All women who fulfil the criteria, have a participating GP, and who attend hospital based booking clinics within the catchment area (ie at Glasgow Royal Maternity and Stobhill Hospitals) are approached to participate. Women are randomly allocated to Midwifery Development Unit or existing care.

Actual sample size:
Recruitment ongoing.

Interventions, Outcomes and Analysis:
Interventions used:
Midwifery led care in the Midwifery Development Unit.
Main outcomes measured:
Economic costs and benefits.
Women's satisfaction.
Continuity of care.
Postnatal depression.
Clinical outcomes.
Complication rates.
General clinical intervention rates.
Analysis:
SPSSPC.
Chi-square test.
Multivariate methods.

Keywords: CONSUMER SATISFACTION, CONTINUITY OF CARE, MIDWIFE'S CARE, MIDWIFERY MANAGED CARE, MIDWIFERY UNIT, SHARED CARE

Turnbull D, McGinley M, Reid M. A methodology for monitoring midwifery process measures. Paper presented to the International Confederation of Midwives 23rd Triennial Congress, Vancouver, May 1993, 1925-1934.

226. BIRTH - HOSPITAL OR HOME?
May - September 1992
C Wright, Community Midwife, C Harries, Research and Development. **Contact:** C Wright, Sandwich Close, St Ives, Huntingdon, Cambridgeshire PE17 6DQ.

Funded as integral or additional part of a job by employer: Hinchingbrooke Hospital. 2 hours/week of own time spent.

Aims of the study: To describe the experiences of a small group of women having births at home, and compare them with a similar group confined in hospital.

Ethics committee approval gained: No

Research design: Descriptive – Qualitative – Descriptive comparison

Data collection:
Techniques used:
Semi-structured interview.
Time data were collected:
Retrospectively for previous year, ie from a few days to several months after delivery.

Testing of any tools used:
No.
Topics covered:
Experience of making a decision about home or hospital delivery.
Birth experience.
Reflections.
Setting for data collection:
Community.

Details about sample studied:
Planned size of sample:
All home births in one community patch, plus matching number of hospital births.
Rationale for planned size:
This particular community patch is the one in which most home births occur.
Entry criteria:
Home birth group - delivering in one community patch.
Hospital birth group - matched by parity, marital status, partner's employment, type of accommodation, length of residence in area.
Sample selection:
Convenience.
Actual sample size:
45 (22 home birth mothers, 23 hospital birth mothers).
Response rate:
98%

Interventions, Outcomes and Analysis:
Analysis:
Content analysis.

Results: All mothers in this study were multiparous except one in each group. All the pregnancies were wanted and all the women had help at home. Many women felt that they had had no choice about the place of birth, and had merely complied with what they saw as the existing system of hospital births - there had been no discussion on the subject with health care workers. While those having hospital deliveries talked about perceived risks and safety, those who had home births identified specific reasons for their choice and retrospectively emphasised the fulfilling and satisfying process. Both groups felt their choice had been right for them. For the majority delivering at home, their decision had been determined by a previous unexpected home birth which had been a good experience. The perceived lack of choice raises important questions about the way in which information is given to women in pregnancy.

Keywords: EXPERIENCE (WOMEN'S), HOME BIRTHS, HOSPITAL BIRTHS, PLACE OF BIRTH

227. SOCIOLOGICAL ASPECTS OF THE MOTHER/COMMUNITY MIDWIFE RELATIONSHIP
October 1989 - January 1993
R Wilkins, Researcher. **Contact:** R Wilkins, Waltham Avenue, Guildford, Surrey GU2 6QE.

Funded by Economic and Social Research Council (ESRC).

Aims of the study: To answer two questions:
1. What is 'special' about mother/community midwife relationships?
2. What is distinctive about the community midwife's role (compared to GPs, Health Visitors and hospital based midwives)?

Ethics committee approval gained: Yes

Research design: Descriptive – Qualitative – Ethnography/Case Study

Data collection:
Techniques used:
Informal, indepth interviews.
Participant observation.
Observation.
Time data were collected:
Interviews:
a) Mothers: late pregnancy (35-38 weeks), 2-3 weeks postnatally.
b) Midwives: mostly during off duty hours.
Observation: range of antenatal and postnatal contact up to 10 days. Limited intranatal contact.
Testing of any tools used:
Interview based pilot study conducted Summer 1989.
Topics covered:
Definitions of the community midwife's role.
Mother/community midwife interaction.
Personal factors influencing relationship outcome.
The impact of different community settings (eg clinic vs home).
The impact of 1:1 continuity of care on the mother's experience.
Setting for data collection:
Predominantly in the community setting, both clinical and the mother's own home.

Details about sample studied:
Planned size of sample:
Observation: 18 community midwives, unspecified number of mothers.
Interviews: 24 mothers, 6 community midwives.
Rationale for planned size:
Observation: all community midwives within the District Health Authority.

To permit analysis of variability.

Feasibility.

Entry criteria:

Midwives: currently practising in the community.

Mothers: 30-37 weeks pregnant. GP had consented.

Sample selection:

Midwives: by invitation.

Mothers: consecutive.

Actual sample size:

Midwives - 12.

Mothers - 200.

43 in interview based study.

Response rate:

Midwives - 66%

Mothers - 100%

Interviews - 95%

Interventions, Outcomes and Analysis:

Analysis:

Content analysis.

Simple percentages and frequencies.

Results: 1. Approximately one third of relationships emerged as routine, appreciative and special respectively.

2. Routine relationships were instrumentally defined by the mother and clinically oriented. Special relationships were woman-centred, supportive and emotionally invested. Appreciative relationships were a blend of both: a supportive relationship but with instrumental boundaries.

3. Approximately two thirds of mothers valued the supportive aspect of community midwifery and developed emotional attachments to the community midwife.

4. The distinctive role of the community midwife lies in the '3R's' of relationship, role and real social context. Firstly, women seek a personal rather than a professional relationship with their community midwife. Secondly, the community midwife's role is psychosocially oriented. Thirdly, the community is the appropriate context for midwifery care thus defined, facilitating both relationship and role.

Recommendations for further research: More research needed on:

1. The impact of the community setting;

2. Variability within a role; personal factors influencing professional practice;

3. A distinctive philosophy of midwifery practice and research.

Keywords: COMMUNICATION, COMMUNITY MIDWIVES, CONTINUITY OF CARE, EXPERIENCE (WOMEN'S), GENERAL PRACTITIONERS, HEALTH VISITORS, MIDWIFE'S ROLE, MIDWIFE-MOTHER RELATIONSHIP

Wilkins R. Sociological aspects of the mother/community midwife relationship. University of Surrey. Unpublished PhD thesis 1993.

Wilkins R. Taking it personally: a note on emotion and autobiography. Sociology 1993;27:93-100.

228. A NATIONAL STUDY OF LABOUR AND BIRTH IN WATER
August 1993 - October 1994

Jo Garcia, Social Scientist, Fiona Alderdice, Survey Researcher, Sally Marchant, Research Midwife, Pam Hughes, Project Secretary, Mary J Renfrew, Director, Midwifery Research Programme, Georgina Berridge, Computer Programmer. **Contact:** Fiona Alderdice, National Perinatal Epidemiology Unit, Radcliffe Infirmary, Oxford OX2 6HE. Tel: 0865 224118

Funded as integral or additional part of a job by Department of Health. 2 hours/week of own time spent.

Aims of the study: To ascertain the extent to which immersion during labour and/or birth is available to maternity service users in England, and to provide estimates of the numbers of labours and deliveries where this form of care is used.

Ethics committee approval gained: No

Research design: Descriptive – Qualitative and Quantitative – Survey/Case Study

Data collection:
Techniques used:
A preliminary questionnaire to heads of midwifery in England and Wales. Telephone interviews with care providers for additional information. Observation.
Time data were collected:
November 1993 - June 1994.
Testing of any tools used:
Questionnaires and interview schedules piloted in Scotland and Wales.
Topics covered:
Practice of water births.
Numbers of women interested in waterbirths.
Cost.
Problems associated.
Setting for data collection:
England and Wales.

Details about sample studied:
Planned size of sample:
Heads of midwifery in all districts in England and Wales.
Rationale for planned size:
A complete national sample.
Entry criteria:
All NHS Units, Trust Hospitals and Community Services.
Sample selection:
Inclusive.
Actual sample size:
Recruitment ongoing.

Interventions, Outcomes and Analysis:
> **Analysis:**
>> SPSS/PC.
>> Frequencies and crosstabs.

Keywords: HYDROTHERAPY, LABOUR, WATER BIRTH

McCandlish R, Renfrew M. Immersion in water during labour and/or birth: The need for evaluation. Birth 1993;2:79-85.

Alderdice F, Renfrew M, Garcia J, McCandlish R. Labour and birth in water. Lancet 1993;342:1563.

Alderdice FA, Renfrew MJ, Garcia J, McCandlish RM. A National Study of Labour and Birth in Water. Modern Midwife 1993;4:14.

229. BATHING NEWBORNS - IS HYPOTHERMIA INDUCED BY BATHING BABIES IMMEDIATELY AFTER DELIVERY?

May - August 1993

C K Bates, Staff Midwife, J Driver, Midwife. **Contact:** C K Bates, Tittleshall, Kings Lynn PE32 2PJ.

6-12 hours/week of own time spent.

Aims of the study: To establish whether babies become hypothermic if bathed immediately after delivery.

Ethics committee approval gained: Yes

Research design: Experimental – Quantitative – Randomized Controlled Trial

> **Data collection:**
>> **Techniques used:**
>>> Records of observation.
>> **Time data were collected:**
>>> At time of delivery.
>>> Approximately 2 hours after delivery.
>> **Testing of any tools used:**
>>> Piloted with 20 people.
>> **Topics covered:**
>>> Temperature changes.
>> **Setting for data collection:**
>>> Hospital.

> **Details about sample studied:**
>> **Planned size of sample:**
>>> 150

Rationale for planned size:

Represents one month's delivery numbers. One month chosen to prevent staff becoming de-motivated.

Entry criteria:

Inclusion: Gestational age of 37+ weeks.

Birthweight between 2500 gms - 4500 gms.

Apgar of 7 or more at one minute.

Exclusion: Any baby with initial rectal temperature of <36˚

Sample selection:

Random.

Actual sample size:

200

Response rate:

Ongoing

Interventions, Outcomes and Analysis:

Interventions used:

Bathing the study group.

Main outcomes measured:

Rectal temperature change.

Analysis:

Computer software - analysis in process.

Results: Not yet available.

Keywords: BATHING, HYPOTHERMIA, INFANT NEWBORN, NEONATE

230. THE RESOURCE IMPLICATIONS OF DIFFERENT APPROACHES TO THE MANAGEMENT OF PERINEAL TRAUMA
November 1991 - October 1994

Sarah Howard, Health Economics Researcher, Miranda Mugford, Economist, Denise Mickell, Student. **Contact:** Sarah Howard, National Perinatal Epidemiology Unit, Radcliffe Infirmary, Oxford OX2 6HE. Tel: 0865 224126

Funded as integral or additional part of a job by employer: Department of Health.

Aims of the study: To provide information on the cost effectiveness of preventative and treatment interventions for perineal trauma.

Ethics committee approval gained: No

Research design: Descriptive – Secondary use of Experimental data – Quantitative Survey/Cost effectiveness analysis

Data collection:

Techniques used:

Interviews.

Questionnaires.

Reviewing any evidence on resource use from systematic reviews of RC trials.

Time data were collected:

Prospectively alongside an RCT. Also retrospectively.

Testing of any tools used:

No.

Topics covered:

Resources involved in the process of perineal suturing, removal of sutures, resuturing, and associated perineal pain.

Setting for data collection:

Hospital and community setting.

Details about sample studied:

Planned size of sample:

110 (100 removal of sutures, 10 resuturing).

Rationale for planned size:

Practical.

Entry criteria:

Any women having stitches removed from their perineum after childbirth by midwives based at the Ipswich Hospital.

Any women having their perineum resutured for whatever reason, at the Ipswich Hospital.

Sample selection:

Convenience.

Actual sample size:

Recruitment ongoing.

Interventions, Outcomes and Analysis:

Interventions used:

So far comparing:

1. Absorbable versus non-absorbable perineal skin sutures.
2. Continuous versus interrupted perineal sutures.
3. Apposing the perineal skin versus suturing.

Main outcomes measured:

Long term pain (3 months).

Short term pain (10 days).

Dyspareunia at 3 months.

Need for removal of sutures.

Need for resuturing.

Analysis:

Not yet completed.

Keywords: COST EFFECTIVENESS, DYSPAREUNIA, ECONOMIC EVALUATION, PAIN, PERINEAL REPAIR, SUTURE MATERIALS, SUTURING

231. CLEANSING AND LUBRICATING PRIOR TO VAGINAL EXAMINATION AND VAGINAL PROCEDURES IN LABOUR. A COMPARISON OF THE USE OF CHLORHEXIDINE BASED SOLUTIONS AND CREAMS, LUBRICATING JELLY AND STERILE WATER

May 1993 - April 1995

Wendy C Jessiman, Research Midwife. **Contact:** Wendy C Jessiman, Delivery Suite, Maternity Department, John Radcliffe Hospital, Headington, Oxford OX3 9DU. Tel: 0865 221974 BLP 1989

Funded by locally organised research scheme and District Research Committee.

Aims of the study: 1. To describe the range of midwifery practices in the United Kingdom with regard to the cleansing and lubricating agents used prior to vaginal examination and vaginal procedures.

2. To compare differing cleansing and lubricating agents used prior to vaginal examinations and vaginal procedures.

The following hypothesis will be tested: There will be no difference in perineal healing, neonatal and maternal infection between the groups using any chlorhexidine products and the group using only sterile water and lubricating jelly.

Ethics committee approval gained: Yes

Research design: Descriptive/Experimental – Qualitative and Quantitative – Survey/ Randomized Controlled Trial

    Data collection:
        Techniques used:
            Telephone survey.
            Questionnaires.
        Time data were collected:
            During labour, 24-28 hours post-partum and at ten days post-partum.
        Testing of any tools used:
            The telephone questionnaire has been piloted.
            All data collection tools in the randomised controlled trial will be piloted.
        Topics covered:
            Experiences of internal examinations
            Perineal healing
            Neonatal and maternal infection.
        Setting for data collection:
            Hospital and community.

    Details about sample studied:
        Planned size of sample:
            Telephone survey:
            35 consultant units, 15 GP and midwife units.
            Randomized controlled trial:
            1,000 women in 4 groups (total 4,000 women).

Rationale for planned size:

Sample size is based on a power calculation when the incidence of neonatal and maternal infection is 5%. The sample size of 1000 in each group will be sufficient to detect a 50% difference in infection in the groups.

Entry criteria:

Exclusion:

1. Not in spontaneous labour.

2. For elective Caesarean Section.

3. Presence of prolonged rupture of membranes (greater than 24 hours).

4. Overt clinical infection (a temperature above 37.2 degrees Celsius), abnormal vaginal discharge or on current antibiotic therapy.

5. Less than 37 completed weeks.

6. Having or suspecting any sensitivity/allergy to chlorhexidine or cetrimide preparations.

Sample selection:

Random.

Actual sample size:

Recruitment ongoing.

Interventions, Outcomes and Analysis:

Interventions used:

Women will be allocated to one of four groups using either Hibitane obstetric cream and Tisept, Hibitane obstetric cream and sterile water, lubricating jelly and sterile water or lubricating jelly and Tisept.

Main outcomes measured: Perineal healing.

Neonatal and maternal infection.

Keywords: CETRIMIDE, CHLORHEXIDINE, EXPERIENCE (WOMEN'S), INFECTION RATES, LUBRICATING JELLY, MATERNAL INFECTION, NEONATAL INFECTION, STERILE WATER, VAGINAL EXAMINATIONS

232. A COMPARATIVE STUDY OF HAND AND MECHANICALLY EXPRESSED HUMAN MILK - NUTRITIONAL CONTENT AND EFFECT ON BABIES' WEIGHT AND GROWTH

April 1992 - June 1993

S Lang, Research Midwife, R Orme, Consultant Paediatrician, C Lawrence, Senior Lecturer in Statistics. **Contact:** S Lang, St Leonards Avenue, Exeter, Devon EX2 4DL.

Funded as integral part of a job by funding agency(ies): Northcott Devon Medical Foundation. 12-20 hours/week of own time spent.

Aims of the study: 1. To establish whether different methods of expressing breast milk, using either manual or mechanical expression, affect the constituents and nutritional value of the milk.

2. To assess whether breast milk expressed by these two methods affects weight gain and growth of babies fed their own mothers' breast milk in a neonatal unit.

3. To use the results of this study to form the basis of an educational training programme for neonatal nursing staff in methods of human milk expression.

Ethics committee approval gained: Yes

Research design: Experimental – Qualitative and Quantitative – Controlled study, Cross over design

Data collection:
Techniques used:
Case note review.
Parent interview (structured).
Records of observations.
Milk sampling.
Time data were collected:
Admission and discharge data collected when appropriate.
Feeding data collected daily.
All body measurements collected every 2 days, except skinfold thickness and body composition analysis, which were collected every 4 days.
Milk sampling undertaken every six days, at each expression over a 24 hour period.
1 sample from each complete expression or 3 samples from each expression ie. fore, mid and hind milk.
Testing of any tools used:
Tested in previous study.
Baby measurement questionnaire with 60 infants.
Milk questionnaire with 20 mothers.
Topics covered:
The infant - admission and discharge details: weight, head circumference and length, upper arm and lower leg circumferences, leg arm and foot length. Skin fold thickness at two sites and body composition analysis. Blood and urine results.
Daily feeding details including type of milk, amount, frequency, type of oral/tube/IV feeding, output, actual and prescribed intake.
Mothers - Milk samples: time of expression, total volume of milk expressed, method of expression, any problems.
Parents - Demographic information.
Setting for data collection:
Neonatal Unit.

Details about sample studied:
Planned size of sample:
70 mother/infant pairs to be selected according to gestational age (28 at 24-30 weeks, 28 at 30-36 weeks, 14 at term).

Rationale for planned size:

Based on figures from a previous study. To show any statistically significant differences in milk composition it was necessary to have a minimum of 6 mothers in each group.

Entry criteria:

Babies admitted to the Neonatal Unit on the day of birth.

Mother initially resident in the hospital.

Mother wishing to breastfeed.

Expression of milk necessary.

Sample selection:

Consecutive admissions.

Actual sample size:

20 mothers, 36 mother/infant pairs.

Response rate:

100%

Interventions, Outcomes and Analysis:

Interventions used:

There were two groups A and B.

Group A consisted of 20 mothers only, divided into two smaller groups of 10. One group of 10 expressed by hand then pump and repeated this sequence for 24 days, each method of expression being carried out for 6 days before changing. In this way each mother was her own control. On day 6, 12, 18 and 24 samples of milk from each expression over a 24 hour period were taken from the fore, mid and hind milk. The second group of 10 mothers began expression by pump and then hand.

Group B consisted of 50 mother and baby pairs. The mothers expressed their milk using only one of 3 methods: hand, pump, pump for hind milk regime. The milk was fed to their own infants who were measured every second day for their entire hospital stay.

Main outcomes measured:

1. Differences in the constituents of milk in hand and machine expression, ie sodium and potassium triglycerides, protein, chloride, calcium.

2. Differences in volumes of milk produced by hand and machine expression.

3. Weight gain and skin fold thickness in the babies.

Analysis:

Paradox 3.

SPSSx.

Regression and multivariate analysis.

'Balaams' design.

Linear model analysis.

Results: Sodium content was analysed in the expressed breastmilk from 30 mothers. Measurements were taken up to 24 days postpartum, during which period the mothers expressed manually or by means of a pump. Statistical analysis has confirmed not only the known decline in sodium levels postpartum but has also shown a significantly higher sodium content in manually expressed milk compared to that from pump expressed milk. In addition there is a significant difference in milk volume between two methods of expression, with less milk produced by manual expression than by mechanical expression.

Keywords: BREAST EXPRESSION, BREAST EXPRESSION (MANUAL), BREAST EXPRESSION (MECHANICAL), BREASTMILK, INFANT WEIGHT GAIN, NEONATAL CARE

233. ARE YOU SITTING COMFORTABLY? THE DEVELOPMENT OF A PERINEAL AUDIT SYSTEM ENABLING MIDWIVES TO FOLLOW THEIR PERINEAL MANAGEMENT UP TO 13 MONTHS FOLLOWING DELIVERY

February 1993 - March 1995

Lucy Lewis, Research Midwife, Katherine Rounce, Course Director, Womens Health, Lai Y Polenz, Midwifery Tutor, Judi Keshet-Orr, Counsellor. **Contact:** Lucy Lewis, Womens Health, Maternity Department, Whittington Trust, Highgate Hill, London N19 5NF. Tel: 071 288 5436

Funded as integral or additional part of a job by employer: Whittington Hospital Trust. Additional funding from North East Thames Regional Health Authority (NETRHA) under their 'Locally Organised Research' scheme (LORS). 2-6 hours/week of own time spent.

Aims of the study: 1. To develop a perineal audit system to enable midwives to follow their perineal management up to 13 months following delivery in order to improve their practice.
2. To examine women's experience of the effects of perineal laceration.

Ethics committee approval gained: Yes

Research design: Descriptive – Qualitative and Quantitative – Action Research

> **Data collection:**
> > **Techniques used:**
> > > 1. Questionnaires.
> > > 2. Semi-structured diaries (proforma).
> > **Time data were collected:**
> > > 1. 10 days, 6 weeks, 8 months and 13 months postnatally for the proforma.
> > > 2. Questionnaire 1 prior to proforma and following return of all proforma.
> > > 3. Questionnaire 2 following delivery.

Testing of any tools used:

All tools were piloted with midwives/women attending University College Hospital, London.

Topics covered:

Care of the perineum.

Type of suturing.

Decision not to suture.

Advice given to women.

Action taken.

Women's perceptions of the care they received in relation to the perineum.

Women's perceptions of the effect of perineal trauma on specific postnatal problems.

Episiotomy rate.

Suturing rate.

Non-suturing rate.

Setting for data collection:

Community for proforma. Hospital for questionnaires.

Details about sample studied:

Planned size of sample:

120 women.

70 midwives.

Rationale for planned size:

All midwives practising in a certain catchment area (Whittington Hospital).

Entry criteria:

Midwives - practising in the Whittington Hospitals catchment area. Women - cared for by these midwives having a first or second degree perineal tear or episiotomy; a singleton cephalic presentation; at least 36 weeks gestation.

Sample selection:

Convenience.

Actual sample size:

106 women.

110 midwives invited to participate.

70 responded.

Response rate:

Recruitment ongoing for women.

Midwives - 64%

Interventions, Outcomes and Analysis:

Analysis:

Simple statistics (eg frequencies and percentages).

Turner's nine stage framework for qualitative analysis.

Keywords: AUDIT, EXPERIENCE (WOMEN'S), PERINEAL AUDIT SYSTEM, PERINEAL TRAUMA, PERINEUM, SEXUAL INTERCOURSE

234. ECONOMIC ASPECTS OF CARE OF WOMEN DURING NORMAL LABOUR

September 1986 - October 1994

Miranda Mugford, Economist, Gerard Breart, Director, Inserm, James Thornton, Senior Lecturer in Obstetrics, Ethel Burns, Midwifery Lecturer Practitioner, Najoua Mlika-Cabanne, Epidemiology Researcher, Shane Kavanagh, Student. **Contact:** Miranda Mugford, National Perinatal Epidemiology Unit, Radcliffe Infirmary, Oxford OX2 6HE. Tel: 0865 224187

Funded as integral or additional part of a job by Department of Health.

Aims of the study: To determine how different policies for care of women during labour affect the cost of care.

Ethics committee approval gained: Yes

Research design: Descriptive – Secondary use of Experimental data – Quantitative Survey/Cost Effectiveness Evaluation

Data collection:
Techniques used:
Interviews with clinicians (midwives) to establish important resources.

Observational data collected:

1. By midwives during provision of care on data collection forms specially designed for the study.

2. By survey of senior labour ward midwives.

Time data were collected:
Prospectively for provision of care during labour.

Outcome data from RCTs - up to 3 months retrospectively.

Testing of any tools used:
Survey of labour ward midwives was piloted.

Topics covered:
Staff input to procedures during labour.

Overall staffing in the labour ward.

Materials and equipment used for procedures during labour.

Cost-effectiveness evaluation will be of:

1. Early versus delayed rupture of the membranes.

2. Continuous presence of a midwife with a woman in labour.

3. Routine use of electronic fetal monitoring.

Labour ward resource use.

Women's health outcomes.

Setting for data collection:
Hospital labour wards.

Details about sample studied:
Planned size of sample:
Survey: 21 hospital and maternity departments participating in the

European trial.

Observation: all women admitted to the labour ward for consultant obstetric care over a 2 week period, estimated to be about 180.

Rationale for planned size:

Units involved in randomized controlled trials;

1. Set by collaboration in European trial.

2. Observation - pilot study, to allow sufficient numbers of unusual procedures to be included.

Entry criteria:

Survey: all 21 units taking part in the two European randomized controlled trials of alternative approaches to care during labour.

Sample selection:

Survey:

Convenience.

Determined by trial participation.

Observation:

Sufficient numbers of cases to include all procedures of interest.

Actual sample size:

Survey - 21 units.

Observational study - data were collected for 166 women who were admitted during the study period.

Response rate:

Survey - 100%

Observation - 92%

Interventions, Outcomes and Analysis:

Analysis:

Use of database and spreadsheet software (Reflex, Planperfect, Quattro-Pro).

T-test.

Chi-square.

Keywords: ARTIFICIAL RUPTURE OF THE MEMBRANES, COST EFFECTIVENESS, ECONOMIC EVALUATION, FETAL MONITORING (ELECTRONIC), LABOUR, MIDWIFE'S CARE

235. THE HINCHINGBROOKE THIRD STAGE TRIAL
April 1993 - August 1996

J Rogers, Midwife, J Wilson, Midwife, D Elbourne, Deputy Director Perinatal Trials Service, R McCandlish, Research Midwife, A Truesdale, Research Administrator. **Contact:** J Rogers, Carisbrooke Road, Cambridge CB4 3LP.

Funded by funding agency: Public Health and Operational Research Award and East Anglia Regional Health Authority.

Aims of the study: To determine whether in terms of maternal and neonatal morbidity, it is justifiable to continue with the current option of employing expectant rather than active management of the third stage of labour for women considered to be at low risk of postpartum haemorrhage (PPH) in a setting in which both managements are commonly practised.

The primary hypothesis is that the active management of the third stage of labour reduces the incidence of postpartum haemorrhage, even in a setting in which both expectant and active management are routinely practised for women thought to be at low risk of postpartum haemorrhage.

Ethics committee approval gained: Yes

Research design: Experimental – Qualitative and Quantitative – Randomized Controlled Trial

Data collection:
Techniques used:
Questionnaires.
Case note review.
Records of observation.
Time data were collected:
Immediately after delivery.
At transfer from hospital to home.
Six weeks postnatally.
Testing of any tools used:
Small pilot of questionnaires prior to trial.
Sample of Edinburgh postnatal depression scale scores used to validate part of 6 week questionnaire.
Topics covered:
Obstetric and medical history.
Delivery details.
Management of third stage: technique; timing; manual removal of placenta; estimated blood loss; side effects and use of oxytocics.
Postnatal maternal morbidity (anaemia, blood transfusion, iron therapy, ERPOC, positive Kleihauer test, fatigue, depression, feeding difficulties).
Neonatal jaundice treated with phototherapy.
Admission to SCBU.
Women's and staff views of participation in the trial.
Economic/resource outcomes.
Setting for data collection:
Maternity Unit in District General Hospital, rural and urban surgeries and mothers' homes.

Details about sample studied:
Planned size of sample:
2000
Rationale for planned size:
To reach statistical significance.

Entry criteria:

Inclusion: Women at low risk of post-partum haemorrhage.

Exclusion: placenta praevia; previous postpartum haemorrhage; APH after 20 weeks; gestation; haemoglobin <10 gdl or mean cell volume <75; multiple pregnancy; intrauterine death; epidural; parity >5; uterine fibroid; syntocinon infusion for induction/augmentation of labour; anti-coagulant therapy; instrumental/operative delivery; <32/40 gestation. Any other circumstances where the clinician feels there are overwhelming contra-indications to any of the forms of management.

Sample selection:

All eligible mothers.

With consent, randomized to one of four groups.

Actual sample size:

Recruitment ongoing.

Interventions, Outcomes and Analysis:

Interventions used:

Four management groups:

1. Active management, upright position.
2. Active management, semi-recumbent position.
3. Expectant management, upright position.
4. Expectant management, semi-recumbent position.

Active management = 1ml syntometrine, (usually 1M), with delivery of baby or 10iu syntocinon (usually 1M), if mother is hypertensive.

Main outcomes measured:

Postpartum haemorrhage rate.

Estimated blood loss.

Hb and MCV (32 weeks and day 2 postnatal).

Length of 3rd stage.

Manual removal of placenta.

Blood transfusion.

Maternal fatigue and depression.

Analysis:

SPSS

Keywords: ACTIVE MANAGEMENT, MATERNAL MORBIDITY, NEONATAL MORBIDITY, POSTPARTUM HAEMORRHAGE, THIRD STAGE

236. FOREST HEALTHCARE: EVALUATION OF MIDWIFERY GROUP PRACTICE

January 1993 - April 1994

B Bryans, Care Group Director (Women & Children), W Sykes, Research Consultant, B Lynch, Midwife Manager. **Contact:** W Sykes, Midhurst Avenue, London N10 3EP.

Funded as integral or additional part of a job by Regional Health Authority. 2-6 hours/week of own time spent.

Aims of the study: Evaluation of a pilot midwifery group practice providing continuity of carer to high and low risk women

Ethics committee approval gained: No

Research design: Descriptive/Experimental – Qualitative and Quantitative – Survey

Data collection:
Techniques used:
In depth interviews and group discussion.
Questionnaires.
Case note review/analysis.
Time data were collected:
Qualitative interviews - 6 months after start of pilot.
Questionnaires: 4-6 weeks postnatally.
Case notes: retrospective.
Testing of any tools used:
Questionnaires - piloted on small sample of women.
Topics covered:
Experience - antenatal, intrapartum and postnatal; continuity of carer;
clinical outcomes;
satisfaction - mothers' and midwives';
costs.
Setting for data collection:
Urban hospital and community.

Details about sample studied:
Planned size of sample:
280-300 in pilot scheme.
280-300 in control caseload.
Rationale for planned size:
8 midwives each with a caseload of 35 women.
Entry criteria:
Pilot scheme - all women attending four GP practices selected for proximity to the hospital and representativeness.
Control caseload - women attending GP practices covering similar population mix (ethnic, socio economic etc).
Sample selection:
GPs - purposive.
Actual sample size:
Recruitment ongoing.

Interventions, Outcomes and Analysis:
Interventions used:
For scheme: Midwives taking responsibility for case load.
Midwives working in hospital and community to provide continuity of carer throughout.

Main outcomes measured:
    Clinical outcomes.
    Satisfaction (women and midwives).
    Costs.
Analysis:
    SPSSx - questionnaires and medical records.

Keywords: CONSUMER SATISFACTION, CONTINUITY OF CARE, COST-BENEFIT ANALYSIS, EXPERIENCE (WOMEN'S), MIDWIFERY GROUP PRACTICE, MIDWIFERY UNIT, OUTCOMES (MATERNAL)

Sykes W. Forest Midwifery Group: Phase I Evaluation. Maternity Unit. Whipps Cross Hospital. Forest Healthcare Trust 1993.

237. INVESTIGATION OF ETHICAL DECISION MAKING BY MIDWIVES
September 1993 - ongoing
F M Telfer, Midwife Teacher. **Contact:** F M Telfer, Lincoln Circus, Nottingham NG7 1BG.
DETAILS TO BE CONFIRMED.

238. RANDOMIZED CONTROLLED TRIAL MEASURING THE EFFECTS ON LABOUR OF OFFERING A LIGHT, LOW FAT DIET
February - July 1992
Katie Yiannouzis, Midwife Teacher, Christopher Parnell, Consultant Anaesthetist. **Contact:** Katie Yiannouzis, Midwife Teacher, Department of Nursing and Midwifery, Christchurch College, Canterbury CT1 1QU. Tel: 0227 767700 Ex 622

Funded as integral or additional part of a job by employer: Medway Health Authority. 2-6 hours/week of own time spent.

Aims of the study: To test the hypothesis that labour outcomes would be improved if women were offered nourishment during labour.

Ethics committee approval gained: Yes

Research design: Experimental – Quantitative – Randomized Controlled Trial

    Data collection:
        Techniques used:
            Labour ward records.
        Time data were collected:
            At end of labour.
        Testing of any tools used:
            No.

Topics covered:
Mother - consumption of food and drink; vomiting; need for syntocinon; pain relief; type of delivery; length of labour.
Baby - need for admission to SCBU/TCU; Apgar scores.

Setting for data collection:
Consultant unit serving mixed urban and rural population.

Details about sample studied:

Planned size of sample:
297

Rationale for planned size:
Convenience sample.

Entry criteria:
All women admitted to delivery suite who were of 34 weeks gestation or more, with a single fetus, cephalic presentation, who had not had a previous Caesarean Section and were not at greater risk of Caesarean Section than the general pregnant population.

Sample selection:
Random allocation to study group or control group.

Actual sample size:
297
154 in study group.
143 controls.

Response rate:
Unknown.

Interventions, Outcomes and Analysis:

Interventions used:
Study group offered light low fat diet during labour. Food taken was as much as women desired, as often as they wished for duration of labour.

Main outcomes measured:
1. Requirement for syntocinon.
2. Pain relief.
3. Length of labour.
4. Type of delivery.
5. Vomiting.
6. Apgar scores of babies.
7. Admission to SCBU or TCU.

Analysis:
For all outcome measures, except the length of labour - Chi-square test. For the length of labour - t-test.

Results: Four women in the study group required Caesarean Section, three of which were performed under general anaesthesia with no adverse outcomes.

Observations of women in the study group suggest that most do not crave large amounts of food especially when in active labour. However, some women in this study were already in active/advanced labour on admission. Whatever they had eaten at home might have had an impact on labour outcomes.

There were no statistical differences between the two groups in the outcomes of labour except in the occurrence of vomiting and in the length of labour. Women in the study group were twice as likely to vomit as those in the control (chi^2 = 6.069 P = 0.05).

Vomiting is an extremely common feature of labour. Some women commented that vomiting is less unpleasant if the stomach is not empty.

With regard to the length of labour the mean in the study group was one hour and 34 minutes longer than in the controls (P = 0.05).

The increased length of labour may not have been perceived as totally negative for the women in the study group. Comments applauded the availability of choice and the improvement in the social context of labour when food was offered.

The hypothesis therefore was not proven.

Recommendations for further research: A study of the types and quantities of food women choose to eat in 24 hours prior to delivery.

Keywords: DIET (LOW FAT), FASTING, HYDRATION (LABOUR), LABOUR, NUTRITION (LABOUR), OUTCOMES, VOMITING

239. PRELIMINARY EVALUATION OF HYDROTHERAPY IN LABOUR, USING HARD INDICATORS
December 1989 - January 1994

Dianne Garland, Senior Midwife Practice and Research, Keith Jones, Honorary Research Fellow. **Contact:** Dianne Garland, Maidstone Hospital, Hermitage Lane, Maidstone, Kent ME16 9QQ. Tel: 0622 729000 X 4421

Funded as integral or additional part of a job by employer: Maidstone Hospital.

Aims of the study: To compare three groups of women in 'normal' labour:-
a) those who did not use hydrotherapy.
b) those who used hydrotherapy during labour but left the water prior to delivery.
c) those who delivered in water.

Ethics committee approval gained: No

Research design: Descriptive – Qualitative and Quantitative – Retrospective Analysis of Activity Data

    Data collection:
        Techniques used:
            Extraction of data from daily activity records in delivery suite.
        Time data were collected:
            Retrospectively.
        Testing of any tools used:
            No special tools used.
        Topics covered:
            Use of drugs.
            Instrumental delivery.

Operative delivery.
Duration of labour.
Naturally occurring genital trauma.
Post-partum haemorrhage.
Setting for data collection:
Hospital maternity department.

Details about sample studied:
Planned size of sample:
600 (200 in each of the three groups).
Rationale for planned size:
Availability of information on waterbirths.
Entry criteria:
More than 37 weeks gestation.
Singleton.
Cephalic presentation.
No known or envisaged problems.
Sample selection:
Convenience.
Actual sample size:
600 (200 in each of the three groups)

Interventions, Outcomes and Analysis:
Analysis:
SPSS SYSTAT

Results: Details to be confirmed.

Keywords: HYDROTHERAPY, LABOUR, WATER BIRTH

241. AN EVALUATION OF THE BREAST FEEDING SUPPORT GROUP AT QUEEN CHARLOTTE'S AND CHELSEA HOSPITAL
October 1991 - June 1992
J Andrews, Midwifery Sister, V T Dugbartey, Infant Feeding Specialist. **Contact:** J Andrews, Twining Avenue, Twickenham, Middlesex TW2 5LP.

Formed part of a course. 2 hours/week of own time spent.

Aims of the study: To evaluate the breastfeeding support group run by the Queen Charlotte's and Chelsea Hospital.
Ethics committee approval gained: Yes

Research design: Descriptive – Qualitative – Survey

Data collection:
Techniques used:
Questionnaires

Time data were collected:
2 days - 3 months after the commencement of breastfeeding.
Testing of any tools used:
Questionnaires were piloted with 5 mothers.
Topics covered:
Demographic details.
Clients' opinions of the benefits derived from the group.
Setting for data collection:
Hospital.

Details about sample studied:
Planned size of sample:
50
Rationale for planned size:
Advised sufficient to give adequate response.
Entry criteria:
All members of the group were breastfeeding mothers who attended the support group based at the hospital and co-ordinated by the infant feeding specialist working there.
Sample selection:
Randomly.
Actual sample size:
50
Response rate:
84%

Interventions, Outcomes and Analysis:
Analysis:
Content analysis.

Results: Not yet available.

Keywords: BREASTFEEDING, BREASTFEEDING (SUPPORT), CONSUMER SATISFACTION, POSTNATAL SUPPORT, SUPPORT GROUPS

242. PROSTAGLANDIN INDUCTION: A RANDOMIZED CONTROLLED TRIAL

June 1993 - June 1994
Ethel Burns, Lecturer Practitioner, Ian Z MacKenzie, Clinical Reader. **Contact:** Ethel Burns, Delivery Suite, John Radcliffe Hospital, Headley Way, Headington. Tel: 0865 221988/7

Funded as integral or additional part of a job. 2-6 hours/week of own time spent.

Aims of the study: To compare the effect of single versus repeat vaginal prostaglandin gel E2 to induce labour.

Ethics committee approval gained: Yes

Research design: Experimental – Qualitative and Quantitative – Randomized Controlled Trial

    Data collection:
        Techniques used:
            Questionnaires.
        Time data were collected:
            Contemporaneously with each case.
        Testing of any tools used:
            No.
        Topics covered:
            Mother:
            Obstetric history.
            Augmentation of labour.
            Monitoring.
            Vaginal examinations.
            Pain relief.
            Type of delivery.
            Perineal trauma.
            Length of labour.
            Baby:
            Apgar score.
            Weight.
            Transfer to SCBU.
        Setting for data collection:
            Delivery suite - hospital.

    Details about sample studied:
        Planned size of sample:
            1000 women and babies
        Rationale for planned size:
            Power statistics.
        Entry criteria:
            Inclusion: women scheduled for induction of labour.
            Exclusion: high risk eg marked IUGR, diabetes, high blood pressure and pre-eclampsia.
        Sample selection:
            Women are randomly allocated to a group.
        Actual sample size:
            Recruitment ongoing.

    Interventions, Outcomes and Analysis:
        Interventions used:
            Women given vaginal prostaglandin a) single gel b) repeat gel.
        Main outcomes measured:
            Length of labour.

Length of time on delivery suite.
Baby outcomes.
Analysis:
Not yet undertaken.

Keywords: LABOUR, LABOUR (INDUCTION), PROSTAGLANDIN E2

243. AN OBSERVATIONAL STUDY ON THE EFFECT OF THE TECHNIQUE "MOXIBUSTION FOR BREECH PRESENTATION" ON MOTHER AND FETUS
July 1992 - August 1993
Sarah Budd, Midwifery Sister/Acupuncturist, Keith Greene, Clinical Director and Consultant Obstetrician, Karl Rosen, Dean of Post-Graduate Medical Centre, Rekha Shesthra, Registrar, Paul Dubbins, Consultant in Ultrasound, Sharon Yelland, Midwifery Sister/ Acupuncturist. **Contact:** Sarah Budd, Maternity Unit, Derriford Hospital, Plymouth, Devon. Tel: 0752 763689/777111

Funded as integral or additional part of a job by employer. Additional funding by J Scarborough & Sons. Formed part of a course. 2 hours/week of own time spent.

Aims of the study: To show what effect the technique "moxibustion" has on mother and fetus which may explain the apparent increase in spontaneous version of breech presentation fetuses with this technique.

Ethics committee approval gained: Yes

Research design: Experimental – Qualitative and Quantitative – Serial, observational Study

Data collection:
Techniques used:
Records of observation - video tape of ultrasound scan, CTG recording
Time data were collected:
During the 34th week of pregnancy.
Testing of any tools used:
Maternal record of fetal movements on "kick chart" before intervention.
Topics covered:
Fetal movement.
Fetal heart pattern.
Fetal behaviour.
Changes in maternal observations.
Maternal BP.
Pulse.
Blood-sugar level.

Setting for data collection:
Hospital Maternity Unit.

Details about sample studied:
Planned size of sample:
10
Rationale for planned size:
Based on statistical advice.
Pilot study.
Entry criteria:
Inclusion: primigrivid and multigravid women in 34th week gestation of pregnancy booked to deliver in Plymouth Health District.
Exclusion: Those women with the following conditions:
1. Placenta previa.
2. History of ante partum haemorrhage.
3. Multiple pregnancy.
4. Known abnormality of uterus or pelvis.
5. History of premature labour and premature rupture of membranes.
6. Previous Caesarean Section.
7. Oligohydramnios.
8. Rhesus antibodies.
9. Known hydrocephalic fetus.
10. Patients on drug therapy eg betablockers, betamemetics etc.
Sample selection:
Convenience.
Actual sample size:
Recruitment ongoing.

Interventions, Outcomes and Analysis:
Interventions used: "Moxibustion" - a Chinese medical technique which involves heating specific acupuncture points on the feet using a herb "artemesia vulgaris" or mugwort ("moxa") for 15 minutes daily at 34 weeks gestation up to 10 times. Treatment stops when version has been achieved.
Main outcomes measured:
Changes in fetal heart rate and pattern.
Changes in fetal breathing and limb movements on ultrasound scan.
Changes in maternal observation.
Analysis:
Observational difference on fetal movement charts and ultrasound scans.

Results: Not yet available.

Keywords: BREECH PRESENTATION, COMPLEMENTARY THERAPIES, MOXIBUSTION

244. A COMPARATIVE STUDY ON TREATMENT VERSUS NON TREATMENT OF THE UMBILICAL CORD

January - April 1993

C Bradshaw, Midwifery Sister. **Contact:** C Bradshaw, Brownswood Road, Finsbury Park, London N4 2XP.

Formed part of a course. Over 20 hours/week of own time spent. Funded by employer and by funding agency(ies): Hospital Savings Association Scholarship and St Bartholomew's Hospital.

Aims of the study: To test the hypothesis: the use of sterzac hexachlorophane powder in combination with alcohol swabs would cause delay in umbilical cord separation and healing, until day 10 postpartum or later, when compared to no routine treatment of the cord other than general hygiene measures.

Ethics committee approval gained: Yes

Research design: Experimental – Quantitative – Randomized Controlled Trial

> **Data collection:**
>> **Techniques used:**
>>> Data collection sheets completed daily by the midwives.
>> **Time data were collected:**
>>> Immediately following delivery and until the umbilical cord had completely separated and healed.
>> **Testing of any tools used:**
>>> Data collection sheet was a modified version of the one used by Mugford and colleagues (1986) in the West Berkshire Cord Trial. A two week pilot study was also undertaken.
>> **Topics covered:**
>>> Maternal age.
>>> Maternal ethnic group.
>>> Baby's sex.
>>> Birthweight.
>>> Type of delivery.
>>> Day of hollister clamp removal.
>>> Condition of cord on daily basis (eg, dry, sticky, moist, infected).
>>> Day of cord separation.
>>> Treatment given to the cord.
>> **Setting for data collection:**
>>> Inner city setting (hospital and community).

> **Details about sample studied:**
>> **Planned size of sample:**
>>> 396
>> **Rationale for planned size:**
>>> Based on a pre-trial audit of cord separation times and to be 90% sure of a statistically significant difference at the 5% level (2 tailed test), required 198 babies in each treatment group.

Entry criteria:

Babies of 37 weeks gestation or more.

Birthweight of 2.4kg or more.

Apgar of 8 or more at 5 minutes.

Clinically well babies.

Informed parental consent.

Sample selection:

Babies delivered concurrently - April 1993.

Actual sample size:

396

Response rate:

96% (388)

Interventions, Outcomes and Analysis:

Interventions used:

Babies were randomly allocated to one of two treatments:

a) No routine treatment to the cord unless soiled. If soiled the cord was cleaned with warm tap water and dried with cotton wool (intervention).

b) The cord was cleaned with alcohol swabs and dusted with hexachlorophane (sterzac) powder at each napkin change (conventional cord care policy).

Main outcomes measured:

Day of cord separation and healing.

The number of visits required by the midwife beyond the 10th postpartum day, according to treatment group.

Infection rates.

Analysis:

SAS Statistical system.

Tests used:

2 tailed test;

Chi-square test;

Student t-test;

Fishers Exact test.

Results: The two groups were comparable in terms of maternal age, birthweight, sex, mode of delivery and maternal ethnic group. No significant difference in cord separation and healing was found between the two treatment groups ($p > 0.2$).

Other observations:

1. A significant relationship was found between day of cord clamp removal and day of cord separation. Where the cord clamp was removed on or before day 2, the cord was more likely to separate on or before day 10 ($p < 0.05$).

2. The cords of babies delivered by Caesarean Section (39) took significantly longer to separate than babies delivered vaginally regardless of treatment group ($p < 0.001$).

Recommendations for further research: 1. To test the effects of other common cord treatments in use and "non treatment" on cord separation and healing.

2. Exploration of delayed cord separation associated with Caesarean Section.

Keywords: CORD CARE, CORD HEALING, CORD SEPARATION, HEXACHLO-
ROPHANE POWDER, STERZAC, UMBILICAL CORD

245. EVALUATION OF ONE TO ONE MIDWIFERY PRACTICE
October 1993 - September 1996
Lesley Page, Professor of Midwifery, Agneta S Bridges, Midwifery Research Fellow,
Richard Lilford, Professor of Obstetrics and Gynaecology, James Piercy, Research Fellow, Ruth Wilkins, Research Adviser, Trudy Stevens, Research Associate, Sarah Beake,
Project Assistant. **Contact:** Agneta S Bridges, Queen Charlotte's and Chelsea Hospital,
Goldhawk Road, London W6 OXG. Tel: 081 748 4666 Ex 5131
For full details see under Management Studies (Record No. 245).

246. DOUBLE BLIND PROSPECTIVE STUDY OF THE EFFECT OF GAMMA LINOLENIC ACID IN THE MANAGEMENT OF POSTNATAL DEPRESSION
February 1992 - February 1994
Gail Chapman, Research Midwife, John Cox, Professor of Psychiatry, Shaughn O'Brien,
Professor of Obstetrics & Gynaecology. **Contact:** Gail Chapman, North Staffs Maternity Hospital, Hilton Road Sciences, Harpfields, Stoke on Trent ST4 6SD. Tel: 0782
718449/472

Funded as integral or additional part of a job, and by funding agency: Scotia Pharmaceuticals Ltd.

Aims of the study: To test the hypothesis that gamma linolenic acid (GLA - Evening
Primrose Oil) will reduce severe postnatal blues and postnatal depression.

Ethics committee approval gained: Yes

Research design: Experimental – Quantitative – Double Blind Prospective Study.

> **Data collection:**
> > **Techniques used:**
> > > Self report questionnaires.
> > > Interviews.
> > **Time data were collected:**
> > > 38 weeks gestation.
> > > 2, 6 and 26 weeks postnatally.
> > **Testing of any tools used:**
> > > EPQ (Eysenyck's Personality Quotient).
> > > EPDS (Edinburgh Postnatal Depression Scale).
> > > Kennerly and Gath Maternity Blues Questionnaire.
> > > Visual analogue scale.
> > > Standard Psychiatric interview.
> > **Topics covered:**
> > > Postnatal blues.

Personality.
Postnatal depression.
Depression diagnosis.
Setting for data collection:
Community.
Recruitment in hospital ANC.

Details about sample studied:
Planned size of sample:
120
Rationale for planned size:
Time allowed.
Entry criteria:
Inclusion: Understanding the English Language.
Exclusion: Known epileptics.
Sample selection:
Convenience.
Actual sample size:
Recruitment ongoing.

Interventions, Outcomes and Analysis:
Interventions used:
8 capsules a day for 14 weeks commencing at 38 weeks gestation.
Two groups:
1. Evening Primrose Oil.
2. Sunflower Oil.
Main outcomes measured:
Postnatal "Blues" and depression rate in both groups.
Analysis:
NCSS statistics package.

Keywords: COMPLEMENTARY THERAPIES, EVENING PRIMROSE OIL, GAMMA LI-NOLENIC ACID, POSTNATAL DEPRESSION

247. DOES MENSTRUAL CYCLE AFFECT THE EDINBURGH POSTNATAL DEPRESSION SCALE SCORE?
February - July 1993

Gail Chapman, Research Midwife, Carol Henshaw, Research Fellow, John Cox, Professor of Psychiatry, Shaughn O'Brien, Professor of Obstetric and Gynaecology, Imad Abukhalil, Research Fellow. **Contact:** Gail Chapman, North Staffs Maternity Hospital, Hilton Road Sciences, Harpfields, Stoke on Trent ST4 6SD. Tel: 0782 718449/472

Funded as integral or additional part of a job.

Aims of the study: To determine whether the Edinburgh Postnatal Depression Scale score is affected by the menstrual cycle and whether it has relevance in the clinical practice of midwives.

Ethics committee approval gained: Yes

Research design: Descriptive – Quantitative – Survey

Data collection:
    Techniques used:
        Daily self report questionnaires.
    Time data were collected:
        For 2 months luteal and follicular phases.
    Testing of any tools used:
        Moos Menstrual Distress Questionnaire used.
    Topics covered: Menstrual cycle.
        Postnatal depression.
    Setting for data collection:
        Hospital based and home.

Details about sample studied:
    Planned size of sample:
        50
    Rationale for planned size:
        Availability of subjects.
    Entry criteria:
        Referred for pre-menstrual syndrome.
        Aged 18 or over.
    Sample selection:
        Convenience.
    Actual sample size:
        32
    Response rate:
        21 (65%)

Interventions, Outcomes and Analysis:
    Analysis:
        Statistical package - NCSS.
        Non parametric tests.
        Mann-Whitney Two sample (non matched) test.
        Descriptive statistics.

Results: Details to be confirmed.

Keywords: EDINBURGH POSTNATAL DEPRESSION SCALE, MENSTRUAL CYCLE, PRE-MENSTRUAL SYNDROME

248. WEST MIDLANDS REGIONAL HEALTH AUTHORITY - MIDWIVES' VENTOUSE EXTRACTION SURVEY

June - August 1993

Imad Abukhalil, Senior Registrar, Gail Chapman, Research Midwife, Madurima Rajkhowa, Research Fellow, Shaughn O'Brien, Professor of Obstetrics and Gynaecology. **Contact:** Gail Chapman, North Staffs Maternity Hospital, Hilton Road Sciences, Harpfields, Stoke on Trent ST4 6SD. Tel: 0782 718449/472

Funded as integral or additional part of a job.

Aims of the study: To explore the perceptions of consultants, senior registrars, senior midwives and labour ward managers in the West Midlands Regional Health Authorities in relation to midwives' performance of ventouse extractions.

Ethics committee approval gained: No

Research design: Descriptive – Quantitative – Survey

Data collection:
Techniques used:
Questionnaires.
Time data were collected:
Prospectively.
Testing of any tools used:
Questionnaires piloted with colleagues.
Topics covered:
Whether or not midwives are allowed to perform ventouse extraction.
Type of ventouse.
Indications.
Medico-legal aspects.
Setting for data collection:
Hospital.

Details about sample studied:
Planned size of sample:
235
Rationale for planned size:
Total population.
Entry criteria:
All consultants, senior registrars, senior midwives and labour ward managers working in West Midlands Regional Health Authority in 1993.
Sample selection:
Inclusive.
Actual sample size:
134

Response rate:
57%

Interventions, Outcomes and Analysis:
Analysis:
Microstar.
Fishers.
Hearns.

Results: Details to be confirmed.

Recommendations for further research: Pilot trial in selected centre(s) with specially trained midwives carrying out ventouse extractions.

Keywords: ASSISTED DELIVERY, LABOUR, MIDWIFE'S ROLE, MIDWIVES, STAFF ATTITUDES, VENTOUSE EXTRACTIONS

249. THE USE OR MISUSE OF THE EDINBURGH POSTNATAL DEPRESSION SCALE IN THE FIRST WEEK POSTPARTUM
February 1992 - January 1994
Gail Chapman, Research Midwife, John Cox, Professor of Psychiatry, Shaughn O'Brien, Professor of Obstetrics & Gynaecology, Carol Henshaw, Lecturer/Senior Registrar.
Contact: Gail Chapman, North Staffs Maternity Hospital, Hilton Road Sciences, Harpfields, Stoke on Trent ST4 6SD. Tel: 0782 718449/472

Funded as integral or additional part of a job.

Aims of the study: To validate the Edinburgh Postnatal Depression Scale against the Kennerley and Gath Maternity Blues Questionnaire during the first week postnatally.

Ethics committee approval gained: No

Research design: Descriptive – Quantitative – Survey
Data collection:
Techniques used:
Questionnaires.
Time data were collected:
Day 3, 5 and 8 postnatal.
Testing of any tools used:
Tools already validated.
Topics covered:
Postnatal blues and depression.
Setting for data collection:
Community and Hospital.

Details about sample studied:
 Planned size of sample:
  500
 Rationale for planned size:
  Collected from ongoing studies of 120 + 1000.
 Entry criteria:
  Understanding of written English.
 Sample selection:
  Convenience.
 Actual sample size:
  Recruitment ongoing.

 Interventions, Outcomes and Analysis:
  Analysis:
   NCSS

Keywords: EDINBURGH POSTNATAL DEPRESSION SCALE, POSTNATAL CARE, POST-NATAL DEPRESSION, PUERPERIUM

250. WOMEN'S PERCEPTIONS OF THE CARING ROLE OF THE MIDWIFE DURING CHILDBIRTH WITH REFERENCE TO THE EXPERIENCE OF PAIN

September 1992 - June 1993
L Choucri, Part time Midwife. **Contact:** L Choucri, Parkfield Drive, Triangle, Sowerby Bridge, West Yorks.

Formed part of a course. 12-20 hours/week of own time spent.

Aims of the study: To examine the subjectivity and the physical, emotional and cultural context of the birth experience within the prevailing model of care in one maternity unit.
The main objective: to examine the birth experience and the experience of midwife care as they are consciously lived through by women.

Ethics committee approval gained: Yes
Research design: Descriptive – Qualitative – Phenomenology

 Data collection:
  Techniques used:
   Taped interviews.
  Time data were collected:
   Three to six days postnatally.
  Topics covered:
   Women's experience of birth.
   Perception of the midwives' caring role.
   Women's expectations of midwives.
   Experience of pain in labour.

Setting for data collection:
Hospital.

Details about sample studied:
Planned size of sample:
10
Rationale for planned size:
Time and resource factors.
In depth nature of the data.
Entry criteria:
Primigravidae only.
Normal birth attended by a midwife in the hospital delivery suite.
Able to speak and understand English.
Sample selection:
Convenience.
Actual sample size:
7
Response rate:
100%

Interventions, Outcomes and Analysis:
Analysis:
Each transcript of the mother's descriptions of their birth experiences was analysed using Colaizzis (1978) phenomenological method involving conceptual labelling and sorting into themes.

Results: Six themes emerged from the data:
1. The sense of having "mastery" is essential to the woman's perception of a successful birth experience ie the woman feels that she is really giving birth in an active sense. The midwife attending each woman enabled or disabled the sense of mastery.
2. "Being with"/"Being there": Interaction between mother and midwife was paramount, authentic personal relationships, knowing women subjectively rather than as objects.
3. "Being valued as an individual"/"Being believed": Not demeaning each woman's need for help.
4. "The mind and body experiences a sense of fragmentation": A feeling of the mind being detached from the pain in the body.
5. "The value of involving significant others is viewed as a caring skill": Those midwives who used the support of the partner therapeutically to enhance the woman's ability to give birth were viewed as giving good care.
6. "The significance of the sensations of birth make the wholeness of the experience": The women spoke spontaneously regarding the uniqueness of the sensations of their baby moving through their pelvis towards birth.

Recommendations for further research: 1. Observational research on caring interactions between mothers and midwives.
2. Clarification by midwives of caring skills in order to enhance midwifery practice.
3. Further exploration of the concept of "mastery" in order that midwives and women

may plan care based on concept of control of decision making, taking responsibility, encouragement of self esteem needs and choices of care.

Keywords: COMMUNICATION, EXPERIENCE (WOMEN'S), LABOUR, MASTERY, MID-WIFE'S ROLE, MIDWIFE-MOTHER RELATIONSHIP, PAIN, PERCEPTIONS OF CHILD-BIRTH (WOMEN'S)

251. AN ASSESSMENT OF ANTENATAL CARE IN TOWER HAMLETS
January 1989 - July 1991
Ruth Cochrane, Part time Senior Registrar, Wendy Savage, Consultant. **Contact:** Ruth Cochrane, Department of Obstetrics and Gynaecology, St Mary's Hospital, Praed Street, London W2. Tel: 071 725 6666

Funded as integral or additional part of a job and by funding agency: Womanschoice. 2-6 hours/week of own time spent.

Aims of the study: To assess women's expectations and experiences of antenatal care in Tower Hamlets and to ascertain whether community based antenatal care should be offered on a wider scale where practicable.

Ethics committee approval gained: Yes

Research design: Descriptive – Qualitative and Quantitative – Survey

> **Data collection:**
> > **Techniques used:**
> > > Questionnaires.
> > **Time data were collected:**
> > > 16-20 weeks antenatally.
> > > 1-2 days postnatally.
> > **Testing of any tools used:**
> > > Pilot study carried out for both antenatal and postnatal question-naires.
> > **Topics covered:**
> > > All aspects of antenatal care.
> > **Setting for data collection:**
> > > Hospital antenatal clinics.
> > > Community antenatal clinics.
> > > GPs surgeries.
> > > Postnatal wards.

> **Details about sample studied:**
> > **Planned size of sample:**
> > > 2000
> > **Rationale for planned size:**
> > > All English speaking Tower Hamlets residents booking over 1 year.

Entry criteria:
> *Exclusion:* non-English speakers, late bookers.

Sample selection:
> Convenience - depending on access to clinics.

Actual sample size:
> 955 (Reduced for logistical reasons).

Response rate:
> 100%

Interventions, Outcomes and Analysis:
> **Analysis:**
>> SPSS-PC
>> Biomedical Data Programmes.
>> Chi-square.
>> Logistical regression.

Results: Women were studied in the light of the experience they had. Although the groups were not numerically equivalent, they were comparable in terms of their demographic characteristics.

Women were most satisfied with community based antenatal care compared with hospital based care or shared care. Reasons for this were that they valued the continuity of people and felt better able to communicate with the community staff. Obstetric outcomes did not differ for the 3 main types of care except that the community based women had less pre-term deliveries and low birth weight babies (p <0.05).

Recommendations for further research: Similar study in Tower Hamlets Bangladeshi community.

Keywords: ANTENATAL CARE, COMMUNITY CARE, CONSUMER SATISFACTION, EXPECTATIONS (WOMEN'S), EXPERIENCE (WOMEN'S)

Cochrane R. An assessment of antenatal care in Tower Hamlets. Journal of Advances in Health and Nursing Care (details not confirmed).
Cochrane R. An assessment of antenatal care in Tower Hamlets. In: McKie L (ed). Researching Women's Health. Quay Publishing (details not confirmed).

252. BATH ADDITIVE TRIAL
January 1990 - June 1991
S Cornwell, Midwifery Sister, A Dale, Midwifery Sister. Contact: A Dale, Green Leys, St Ives, Cambridgeshire PE17 4SB.

Funded as integral or additional part of a job by East Anglian Regional Health Authority. 2 hours/week of own time spent.

Aims of the study: The role of Lavender Oil in relieving perineal discomfort following childbirth.

Ethics committee approval gained: Yes

Research design: Experimental – Qualitative and Quantitative – Randomized Controlled Trial

Data collection:
Techniques used:
Questionnaires, Visual Analogue Scale (VAS).
Time data were collected:
1-10 days postnatally.
Testing of any tools used:
Pilot study.
Topics covered:
Mood.
Discomfort.
Comments.
Setting for data collection:
Hospital and community

Details about sample studied:
Planned size of sample:
636
Rationale for planned size:
120 women in each of these groups.
Even distribution of variables.
Entry criteria:
Inclusion: All women with perineal damage following childbirth.
Exclusion:
Women with active skin disorders;
Women having stillbirths or sick neonates;
Women without baths at home;
Anyone not wishing to participate.
Sample selection:
Random self-selection of envelope containing bath additive bottle number.
Actual sample size:
360
Response rate:
60.8%

Interventions, Outcomes and Analysis:
Interventions used:
The women each had a bottle of bath additive:
1. pure Lavender Oil.
2. synthetic Lavender Oil.
3. placebo - distilled water containing 'GRAS' compound (smell).
They used 6 drops in a bath daily and half an hour later recorded their mood and discomfort levels on a VAS scale.

> **Main outcomes measured:**
>> Mood.
>> Discomfort.
> **Analysis:**
>> SPSS/PC+ Version 3.1.
>> Analysis of variance.
>> Chi-square.

Results: No statistical difference was found, although the women using Lavender Oil as an additive showed lower mean discomfort scores on days three to five following childbirth. Also, those using the lavender made gratituous comments indicating that it was pleasant to use. No side effects at all were identified.

Recommendations for further research: Replication study to explore the effect of varying the amount of oil used as an additive and/or the mode of application.

Keywords: AROMATHERAPY, BATH ADDITIVES, BATHING, COMPLEMENTARY THERAPIES, ESSENTIAL OILS, LAVENDER OIL, PERINEAL DISCOMFORT, PERINEUM, PUERPERIUM

Cornwell S. The role of lavender oil in relieving perineal discomfort following childbirth: a blind randomized clinical trial. Journal of Advanced Nursing 1994;19:89-96.

253. BREAST FEEDING SUPPORT GROUP IN HOSPITALS
April 1986 - June 1992
V T Dugbartey, Infant Feeding Specialist (Midwife). **Contact:** V T Dugbartey, Longstone Avenue, Harlesden, London NW10 3UD. Tel: 081 740 3580 (W)

Formed part of a course. 2 hours/week of own time spent. Funded by employer: Queen Charlotte's and Chelsea Hospital.

Aims of the study: To assess the effect on women's breast feeding of continuing support with particular reference to the problems encountered, advice given and the attitudes of health professionals.
Ethics committee approval gained: Yes

Research design: Descriptive – Qualitative – Survey

> **Data collection:**
>> **Techniques used:**
>>> Questionnaires.
>>> Interviews.
>>> Discussions.
>> **Time data were collected:**
>>> Within the first 5 days post delivery.
>> **Testing of any tools used:**
>>> Tested with 5 women.

Topics covered:
> Personal feelings of clients.
> Clients' opinions of the support system.
> Participation in the study and survey.
> How services could be improved.

Setting for data collection:
> Hospital.

Details about sample studied:
Planned size of sample:
> 50 (25 primipara, 25 multipara).

Rationale for planned size:
> Time constraints.

Entry criteria:
> No exclusions.

Sample selection:
> Random.

Actual sample size:
> 50

Response rate:
> 100%

Interventions, Outcomes and Analysis:
Analysis:
> Simple frequencies.

Results: Many mothers felt they were obtaining needed information but midwifery staff were perceived as lacking time to assist with breast feeding. 44% felt they had received conflicting advice and 96% wished for a more individualised approach. There was a consensus view that first-time mothers would benefit from a support group in the first postnatal days to discuss breast feeding and gain reassurance.

Keywords: BREASTFEEDING, BREASTFEEDING (SUPPORT), CONSUMER SATISFACTION, POSTNATAL SUPPORT, SUPPORT GROUPS

255. THE ANTENATAL CARE PROJECT: A RANDOMIZED CONTROLLED TRIAL OF A REDUCTION IN THE NUMBER OF ROUTINE ANTENATAL VISITS FOR LOW RISK WOMEN
February 1993 - August 1995
Jim Sikorski, Honorary Research Fellow, Jenny Fleming, Research Midwife, Sarah Fields, Research Midwife, Sarah Clement, Research Fellow. **Contact:** Jenny Fleming, The Antenatal Care Project, Dept of General Practice UMDS, Guy's Campus, St Thomas' Street, London Bridge London SE1 9RT. Tel: 071 955 5000 Ex 3159

Funded as integral or additional part of a job and by funding agency(ies): Primary Care Development Fund, Lambeth Southwark and Lewisham FHSA.

Aims of the study: To assess the acceptability and clinical and psychosocial effectiveness of a reduction in the number of routine antenatal visits for low risk women.

Ethics committee approval gained: Yes

Research design: Experimental – Qualitative and Quantitative – Survey/Randomized Controlled Trial

> **Data collection:**
> > **Techniques used:**
> > > Case note review.
> > > Questionnaires - health care professionals, mothers.
> > **Time data were collected:**
> > > Case note review - retrospectively.
> > > Questionnaires - for health care professionals at start of project and approximately one year later;
> > > - for mothers at 35 weeks gestation and 6 weeks postnatally.
> > **Testing of any tools used:**
> > > Questionnaires to be piloted.
> > **Topics covered:**
> > > Maternal satisfaction.
> > > Emotional wellbeing (Edinburgh Postnatal Depression Scale).
> > > Maternal fetal attachment (Attitudes towards pregnancy and baby scale).
> > > Locus of control.
> > > Worry (Cambridge Worry Scale).
> > **Setting for data collection:**
> > > Hospital and community.
>
> **Details about sample studied:**
> > **Planned size of sample:**
> > > 2800
> > **Rationale for planned size:**
> > > To detect an increase in the Caesarian Section rate for hypertensive disorders, from 1% to 2% in the intervention group (5% significance, 80% power).
> > **Entry criteria:**
> > > Women of less than 22 weeks gestation at booking;
> > > - who are registered with GPs of Lambeth, Lewisham and Southwark FHSA;
> > > - and are booked for delivery at Guy's, Lewisham or St Thomas's Hospitals;
> > > - and are not excluded by predefined medical/obstetric conditions ie are "low risk".
> > **Sample selection:**
> > > Inclusive.
> > **Actual sample size:**
> > > Recruitment ongoing.

Interventions, Outcomes and Analysis:
> **Interventions used:**
>> Women are randomly allocated to either:
>> - study group with a reduced antenatal visit schedule or
>> - control group with traditional antenatal visit schedule.
>
> **Main outcomes measured:**
>> Clinical outcomes for mother and baby.
>> Psychosocial outcomes.
>
> **Analysis:**
>> Yet to be finalised.
>> SPSS-PC to be used.

Keywords: ANTENATAL CARE, ANTENATAL CARE (FREQUENCY), CONSUMER SATISFACTION

257. PRIMIGAVIDAES' EXPERIENCE OF THE ANTENATAL BOOKING INTERVIEW
December 1992 - April 1993
U Kelly, Student Midwife. **Contact:** U Kelly, Drayton Bridge Road, Hanwell, London W7 1EX.

Formed part of a course. Funded by employer: King's College.

Aims of the study: The study focused on two main areas:
1. A replication of some of Methven's study (1989) looking specifically at the views of primigravidae in relation to their social circumstances.
2. The recommendations of the Health Committee's second report (1992) with questions related to consumer choice about carer and place of birth and whether the majority of consumers 'regard midwives as the group best placed to provide this care'.

Ethics committee approval gained: No

Research design: Descriptive – Qualitative and Quantitative – Survey
> **Data collection:**
>> **Techniques used:**
>>> Questionnaires.
>>
>> **Time data were collected:**
>>> 1-3 days following booking interview.
>>
>> **Testing of any tools used:**
>>> Questionnaires were piloted.
>>
>> **Topics covered:**
>>> Age.
>>> Marital status.
>>> Ethnic origin.
>>> Housing tenure.
>>> Educational attainment.
>>> Choice of carer.

Place of delivery.
Perceptions of the midwife.
Perceptions of midwife/client relationship.

Setting for data collection:
Hospital setting.

Details about sample studied:
Planned size of sample:
60
Rationale for planned size:
Financial and time constraints.
Entry criteria:
Primigravidae.
Sample selection:
A convenience sample taken from one hospital's booking list.
Actual sample size:
58
Response rate:
69%

Interventions, Outcomes and Analysis:
Analysis:
Minitab package
Cross tabulations.

Results: 1. The majority of respondents in the study were happy with the treatment they received in the antenatal booking interview. Unfamiliar words were explained, the interviewer listened and the majority of respondents felt free to ask questions. There were however no significant links between respondents' replies and their social circumstances except that women from ethnic minorities were more likely to feel free to ask questions.

2. The majority of respondents were happy with the relationship formed with the midwife, the speed at which the interview was conducted and the way in which the interview was brought to an end. However a significant minority indicated that they were not satisfied with these particular aspects of the antenatal booking interview.

3. 77.5% were happy with where they were booked. One hundred percent of respondents felt they did not have a choice of consultant. 60% of the respondents did not know whether they would have wanted someone else and 85% of the women did not know whether they could change consultants during pregnancy. The two women who felt they could not change consultants belonged to the Asian community. Education or other circumstances was not significantly linked to either choice of consultant or knowledge as to whether or not the consultant could be changed during pregnancy if desired.

4. 23 respondents replied that they would be happy for a midwife to provide all care supporting the Health Committees second report, para 49. However 10 respondents were equally emphatic that they would not be happy with such a situation and 7 were unsure. There was a link between respondents who were happy for a midwife to provide all care and the level of education. Those who left school at age 19 plus years were more likely to be happy with a midwife providing all care.

Recommendations for further research: 1. The women's perception of the consultant's role in relation to their maternity care.
2. Pregnant women's perception of the midwife's role. Do women see midwives as providing a supporting role to obstetricians or do they see them as capable of giving necessary supervision, care and advice to women during pregnancy, labour and the post partum period as defined by the WHO(1966)?

Keywords: ANTENATAL BOOKING INTERVIEW, ANTENATAL CARE, EXPERIENCE (WOMEN'S), PRIMIGRAVIDAE

260. FACILITATING INFORMED CHOICE IN CHILDBIRTH: A STUDY OF MIDWIVES AND THEIR CLIENTS
September 1993 - September 1997
Valerie A Levy, Principal Lecturer in Midwifery Studies. **Contact:** Valerie A Levy, IANE, Royal College of Nursing, 20 Cavendish Square, London. Tel: 071 409 3333

Formed part of a course. Funded as integral or additional part of a job by employer and funding agency: Smith and Nephew Foundation. 6-12 hours/week of own time spent.

Aims of the study: To investigate issues relating to informed decision making by women during pregnancy. Processes to be explored include:
a) midwives facilitating decision making;
b) women engaging in the processes of facilitation and decision making.

Ethics committee approval gained: Yes

Research design: Descriptive – Qualitative – Ethnography/Grounded Theory

    Data collection:
        Techniques used:
            Observation.
            Taped interviews.
        Time data were collected:
            Booking clinics and later in pregnancy.
        Setting for data collection:
            Hospital and community.

    Details about sample studied:
        Planned size of sample:
            Not planned as using grounded theory.
        Rationale for planned size:
            Theoretical sampling.
        Entry criteria:
            To be decided as study progresses.
        Sample selection:
            In line with emerging themes.

Actual sample size:
Recruitment ongoing.

Interventions, Outcomes and Analysis:
Analysis:
Constant comparative analysis.

Keywords: DECISION MAKING, INFORMATION GIVING, INFORMED CHOICE, PREG-NANCY

261. MIDWIVES' PERCEPTIONS OF WOMEN'S PAIN FOLLOWING CAESAREAN SECTION
October 1993 - July 1994
V M Lewis, Midwife Teacher. Contact: V M Lewis, Station Road, Hanwell, London W7 3JD.

Formed part of a course. 6-12 hours/week of own time spent.

Aims of the study: 1. To assess what priority is given by midwives to pain relief following emergency Caesarean Section.
2. To determine whether a dichotomy exists between midwifery and nursing care following Caesarean Section.

Ethics committee approval gained: No

Research design: Descriptive – Qualitative – Survey

Data collection:
Techniques used:
Interviews.
Time data were collected:
January - February 1994.
Testing of any tools used:
Plans - pilot study with two midwives.
Topics covered:
Perceptions of what influences pain.
Perceptions of need for pain relief.
Perceptions of effectiveness of pain relief.
Assessment of pain.
Setting for data collection:
Hospital post-natal ward.

Details about sample studied:
Planned size of sample:
10 Midwives
Rationale for planned size:
Time constraints.

Entry criteria:
> Qualified for 1 year or more.
> Experience of working in postnatal care.

Sample selection:
> Random selection.

Actual sample size:
> Recruitment ongoing.

Interventions, Outcomes and Analysis:
> **Analysis:**
> > Content analysis.

Keywords: CAESAREAN SECTION, PAIN, PAIN RELIEF (CAESAREAN SECTION), PER-CEPTIONS OF PAIN (MIDWIVES'), PERCEPTIONS OF PAIN (WOMEN'S)

264. MIDWIVES' AND OBSTETRICIANS' PERCEPTIONS OF WATERBIRTHS
March - June 1993
C Newton, Research Midwife, S Clarke, Midwife. **Contact:** C Newton, May Lodge Drive, Rufford Abbey Park, Newark NG21 9DE.

Funded as integral or additional part of a job by employer: City Hospital NHS Trust, University Hospital. 2-6 hours/week of own time spent.

Aims of the study: To determine the attitudes of midwives and obstetricians towards the use of water pools for labour and delivery.

Ethics committee approval gained: Yes

Research design: Descriptive – Qualitative – Survey

Data collection:
> **Techniques used:**
> > Questionnaires.
> **Time data were collected:**
> > March to April 1993.
> **Testing of any tools used:**
> > Questionnaires piloted with five people.
> **Topics covered:**
> > Midwives' attitudes and perceptions.
> > Obstetricians' attitudes and perceptions.
> > Water births.
> **Setting for data collection:**
> > Two hospitals.

Details about sample studied:
Planned size of sample:
258
Rationale for planned size:
Total population.
Entry criteria:
All midwives and obstetricians at both hospitals.
Sample selection:
Total population.
Actual sample size:
166
Response rate:
64%

Interventions, Outcomes and Analysis:
Analysis:
Manual.

Results: An overall 64% response rate was achieved, most of the respondents being F grade midwives. Night staff and obstetricians made up 10% each of the sample. The majority of the sample (72%) had cared for someone in the pool. Most respondents felt that women were well prepared for using the pool and that they would actively encourage anyone interested in having a waterbirth. However, opinion was divided about the timing of the use of water, with about half considering the woman should leave the pool for the second stage.

The major concerns of the sample related to obstetric emergency. Lack of experience, monitoring the fetal heart and neonatal outcome were other areas of concern. Lack of knowledge caused least anxiety in all categories of staff.

98% of respondents agreed that more research into the practicalities and management of waterbirths was necessary.

To improve the care of women labouring and choosing to deliver in water and also to ensure optimum safety for staff it has been suggested:

1. that an underwater sonicaid should be available.
2. workshops be held at each unit on a) back care for midwives, b) strategies for dealing with an obstetric emergency in water.
3. outcomes of waterbirths be carefully audited.
4. women's perceptions of the pool be studied.

Recommendations for further research: Ergonomics - a study of back care for midwives.
Neonatal outcomes for pool deliveries.

Keywords: DELIVERY, HYDROTHERAPY, PERCEPTIONS OF LABOUR (MIDWIVES'), PERCEPTIONS OF LABOUR (OBSTETRICIANS'), WATER BIRTH

266. THE EFFECTS OF A LOW HAEMOGLOBIN ON POSTNATAL WOMEN

May 1990 - February 1992

J A Paterson, Midwifery Sister, M Gregory, Staff Midwife, S J R Holt, Staff Midwife, A Jarrett, Information Officer, A Pachulski, Staff Midwife, D Stamford, Staff Midwife, J B Wothers, Staff Midwife. **Contact:** J A Paterson, Woodstock Road, Bedford MK40 4JY.

Funded as integral or additional part of a job. 2-6 hours/week of own time spent. Additional funding from Knapton Trust Fund for Research.

Aims of the study: To test the hypothesis that a low or reduced haemoglobin will adversely affect a mother's physical and mental state in the early postnatal period.

Ethics committee approval gained: Yes

Research design: Descriptive – Quantitative – Survey
  Data collection:
    Techniques used:
      Questionnaires.
      Case note review.
      Full blood count at 6 weeks post partum.
    Time data were collected:
      Retrospectively
      10 days, 4 weeks and 6 weeks postnatally
    Testing of any tools used:
      Edinburgh Postnatal Depression Scale already validated.
      Pilot study with sample of 250.
    Topics covered:
      Haemoglobin levels in pregnancy and through puerperium.
      Postnatal depression.
      Postnatal physical problems - fatigue, energy, breathlessness, faintness, pain, appetite.
      Iron therapy.
    Setting for data collection:
      Hospital and community.

  Details about sample studied:
    Planned size of sample:
      1000
    Rationale for planned size:
      Statistical basis
    Entry criteria:
      Exclusion:
      Mothers with:
      - existing psychiatric problems,
      - stillbirth,
      - baby remaining in hospital,
      - a hospital stay of more than 7 days.

Sample selection:
All admissions during study period.
Actual sample size:
1010
Response rate:
Response at 10 days - 909 (90%)
Complete dataset on 528 (52.3%)

Interventions, Outcomes and Analysis:
Analysis:
Lotus symphony 2.2 database.
Chi-square.

Results: 29.7% of participating women had a Hb level of less than 10.5gms/dcl on the 3rd postnatal day. Women with a Hb level below 10.5gms/dcl on third postnatal day are likely to:

be under 25 years old (chi^2 = 8.22, df=1, p=0.01)
be primiparous (chi^2=34.24, df=3, p=0.001)
have a low Hb at 34 weeks (chi^2=9.24, df=1, p=0.01)
not to have had a normal delivery (chi^2=47.76, df=2, p=0.0001)
have had a blood loss of more than 250mls at delivery (chi^2=85.73, df=2, p=0.001)
Mothers with a low Hb were slightly more likely to have a high Edinburgh Depression Score, but the relationship was not significant. A significant relationship was identified between a low Hb and breathlessness, faintness, low energy and painful sutures at 10 days post partum. This finding supports the hypothesis that a low Hb does adversely affect a mother's physical and mental state in the early postnatal period.

Recommendations for further research: Further examination of a possible link between postnatal depression and haemoglobin level.

Keywords: ANAEMIA, FATIGUE, HAEMOGLOBIN LEVELS, POSTNATAL CARE, POSTNATAL DEPRESSION, POSTNATAL HEALTH, PUERPERIUM

267. YOUNG MOTHERS' LEARNING THROUGH GROUP WORK: A DESCRIPTIVE STUDY

June 1989 - August 1990
A Rowe, Team Leader, P MacKeith, Midwife, R Phillipson, Midwife/Health Visitor.
Contact: R Phillipson, Cope Street, Hyson Green, Nottingham NG7 5AB.

Funded as integral or additional part of a job by employer: Nottingham Community Health. Addditional funding by The Kings Fund Institute. 2 hours/week of own time spent.

Aims of the study: 1. To describe the circumstances and health needs of young mothers.
2. To evaluate the effectiveness of group work with these young mothers.

Ethics committee approval gained: No

Research design: Descriptive – Qualitative – Case Study

Data collection:
Techniques used:
Interviews and retrospective analysis of data obtained in group work.
Time data were collected:
At point of contact and 6 months later.
Topics covered:
Circumstances of mothers.
Health needs.
Relationship with children.
Self confidence.
Self esteem.
Experience of group work.
Setting for data collection:
Community.

Details about sample studied:
Planned size of sample:
Data collected from June 1989 to August 1990.
Rationale for planned size:
Specific period of time.
Entry criteria:
Referrals from Health Visitor.
Attenders at "Cope Street".
16-25 years of age.
Living in the study area.
Had a child or pregnant.
Sample selection:
All who attended during study period.
Actual sample size:
48 first contact forms.
46 review forms.
46 end of group evaluation forms.
32 end of creche evaluation forms.

Interventions, Outcomes and Analysis:
Analysis:
Content analysis.

Results: The "Cope Street" service offers group work with an available creche. In addition one-to-one work sessions with a keyworker are offered.
Young mothers feel they benefitted from discussing their circumstances and health needs in group work. Where they felt their knowledge and skills were valued, they experienced increased self confidence and self esteem and a more positive relation-

ship with their children. The women learned from each other in the structured group work and valued the social contact. The quality of creche care was important to them. Written evaluations at the end of group sessions demonstrated that the women felt they learned more about children's needs and factors influencing health.

Keywords: ADOLESCENTS, COMMUNICATION, GROUP WORK, HEALTH EDUCA-TION, LEARNING ENVIRONMENT, SELF DIRECTED LEARNING, YOUNG MOTHERS

Billingham K. 45 Cope Street: working in partnership with parents. Health Visitor 1989;62.
Rowe A, MacKeith P. Is 'evaluation' a dirty word? Health Visitor 1991;64:292-3.
Rowe A. Cope Street revisited. Health Visitor 1993;66:358-9.
Rowe A, Billingham K. 45 Cope Street. Working with families in Poverty. 1992 In: Blackburn C (ed). Improving Health and Welfare Work with Families in Poverty. A Handbook. Open University Press, Section 6.
Miles M, Rowe A. Coping strategy. Nursing Times 1994;90:32-4.

268. THE TRIPLE TEST FOR SPINA BIFIDA AND DOWN'S SYNDROME - HOW WOMEN CHOOSE WHETHER OR NOT TO HAVE THE TEST
June 1993 - September 1994
M Stewart, Midwife. **Contact:** M Stewart, Stanley Avenue, St Andrews, Bristol BS7 9AH.

Formed part of a course. 6-12 hours/week of own time spent. Funded by funding agency: Tower Hamlets Education Trust.

Aims of the study: To investigate how women decide whether or not to have the triple test and to identify factors which may influence the decision.

Ethics committee approval gained: Yes

Research design: Descriptive – Qualitative – Survey
> **Data collection:**
>> **Techniques used:**
>>> Tape recorded semi-structured interviews.
>> **Time data were collected:**
>>> At approximately 19 weeks gestation ie. soon after the triple test has been offered.
>> **Testing of any tools used:**
>>> A small pilot study conducted.
>> **Topics covered:**
>>> Gestation.
>>> Parity.
>>> Whether or not the triple test has been offered.
>>> Where woman first heard about the test.
>>> For multiparous women only:
>>> - whether they have been offered test previously.

- what women know of test.
- whether they have had it and why.
- if they discussed test with anyone else.
- religious beliefs.
- women's age, occupation and marital status.

Setting for data collection:
In the women's homes, if possible. The catchment area is largely urban.

Details about sample studied:
Planned size of sample:
20 women.
Rationale for planned size:
Limitations of time.
Entry criteria:
Exclusion:
Non English speaking;
Women aged under sixteen at time of interview.
Sample selection:
Convenience.
Actual sample size:
Recruitment ongoing.

Interventions, Outcomes and Analysis:
Analysis:
Descriptive, using the principles of Agar (1986) - for language.
Znaniecki (1934) - for induction.
Glaser and Strauss (1967) - for theory development.

Keywords: CHOICE, DECISION MAKING, DOWN'S SYNDROME, EXPERIENCE (WOMEN'S), SPINA BIFIDA, TRIPLE TEST

271. EFFECT OF ANTENATAL PERINEAL MASSAGE ON THE INCIDENCE OF PERINEAL TRAUMA IN A NULLIPAROUS POPULATION
December 1992 - April 1995

M Shipman, Staff Midwife (Team Midwifery), K Taylor, Staff Midwife, F McCloghry, General Practitioner. **Contact:** M Shipman, Whippendell Road, Watford, Hertfordshire WD1 7QJ.

Funding under negotiation.

Aims of the study: 1. To provide analysis of perineal outcomes (defined as being intact and for 1 degree tears, or episiotomies and/or 2 degree or 3 degree tears) between those who performed antenatal perineal massage, and those who did not.
2. To analyse the outcomes in the experimental and control groups with regard to instrumental deliveries.

3. To test the hypothesis: that regular antenatal perineal massage in a nulliparous population reduces the incidence of spontaneous perineal trauma and episiotomies at delivery.

Ethics committee approval gained: Yes

Research design: Descriptive/Experimental – Qualitative and Quantitative – Randomized Controlled Trial

Data collection:
Techniques used:
1. Weekly record sheets.
2. Data collection forms.
3. Questionnaires.

Time data were collected:
1. Weekly record sheets - from 34/40 until delivery.
2. Data collection forms - completed following delivery.
3. Questionnaires - following delivery, prior to discharge home.

Testing of any tools used:
1. Information sheets, diagrams and instructions will be piloted with an antenatal class for comprehension.
2. Data collection forms will be piloted, by random selection of antenatal notes.
3. Questionnaires will be piloted with delivered nulliparous population.

Topics covered:
Perineal trauma.
Position in labour.
Perineal massage.
Instrumental delivery rates.

Setting for data collection:
Hospital and community.

Details about sample studied:
Planned size of sample:
616 total.
308 - experimental group.
308 - control group.

Rationale for planned size:
For 80% chance of observing significance, with reduction of 50% to 40% having 2nd degree tears/episiotomies.

Entry criteria:
Inclusion:
Nulliparae,
Singleton pregnancy,
30-32 weeks gestation.
Exclusion: (antenatally): Out of area women, poor English comprehension, known nut allergy, vaginal herpes.
Exclusions (at delivery):

Episiotomies for maternal indication - pre-eclampsia/maternal exhaustion.

Premature delivery less than 36/40 weeks.

Instrumental delivery.

Breech presentation and delivery.

Episiotomy for fetal distress/shoulder dystocia/OP delivery.

Medical delivery.

Intrauterine death.

Sample selection:

Random selection of hospital numbers, as registered on booking.

Allocated alternately to control and experimental group.

Actual sample size:

Recruitment not yet commenced.

Interventions, Outcomes and Analysis:

Interventions used:

Experimental group: antenatal perineal massage for last 6 weeks of pregnancy, at least four times a week for 5 minutes.

Both groups: pelvic floor exercises.

Main outcomes measured:

Perineal outcomes at delivery.

Analysis:

EGRET statistical package.

Chi-square.

Descriptive analysis.

Keywords: ANTENATAL CARE, EPISIOTOMY, OUTCOMES (PERINEAL), PERINEAL MASSAGE, PERINEAL TRAUMA, POSITIONS (DELIVERY)

272. RECENT DEVELOPMENTS IN MATERNITY CARE IN BRITAIN: TOWARDS A SOCIOLOGICAL PERSPECTIVE

September 1990 - September 1991

Jane Sandall, Postgraduate researcher. **Contact:** Jane Sandall, Department of Sociology, University of Surrey, Guildford, Surrey GU2 5XH. Tel: 0483 300800 Ex 2804

For full details see under Management Studies (Record No. 272).

273. CHOICE, CONTINUITY AND CONTROL? : SOCIOLOGICAL ASPECTS OF CONTINUITY OF MIDWIFERY CARE IN ENGLAND AND WALES

October 1993 - October 1996

Jane Sandall, Postgraduate Researcher, Sara Arber, Senior Lecturer, Hilary Thomas, Lecturer. **Contact:** Jane Sandall, Department of Sociology, University of Surrey, Guildford, Surrey GU2 5XH. Tel: 0483 300800 x2804

Over 20 hours/week of own time spent. Funded by funding agency(ies): NHS Management Executive, Department of Health Research Training Programme and Hospital Savings Association.

Aims of the study: 1. To place the current developments in maternity policy and practice in a historical, social and political context.

2. To examine the implications of a professionalisation process in midwifery for midwives and childbearing women.

3. To examine how organisational structures and outcomes influence midwives' practice in terms of occupational autonomy, job satisfaction and stress.

4. To examine the impact of providing continuity of care on midwives' professional and personal lives.

Ethics committee approval gained: No

Research design: Descriptive – Qualitative and Quantitative – Survey/Ethnography/ Case Study

Data collection:
    Techniques used:
        National questionnaire.
        Multiple site case studies.
    Time data were collected:
        April 1994 - October 1996.
    Testing of any tools used:
        To be piloted.
    Topics covered:
        Case studies:
        Midwives' decision making, job satisfaction/stress, occupational autonomy.
        Advantages and disadvantages of providing continuity of care and impact on personal and professional life.
        Professionalisation.
        Questionnaires: Role of midwife, job satisfaction/stress.
    Setting for data collection:
        Case studies: Midwifery practices in London, South East England.
        Questionnaires: Midwives throughout England and Wales.

Details about sample studied:
    Planned size of sample:
        Case studies:
        6 midwives in independent practice,
        6 midwives in group practice in NHS.
        6 community midwives attached to DGH and medical staff, managers, purchasers associated with them.
        Questionnaires: not yet calculated.
    Rationale for planned size:
        Case studies: Theoretical sampling.
        Questionnaires: Statistical grounds.
    Entry criteria:
        Case studies: All staff in each case.
        Questionnaires: Dependent on case studies results.

Sample selection:
Case studies: Theoretical.
Questionnaires: Random, 5% sample of RCM membership and IMA
Actual sample size:
Recruitment ongoing.

Interventions, Outcomes and Analysis:
Analysis:
SPSS PC.
Ethnograph.

Keywords: AUTONOMY, CONTINUITY OF CARE, EXPERIENCE (WOMEN'S), MID-WIFE'S ROLE, PROFESSIONALISM

274. AN EVALUATION OF THE USE OF TENS AS A METHOD OF PAIN RELIEF IN LABOUR
March 1993 - April 1994
R M Reece, District Nurse/Midwife. **Contact:** R M Reece, Eilean Rise, Ellon, Aberdeenshire AB41 9NF.

Formed part of a course. 6-12 hours/week of own time spent.

Aims of the study: 1. To determine demand and uptake of TENS against availability - potential use/ actual use.
2. To determine the effectiveness of TENS.
3. To review the literature regarding the use of TENS.
4. To evaluate the teaching programme on TENS.

Ethics committee approval gained: Yes

Research design: Descriptive – Qualitative and Quantitative – Evaluation.

Data collection:
Techniques used:
Questionnaires.
Time data were collected:
At 38 weeks of pregnancy.
During 1st postnatal week.
Testing of any tools used:
Questionnaire piloted.
Topics covered:
Effectiveness of TENS.
Expectations.
Adequacy of teaching.
Setting for data collection:
Community.

Details about sample studied:
    Planned size of sample:
        All users December to April in our area.
    Rationale for planned size:
        Total population.
    Entry criteria:
        All women using TENS.
    Sample selection:
        Convenience.
    Actual sample size:
        Recruitment ongoing.

Interventions, Outcomes and Analysis:
    Analysis: Not yet undertaken.

Keywords: LABOUR, PAIN RELIEF (LABOUR), TENS

275. CONTINUITY OF CARE FROM COMMUNITY MIDWIVES: A STUDY INTO THE PRESENT SATISFACTION AND FUTURE NEEDS OF WOMEN IN THE AMMAN VALLEY AREA
June 1992 - August 1993
Rose Marx, Community Midwife, Gwyneth R Isaac, Community Midwife, Ann D Jones, Community Midwife, Meinir Rowland, Community Midwife, Rosamund Bryar, Senior Lecturer Teamcare Valleys, Graham Clark, Health Sector Research. **Contact:** Rose Marx, Amman Valley Midwives, c/o Antenatal Clinic, Amman Valley Hospital, Glanamman, Ammanford Dyfed SA18 2BQ. Tel: 0269 822226

Funded as integral or additional part of a job by employer: and by funding agency: Teamcare Valleys.

Aims of the study: To look at the maternity service in the Amman Valley area, prior to implementing a team midwifery scheme, with reference to consumer satisfaction, needs and expectations and preferred choice for delivery.

Ethics committee approval gained: Yes

Research design: Descriptive – Quantitative and Qualitative – Survey

    Data collection:
        Techniques used:
            Self-completion questionnaires.
        Time data were collected:
            Antenatal sample: 25-40 weeks gestation.
            Postnatal sample: 2 months postnatally to 11 months postnatally.
        Testing of any tools used:
            Pilot questionnaire to 10 women.
        Topics covered:
            Antenatal care.

Intrapartum care.

Postnatal care.

Preference for future deliveries.

Consumers' satisfaction, needs and expectations.

Setting for data collection:

Semi-rural community.

Details about sample studied:

Planned size of sample:

216 women:

49 women - antenatal sample.

167 women - postnatal sample.

Rationale for planned size:

All women in the area expecting a baby within three months of the survey: December 1992 to February 1993.

All women in the area who had given birth between January and September 1992.

Entry criteria:

Exclusion:

neonatal deaths and stillbirths,

women moving out of area, and one woman in care.

Sample selection:

Convenience.

Actual sample size:

179 respondents

Response rate:

82.9%

Interventions, Outcomes and Analysis:

Analysis:

SPSS

Interpretation of results by group discussion.

Results: The respondents were highly satisfied with the antenatal and postnatal care they received.

71% of the women who did not know the midwife delivering their babies would have liked a known midwife.

13% of the sample had a DOMINO or a home birth, and expressed a high level of satisfaction with the continuity of care they experienced. 11% of the sample expressed a preference for home birth next time.

A need was demonstrated for women to have appropriate information about choices in childbirth including the options of home birth and the DOMINO system of care.

Recommendations for further research: Evaluation and audit of new systems of maternity care.

Keywords: CHOICE, COMMUNITY MIDWIVES, CONSUMER SATISFACTION, CONTINUITY OF CARE, EXPECTATIONS (WOMEN'S)

277. TO ASSESS THE EFFECT OF INCREASED APPROPRIATE INTERVENTION AND SUPPORT AMONG PREGNANT CIGARETTE SMOKERS AND THEIR FAMILIES
June 1993 - January 1995
Carol Mills, Smoking Information Facilitator, Julia Stallibrass, Research Fellow, Robert West, Reader, H Elsayeh, BSc. Student. **Contact:** Carol Mills, Room 1059 Barnes Ward, First Floor Lanesborough Wing, St George's Healthcare Trust, Blackshaw Road, London SW17 OQT. Tel: 081 784 7855

Funded as integral or additional part of a job by employer and by funding agency: Wandsworth Health Authority.

Aims of the study: To examine the effect on pregnant women of providing:
1. Appropriate information at the time of booking for delivery and at subsequent contacts.
2. Support for those deciding to quit smoking.
3. Study days/workshops for midwives designed to avoid confrontational contacts with clients.
4. Identification of those clients 'ready to change' and offering them various support mechanisms.

Ethics committee approval gained: Yes

Research design: Experimental – Qualitative and Quantitative – Survey/Case Control

    Data collection:
        Techniques used:
            Questionnaires.
            Daily collection of saliva.
        Time data were collected:
            15-20 weeks antenatally.
            8-10 days postnatally.
        Testing of any tools used:
            Questionnaires - piloted with colleagues.
        Topics covered:
            Smoking.
            Smoking related disorders.
            Information re smoking.
        Setting for data collection:
            Community.
            Hospital.

    Details about sample studied:
        Planned size of sample:
            1,500
        Rationale for planned size:
            To include women booking for delivery over a 6 month period.

Entry criteria:
Total pregnant population.
Sample selection:
Inclusive.
Actual sample size:
Recruitment ongoing.

Interventions, Outcomes and Analysis:
Interventions used:
Information pack.
Increased educational input with client group and midwives providing the support.
Adequate support when decision to quit has been made.
Practical minimal advice if client continues to smoke.
Main outcomes measured:
Number of women and their immediate family members who smoke - before, during, after pregnancy.
What influenced them to quit.
Smoking status after delivery.
(Objective verification of nicotine intake using cotinine levels in saliva).
Analysis:
Computer package (not specified).

Keywords: HEALTH EDUCATION, PASSIVE SMOKING, PREGNANCY, SMOKING

278. COMMUNITY TEAM MIDWIFERY CARE: AN ASSESSMENT OF ITS VALUE AND MEANING FOR WOMEN AND MIDWIVES
December 1992 - August 1993
G Lee, Part time staff midwife. **Contact:** G Lee, Kirkstall Road, London SW2 4HF.

Formed part of a course. Funded by University of Sheffield Medical School and by researcher.

Aims of the study: To explore the perceptions of community midwives and their clients concerning those factors which influence the care given.

Ethics committee approval gained: No

Research design: Descriptive – Qualitative and Quantitative – Survey

Data collection:
Techniques used:
Structured interview schedules to parturient women and midwives.
Time data were collected:
Ten or more days postnatally.

Testing of any tools used:
Draft questionnaires were pretested with 6 women and 3 midwives respectively.

Topics covered:
Sociodemographic details.

Perceptions of and values ascribed to, certain aspects of midwifery care.

Continuity of care.

Setting for data collection:
Community.

Inner city.

Details about sample studied:
Planned size of sample:
Women - 36

Midwives - 12

Rationale for planned size:
To include representatives from each team and a variety of experiences.

Entry criteria:
Women - (exclusions) those who had received no antenatal or community based postnatal care from the team of midwives, or who delivered elsewhere.

Midwives - working in community based teams.

Sample selection:
Consecutive, quota.

Actual sample size:
Women - 34. Midwives - 12

Response rate:
Women - 94%

Midwives - 100%

Interventions, Outcomes and Analysis:
Analysis:
SPSS/PC

Frequency counts.

Simple percentages (by hand).

Chi-square test.

Fisher's exact test.

Kendall coefficient of concordance test.

Content analysis.

Results: Community team midwifery care gave a high level of satisfaction to the women and midwives. The bleep system of communication between them was highly rated by both parties but the midwives found the on-call system problematical. However, midwives found relationships with, and support from, colleagues enhanced their enjoyment of work.

There appears to be a need for further research into which caregivers women wish to see during pregnancy; there was a discrepancy between midwives' and womens' views on this. There was no consensus on team size but the most popular choice for women and midwives was 6 midwives or less.

Continuity of carer may be more important postnatally than antenatally and more practical and desirable if it spans one or two stages of maternity care rather than three. Finally, it is suggested that there is some confusion as to whether it is high quality of midwifery care or continuity of carer/knowing the midwife per se, which produces women's satisfaction of care.

Recommendations for further research: Study of:
- women's attitudes to decision making during maternity care.
- the concept of a midwifery team and the concept of an "attitudinal contract".
- women's choices of caregivers during the antenatal period.
- willingness of non-team midwives to convert to team care.
- continuity of carer spanning one or two stages of maternity care only.
- testing an hypothesis as to whether it is quality of care or continuity of carer per se which produces satisfaction.

Keywords: COMMUNITY MIDWIFERY, CONSUMER SATISFACTION, EXPECTATIONS (WOMEN'S), PERCEPTIONS OF TEAM MIDWIFERY (MIDWIVES'), PERCEPTIONS OF TEAM MIDWIFERY (WOMEN'S), TEAM MIDWIFERY

279. AUTONOMY - WHO WANTS IT? AN EVALUATION OF MIDWIFERY LED CARE
July 1992 - June 1994
A Laverty, Midwife. **Contact:** A Laverty, Carter Lane, Mansfield, Notts NG18 3DQ. For full details see under Management Studies (Record No. 279).

280. BOROUGH OF BARNET, STUDY OF BREASTFEEDING UPTAKE AND ITS CONTINUATION
June 1992 - April 1993
Patti M Saha, Community Midwife, Shirley A Smith, Community Midwife. **Contact:** Patti M Saha, Watford Hut, Edgware General Hospital, Edgware, Middlesex HA8 OAD. Tel: 081 732 6206

Funded as integral/additional part of a job by employer: Medical Audit Committee. 12-20 hours/week of own time spent.

Aims of the study: To determine what practices affect the uptake and continuation of breastfeeding in the Borough of Barnet.

Ethics committee approval gained: No

Research design: Descriptive – Qualitative and Quantitative – Survey

   Data collection:
      Techniques used:
         Questionnaires.
      Time data were collected:
         2-3 weeks before expected date of delivery.
         2 and 6 weeks postnatally.
      Testing of any tools used:
         Pilot study of 50 clients in April 1992.
      Topics covered:
         Infant feeding.
      Setting for data collection:
         Hospital and community.

   Details about sample studied:
      Planned size of sample:
         500 clients: 250 primips and 250 multips
      Rationale for planned size:
         25% of mothers who meet selection criteria.
      Entry criteria:
         1. Booked for confinement at Edgware General Hospital.
         2. Resident in the Borough of Barnet.
         3. 32 weeks gestation or more at start of survey.
      Sample selection:
         Consecutive admissions.
      Actual sample size:
         500 questionnaires distributed.
      Response rate:
         62% (307 completed sets returned).

   Interventions, Outcomes and Analysis:
      Analysis:
         DataEase.
         Epi Info.
         Chi-square.

Results: There appears to be a relationship between attending parenthood education and the intention to breastfeed: if mothers attended parentcraft classes they were more likely to intend to breastfeed (P <0.0005).
A mother's choice of feeding method seems to be influenced by how other mothers known to her have chosen to feed their infants (P <0.00001).
There is no significant correlation between the method of delivery and the choice of feeding.
Less than 51% of mothers perceived that they had had discussion with a professional about feeding methods.
Putting the baby to the breast within two hours of birth appears to be related to the continuation of breastfeeding beyond six weeks duration (P <0.05). Mothers who had

a Caesarean Section were more likely to have a time delay of over two hours in putting their baby to the breast.

Where mothers themselves initiated breastfeeding they were less likely to have assistance from a midwife than where the midwife suggested a first feed (P <0.00001).

If assistance was given at the first feed the mothers were less likely to suffer with sore nipples (P <0.05).

Mothers whose expectations of breastfeeding were realized were more likely to be feeding at six weeks (P <0.005).

Recommendations for further research: 1. A study of the significance of the timing of first breast feed.

2. Exploration of the effect of increasing awareness of potential breastfeeding problems in the antenatal period in relation to the continuation rate of breastfeeding.

Keywords: BREASTFEEDING, BREASTFEEDING (DURATION), BREASTFEEDING (INCIDENCE), BREASTFEEDING (INTENTION), BREASTFEEDING (SUPPORT), EDUCATION FOR PARENTHOOD, SORE NIPPLES

281. ABSENT FRIENDS IN HULL - A STUDY OF ATTENDANCE AT PARENTCRAFT CLASSES

March - August 1989

Mary L Beadle, Midwifery Tutor, Linda M Downes, Midwife. **Contact:** Mary L Beadle, Humberside College of Health, East Riding Centre, Beverley Road, Willerby. Tel: 0482 675684

2-6 hours/week of own time spent. Funded by employer: Hull Maternity Hospital.

Aims of the study: To identify problems within the parentcraft service in the Hull District and their possible solutions.

Ethics committee approval gained: Yes

Research design: Descriptive – Qualitative and Quantitative – Survey

> **Data collection:**
> > **Techniques used:**
> > > Self completed questionnaires.
> >
> > **Time data were collected:**
> > > When women attended the antenatal clinic during the period of the survey.
> >
> > **Testing of any tools used:**
> > > A pilot study involving 80 questionnaires was carried out.
> >
> > **Topics covered:**
> > > Reasons for parentcraft non-attendance.
> > > Gravid women's interest in shorter refresher course.
> >
> > **Setting for data collection:**
> > > Antenatal clinics - hospital and community.

Details about sample studied:
Planned size of sample:
500
Rationale for planned size:
Time limit.

Financial restriction.

Approximately 10% of the number of women delivered in Hull Maternity Hospital.
Entry criteria:
Exclusion: Those attending the antenatal clinic for the first time.
Sample selection:
All clinic attenders during one month.
Actual sample size:
382
Response rate:
76%

Interventions, Outcomes and Analysis:
Analysis:
Carried out by other agents - details unknown.

Results: There was found to be a poor uptake of classes, with only 21% primigravidae and 4% of multigravid women attending.

The main reasons for non-attendance for multigravidae were, the care of other children, and the fact that they had attended classes before. These two answers made up for 80% of the reasons given for non-attendance.

Reasons for non-attendance given by primigravid women were more evenly spread between unsuitable time (22%), transport difficulties and partners' inability to attend (17%). Other children (14%) and unhelpful classes (15%) were also cited.

Primigravid women were more likely than multips to perceive classes as unhelpful.

One of the main reasons for undertaking this study was to identify problems in the system of invitation to classes. It was shown however that only 1% of the women did not know about the classes although the class location was unknown to 3%. Lack of information led to 10% of women perceiving the classes as unhelpful. Perhaps the fact that their partner was unable to attend in 9% of the sample may also be included in lack of information, as women are encouraged to bring a partner.

Recommendations for further research: To investigate a link between non-attendance and social class.

Keywords: ANTENATAL EDUCATION, EDUCATION FOR PARENTHOOD, NON ATTENDANCE

282. FETAL MONITORING - MIDWIFERY ATTITUDES
February 1992 - December 1993
S Dover, Midwife Teacher, S Gauge, Clinical Midwife Specialist. **Contact:** S Dover, Hampshire Drive, Edgbaston, Birmingham B15 3NZ.

2-6 hours/week of own time spent.

Aims of the study: To answer 3 questions:
1. What were midwives' preferred methods of fetal monitoring?
2. What were the influencing factors?
3. Was there an educational deficit which needed to be addressed?

Ethics committee approval gained: No

Research design: Descriptive – Qualitative and Quantitative – Survey

Data collection:
Techniques used:
Questionnaires.
Time data were collected:
February to March 1993.
Testing of any tools used:
Questionnaire piloted.
Attitude statements - item analysis.
Topics covered:
Demographic and professional details.
Fetal monitoring - preferred methods/practices.
Attitudes towards fetal monitoring and related midwifery practice/education.
Setting for data collection:
Regional and District Hospitals.
Community.

Details about sample studied:
Planned size of sample:
Total population.
Rationale for planned size:
Representative sample.
Entry criteria:
Midwives in clinical practice.
Sample selection:
Convenience.
Actual sample size:
242
Response rate:
117/242 = 48%

Interventions, Outcomes and Analysis:
    Analysis:
        Descriptive statistics.
        Cross tabulations and correlations.
        ANOVA.
        Factor analysis.

Results: Not yet available.

Keywords: FETAL MONITORING, MIDWIFERY PRACTICE, MIDWIVES' ATTITUDES, STAFF ATTITUDES

283. EPIDURAL ANALGESIA AND POSITION IN THE PASSIVE SECOND STAGE OF LABOUR: OUTCOMES FOR NULLIPAROUS WOMEN

January 1993 - June 1994

S M Downe, Research Midwife. **Contact:** S M Downe, Larges Street, Derby DE1 1DN.

Funded as integral or additional part of a job by employer. Additional funding from SDHA Nurses & Midwives Research Funds. Formed part of a course. 2 hours/week of own time spent.

Aims of the study: To test the null hypothesis:
The use of the lateral position in the passive second stage of labour will have no significant effect on:
a) the rate of instrumental deliveries;
b) the rate of episiotomies;
c) fetal Apgar
and neither staff nor women taking part in the trial will express a preference for either position.

Ethics committee approval gained: Yes

Research design: Descriptive/Experimental – Qualitative and Quantitative – Survey/ Randomized Controlled Trial

    Data collection:
        Techniques used:
            1. Pre and post trial questionnaires to staff.
            2. Pre delivery questionnaires to women.
            3. RCT (including visual analogue pain scales)
            4. Post delivery questionnaires at 2 weeks and 3 months to women postpartum.
        Time data were collected:
            1. 1 month pre trial and 1 month post trial.
            2. At time of consenting.
            3. During labour.
            4. 2 weeks and 3 months.

Testing of any tools used:
1. Tested with 10 midwives.
2. Pre-validated scale (Speilberger State/Trait Anxiety inventory).
4. A composite questionnaire mostly comprising established tools -tested for face validity and comprehension with 10 postnatal women.

Topics covered:
1. Staff preference for position in labour.
2. Anxiety levels (State/Trait) - women.
3. Labour outcomes, intrapartum pain levels and a range of demographic details.
4. Maternal confidence and self image, maternal morbidity, infant feeding method, labour fulfillment, anxiety, difficulty levels.

Setting for data collection:
Consultant Unit.

Details about sample studied:
Planned size of sample:
200 (100 in each group).
Required recruitment of 500 women antenatally.

Rationale for planned size:
Sufficient to demonstrate a significant reduction in forceps rate if it exists based on power calculation.

Entry criteria:
Inclusion:
All nulliparous women who have consented antenatally,
who still consent once an epidural has been sited in labour,
are 36+ weeks gestation,
who have a singleton pregnancy,
cephalic presentation,
live fetus,
Exclusion:
Intrauterine fetal death,
severe maternal hypertension,
severe fetal growth retardation,
breech,
multiple pregnancies,
trial of labour,
trial of uterine scar.

Sample selection:
Women entered as convenience sample then randomized.

Actual sample size:
Recruitment ongoing.

Interventions, Outcomes and Analysis:
Interventions used:
The use of either the sitting or lateral position in the passive 2nd stage of labour.

Main outcomes measured:
>Forceps rate.
>Ventouse rate.
>Perineal trauma rate.
>Fetal Apgar.
>Maternal morbidity.
>Maternal impressions of labour and delivery and their role in it.

Analysis:
>Chi-square.
>T-test.
>Mann-Whitney U.
>Simple frequencies and means.

Keywords: APGAR SCORES, CONSUMER OPINION, EPIDURALS, EPISIOTOMY, LABOUR, OUTCOMES (MATERNAL), OUTCOMES (NEONATAL), POSITIONS (LABOUR), SECOND STAGE

284. DIET IN LABOUR

January 1992 - December 1995

R M Fryer, Labour Ward Sister, Christopher Wilkins, Consultant Anaesthetist. **Contact:** R M Fryer, Labour Ward, North Staffordshire Maternity Unit, Hilton Road, Stoke on Trent. Tel: 0782 718434

Formed part of a course.

Aims of the study: To determine whether allowing oral intake of food and drink during labour in low risk mothers, reduces the need for intervention.

Ethics committee approval gained: Yes

Research design: Experimental – Qualitative and Quantitative – Randomized Controlled Trial

Data collection:
>**Techniques used:**
>>Records of observations.
>
>**Time data were collected:**
>>Following each delivery.
>
>**Testing of any tools used:**
>>Questionnaires not piloted but content discussed with colleagues.
>
>**Topics covered:**
>>Duration of labour.
>>Type of delivery.
>>Need for intervention.
>>Condition of infant.
>>Maternal satisfaction.

Setting for data collection:
Hospital.

Details about sample studied:
Planned size of sample:
800 primigravidae.
Rationale for planned size:
Statistical basis.
Entry criteria:
Exclusion: high risk mothers.
Sample selection:
Random.
Actual sample size:
Recruitment ongoing.

Interventions, Outcomes and Analysis:
Interventions used:
One group offered light diet and high calorie drinks.
Other group denied oral food and liquid but given IV fluids.
Main outcomes measured:
Need for augmentation of labour.
Assisted delivery.
Caesarean Section.
Analysis:
Seeking advice on statistical package for analysis.

Keywords: CONSUMER SATISFACTION, DRINKS (HIGH CALORIE), FASTING, HYDRATION (LABOUR), LABOUR, LABOUR (DURATION), NUTRITION (LABOUR), OUTCOMES (MATERNAL), OUTCOMES (NEONATAL)

285. PERINEAL CLEANSING WITH TAP WATER PRIOR TO NORMAL AND FORCEPS DELIVERY AND PERINEAL SUTURING
November 1992 - July 1993
J Hervé , Department Sister, J Parkin, Infection Control Nurse. **Contact:** J Hervé, Cavendish Close, Green Park, Bawtry, Doncaster DN10 6SD.

Funded as integral or additional part of a job. 2 hours/week of own time spent.

Aims of the study: To test the hypothesis that perineal infections would not increase if tap water was used for perineal cleansing.

Ethics committee approval gained: No

Research design: Experimental – Quantitative – Action Research

Data collection:
    Techniques used:
        Analysis of bacteriological reports.
    Time data were collected:
        November 1992 to April 1993
    Testing of any tools used:
        Procedure tested over a period of one month.
    Topics covered:
        Bacteriological colonisation
        - perineum
        - infants' eyes
    Setting for data collection:
        Hospital and community.

Details about sample studied:
    Planned size of sample:
        All deliveries in 6 month period. Expected number - 1000
    Rationale for planned size:
        Total population.
    Entry criteria:
        Inclusion:
        - all vaginal deliveries
        - all women having perineal suturing.
        Exclusion:
        - women who were catheterised.
    Sample selection:
        Consecutive deliveries.
    Actual sample size:
        1021

Interventions, Outcomes and Analysis:
    Interventions used:
        Tap water for deliveries and perineal suturing.
    Main outcomes measured:
        Perineal infection.
        Eye infection - babies.
    Analysis:
        Simple frequencies.

Results: In the 6 months prior to using tap water there were 927 deliveries, 5 perineal infections, 2 episiotomies and 3 tears.

During the 6 months using tap water, there were 1021 deliveries, 4 perineal infections, 3 episiotomies and 1 tear.

During the study period there was no significant increase in colonization/infection rates of babies' eyes, or in perineal infection. It was concluded that tap water is as effective as chlorhexidine during delivery in terms of control of infection.

Recommendations for further research: To study the effect of using tap water over the period of one year.

Keywords: DELIVERY, FORCEPS, NEONATAL INFECTION, PERINEAL REPAIR, SUTURING, SWABBING, TAP WATER

286. MATERNAL PERCEPTIONS OF HEALTH AND WELL BEING FOLLOWING CHILDBIRTH
November 1993 - December 1994
S Jordan, Lecturer, C Ruby, Midwifery Lecturer. Contact: C Ruby, Norton, Presteigne, Powys ED8 2EL.

Formed part of a course. 2 hours/week of own time spent.

Aims of the study: To ascertain women's perceptions of factors which have affected their health and well being during the postnatal period and to establish whether interventions by partners, relatives, friends or health care professionals were effective in resolving any morbidity present.

Ethics committee approval gained: Yes

Research design: Descriptive – Qualitative – Simple Descriptive Survey

> **Data collection:**
>> **Techniques used:**
>>> Diary - interview method.
>>> Semi-structured interview on completion.
>> **Time data were collected:**
>>> The first four weeks following delivery.
>> **Testing of any tools used:**
>>> Interviews clarify and validate diary entries.
>> **Topics covered:**
>>> Maternal health and well being following childbirth.
>> **Setting for data collection:**
>>> Hospital and community.

> **Details about sample studied:**
>> **Planned size of sample:**
>>> 20
>> **Rationale for planned size:**
>>> Time and resource constraints.
>> **Entry criteria:**
>>> Primiparous women.
>>> Married and/or in a stable relationship.
>>> Literate.
>> **Sample selection:**
>>> Convenience sample.
>> **Actual sample size:**
>>> Recruitment ongoing.

Interventions, Outcomes and Analysis:
Analysis:
Content analysis.

Keywords: PERCEPTIONS OF CHILDBIRTH (WOMEN'S), POSTNATAL HEALTH, POSTNATAL SUPPORT, PUERPERIUM

287. A RANDOMIZED CONTROLLED TRIAL TO COMPARE THREE TYPES OF FETAL SCALP ELECTRODE

January - November 1988
Linda Needs, Midwife, Jennifer Sleep, Research Co-ordinator, Sarah Ayers, Computer Programmer, Gaye Henson, Consultant Obstetrician, Adrian Grant, Epidemiologist.
Contact: Jennifer Sleep, Berkshire College of Nursing and Midwifery, Royal Berkshire Hospital, Craven Road, Reading, Berkshire RG1 5AN. Tel: 0734 877651

Funded by small grant from Oxford Regional Health Authority and conducted as additional part of a job.

Aims of the study: To compare three scalp electrodes in respect of need for reapplication, trace quality and scalp trauma.

Ethics committee approval gained: Yes

Research design: Experimental – Qualitative and Quantitative – Randomized Controlled Trial

Data collection:
Techniques used:
Records of observation and actual practice during labour.
Questionnaires - mothers and midwives.
Time data were collected:
During labour and following delivery.
Scalp trauma reassessed - 10th day postpartum.
Mothers' perceptions - 10th day postpartum.
CTG recordings - at end of study period.
Testing of any tools used:
Tested for reliability and validity - pre-pilot and pilot study.
Topics covered:
Reapplication of electrode.
Quality of CTG tracing.
Scalp trauma.
Setting for data collection:
Maternity Unit, Royal Berkshire Hospital, Reading.

Details about sample studied:
Planned size of sample:
750

Rationale for planned size:

Based on expected reapplication-rate for Rocket-Rolan electrode of 50%.

To give 80% likelihood of identifying reduction to 37.5% associated with one or other electrode.

Entry criteria:

Gestation more than 37 completed weeks.

Cephalic presentation.

Singleton.

Requiring electronic fetal heart rate monitoring.

Sample selection:

Consecutive admissions.

Actual sample size:

750 women entered the study.

Response rate:

83% response rate at 10 days.

Interventions, Outcomes and Analysis:

Interventions used:

Three types of fetal scalp electrode:

Rocket-Rolon (double-helix spiral)

Hewlett Packard (double-helix spiral)

Surgicraft-Copeland (clip)

Main outcomes measured:

Need for more than one electrode.

Reason for replacement.

Trace quality.

Scalp trauma.

Direct financial costs.

Analysis:

Chi-square.

Odds ratio.

Results: Reapplication was significantly least likely in the Surgicraft-Copeland group (odds ratio vs Hewlett-Packard = 0.61, 95% CI 0.41-0.90; odds ratio vs Rocket-Rolon = 0.43, 95% CI = 0.29-0.62). This reflected a much lower rate of replacement because of the detachment. The Hewlett-Packard was, however, least likely to be replaced because of the poor trace quality. Interpretable traces were equally common, but trace quality tended to be superior in the Hewlett-Packard group. There was no serious scalp trauma. Difficulty removing the electrode was least often reported in the Hewlett-Packard group, and a mark on the scalp persisted least often in the Rocket-Rolon group.

The Surgicraft-Copeland performed the best overall, and particularly in respect of attachment to the scalp. It appears to be the electrode of choice of the three tested.

Recommendations for further research: Evaluation of new products before their widespread introduction into care.

Keywords: FETAL MONITORING, FETAL SCALP ELECTRODES, LABOUR

Needs L, Grant A, Sleep J, Ayers S, Henson G. A randomized controlled trial to compare three types of fetal scalp electrode. British Journal of Obstetrics and Gynaecology. 1992;99:302-6.

288. DIASTASIS OF THE SYMPHYSIS PUBIS - ITS DIAGNOSIS AND LONGER TERM SEQUELAE IN A COHORT OF CHILD BEARING WOMEN IN WEST BERKSHIRE

October 1993 - December 1994

Jennifer Sleep, Research Co-ordinator, Jan Baldwin, Staff Midwife, Kate Grayson, Research Assistant. **Contact:** Jennifer Sleep, Berkshire College of Nursing and Midwifery, Royal Berkshire Hospital, Craven Road, Reading, Berkshire RG1 5AN. Tel: 0734 877651

Funded as integral or additional part of a job by Oxford Regional Health Authority. 2 hours/week of own time spent.

Aims of the study: a) To identify potential predictive factors for diastasis of the symphysis pubis and longer term sequelae.
b) To establish duration and progress of the symptoms of women who suffer from diastasis of the symphysis pubis.

Ethics committee approval gained: Yes

Research design: Descriptive – Qualitative and Quantitative – Survey

    Data collection:
        Techniques used:
            Phase 1 - case note review.
            Phase 2 - postal questionnaires.
        Time data were collected:
            Phase 1 - retrospectively.
            Phase 2 - starting March 1994.
        Testing of any tools used:
            Questionnaire not yet developed - will be based on Phase 1 findings.
        Topics covered:
            Symptoms of diastasis of symphysis pubis.
            Degree of separation of symphysis.
            Longer term sequelae.
            Time to full recovery.
        Setting for data collection:
            Royal Berkshire Hospital.
            Community.

Details about sample studied:
    Planned size of sample:
        Unknown number - all cases in defined period.
    Rationale for planned size:
        Total population.
    Entry criteria:
        Any women
        - referred to physiotherapy department following initial diagnosis.
        - with immobilizing pelvic pain.
    Sample selection:
        Inclusive.
    Actual sample size:
        Recruitment ongoing.

Interventions, Outcomes and Analysis:
    Analysis:
        SAS
        DataEase.
        Correlational tests.

Keywords: PELVIC DIASTASIS, PELVIC PAIN, POSTNATAL CARE, SYMPHYSIS PUBIS

290. A DOUBLE BLIND RANDOMISED CONTROLLED TRIAL EVALUATING THE HOMOEOPATHIC REMEDY ARNICA MONTANA FOR THE MANAGEMENT OF PERINEAL PAIN AFTER CHILDBIRTH. REPORT OF A PILOT STUDY

February - August 1993
D L Holwell, Practising Midwife. **Contact:** D L Holwell, Church Road, Mannings Heath, West Sussex RH13 6JE.

Formed part of a course. Over 20 hours/week of own time spent.

Aims of the study: To evaluate the use of Arnica Montana 30c in relief of perineal pain up until the 10th day postnatally.

Ethics committee approval gained: Yes

Research design: Experimental – Quantitative – Randomized Controlled Trial

    Data collection:
        Techniques used:
            Records of observations.
            Pain scales.
        Time data were collected:
            1. The mothers scored perineal pain once a day for the first ten days following delivery.
            2. The midwives assessed the perineum on days 1, 2, 7 and 10.

Testing of any tools used:

The instrument used to record bruising was tested for inter-observer reliability which showed a correlation coefficient value of 0.89.

Topics covered:

Perineal pain.

Bruising.

Oedema.

Setting for data collection:

Hospital and community.

Rural and urban.

Details about sample studied:

Planned size of sample:

Total of 20 subjects.

10 in the experimental group (Arnica).

10 in the control group (placebo).

Rationale for planned size:

Pilot study for main trial.

Entry criteria:

Exclusion: Women who

- could not speak English.
- had stillborn babies or babies in Special Care Baby Unit.
- were under the care of particular consultant who refused permission.
- had Diabetes Mellitus.
- had taken Arnica during pregnancy.

Sample selection:

Double blind random allocation after trial entry.

Actual sample size:

19 subjects were entered and all remained in the allocated group for the purpose of the analysis.

Response rate:

Mothers - 100%

Midwives - 97%

Interventions, Outcomes and Analysis:

Interventions used:

1. The homeopathic remedy Arnica Montana 30c tablet to be taken orally ie one tablet taken six hourly for three days.
2. Matching placebo, identical in weight, size, colour, taste and smell.

Main outcomes measured:

Perineal pain.

Perineal bruising.

Oedema.

Analysis:
> Wilcoxon test.
> Mann-Whitney U test.
> Student t-test.
> Fisher Exact probability test.

Results: The study population was found to be representative of all the vaginal deliveries which required perineal repair and the two groups of women were similar.

This pilot study showed no statistical difference between the groups in relation to bruising and oedema of the perineum.

However perineal pain felt by the Arnica group was significantly greater (p =0.02, p <0.05) than the placebo group. This was also supported by a second analysis of the number of mothers who were pain free by the 10th postnatal day. This analysis showed that 3 out of 10 mothers who received Arnica were pain free on day 10, whereas 8 out of 9 mothers in the placebo group were pain free on day 10 (p =0.015, p <0.05).

Recommendations for further research: Main trial of Arnica montana - will commence at a later date.

A further pilot study using a range of Arnica potencies and matching placebo, to investigate which dilution shows most promise for use in clinical trials of this nature.

Keywords: ARNICA, COMPLEMENTARY THERAPIES, HOMEOPATHY, PERINEAL PAIN

Educational Studies

11. AN EVALUATION OF A NEW UNDERGRADUATE PREPARATION FOR MIDWIVES
April 1989 - July 1992
Sandy Kirkman, Lecturer in Midwifery - Course Leader. **Contact:** Sandy Kirkman, University of Wales College of Medicine, School of Nursing Studies, Heath Park, Cardiff, South Wales CF4 4XN. Tel: 0222 755944 Ex 5339

Funded as integral or additional part of a job by employer: University of Wales School of Nursing Studies. Formed part of a course. 6-12 hours/week of own time spent.

Abstract: (Not updated since 1991) CONFIDENTIAL.

Keywords: INNOVATORY PROGRAMMES, MIDWIFERY EDUCATION, MIDWIFERY EDUCATION (EVALUATION), MIDWIFERY EDUCATION (HIGHER)

17. ASSESSMENT OF ATTITUDES RELATING TO DIRECT ENTRY MIDWIFERY TRAINING AMONG CLINICAL AND TUTORIAL STAFF IN TWELVE HEALTH AUTHORITIES
October 1987 - December 1991
S M Downe, Midwifery Researcher/Practitioner, F Brooks, Research Postgraduate, Chris Gillespie, Head of Psychology Services. **Contact:** S M Downe, Larges Street, Derby DE1 1DN.

Funded as integral or additional part of a job by employer: Southern Derbyshire Health Authority. Additional funding by Iolanthe Trust, Association of Radical Midwives.

Abstract: The purpose of the study is to assess staff attitudes relating to Direct Entry midwifery training, and to determine factors influencing those attitudes. If of value, this information would then be used to promote positive attitudes among staff especially in institutions where Direct Entry (now pre-registration) training is to commence.

The method involved the selection of twelve Health Authorities chosen for diversity of history of Direct Entry midwifery training, and geographical spread. Questionnaires were sent to all midwives and tutors in the Health Authorities followed by validating interviews of a small random selection of respondents. A variety of statistical analyses using SPSSx are being used and are not yet complete.

For a variety of operational reasons, this study did not progress but the data are available from the author.

Keywords: MIDWIFE TEACHERS (ATTITUDES), MIDWIFERY EDUCATION (DIRECT ENTRY), MIDWIFERY EDUCATION (PREJUDICE), STAFF ATTITUDES

28. MIDWIFERY TRAINING IN SCOTLAND: AN OPINION SURVEY
May 1984 - May 1985
Veronica E Pope, Professional Adviser Midwifery. **Contact:** Veronica E Pope, National Board for Nursing, Midwifery, and Health Visiting in Scotland, 22 Queen Street, Edinburgh EH2 1JX. Tel: 031 226 7371

Funded as integral or additional part of a job by employer. Own time spent.

Abstract: The aim of this study was to solicit the opinions of a cohort of students. The students were undertaking the eighteen-month midwifery training, and we wished to find out how they felt about the course. We also sought the opinions of registered midwives in the training institutions who helped the students attain their clinical learning outcomes, and who worked with them following their registration as midwives. Two-hundred and nine questionnaires were issued to the student midwives and 2127 to practising midwives. A postal response was sought. The data were analyzed manually using the Cope Chat Card system.

The findings supported the value of an increased training period, but were critical of elements in the programme which were considered weak. These included management preparation, teaching skills and research-based learning. As a result of the survey, the National Board have issued more precise regulations for the training of midwives, aimed at correcting these faults.

Keywords: CLINICAL TEACHING, MIDWIFERY EDUCATION, MIDWIFERY EDUCATION (EVALUATION), MIDWIFERY EDUCATION (SCOTLAND), MIDWIFERY PRACTICE, OUTCOMES (DEFICIENCIES IDENTIFIED)

Pope VE. Midwifery training in Scotland: An opinion survey. Midwives Chronicle 1986;99:198-200.

33. THE EMPLOYMENT DECISIONS OF NEWLY QUALIFIED MIDWIVES
April 1980 - April 1987
Rosemary Mander, University Lecturer. **Contact:** Rosemary Mander, Department of Nursing Studies, University of Edinburgh, Adam Ferguson Building, 40 George Square, Edinburgh EH8 9LL. Tel: 031 650 3896
For full details see under Management Studies (Record No. 33).

40. SURVEY TO ASSESS ATTITUDES OF SENIOR MIDWIFERY TUTORS TO DIRECT ENTRY MIDWIFERY TRAINING
January - December 1985

S M Downe, Research Midwife, B Kenner, Staff Midwife, W Few, Student Midwife, D Foster, Student Midwife. **Contact:** S M Downe, Larges Street, Derby DE1 1DN.

2-6 hours/week of own time spent. Funded by funding agency(ies).

Abstract: The purpose of the study was to assess the attitudes of tutorial staff to Direct Entry midwifery training prior to the inception of further Direct Entry courses, and also to discover why tutors had ceased, or never even started, training direct entrant midwives.

A questionnaire was sent out to all senior midwifery tutors in England and some in Wales. One hundred and twenty (80%) were returned. Analysis was done by simple percentages. The findings established that key myths abounded about direct entrants (eg their low academic ability). Key obstructions to Direct Entry training were identified, and included lack of tutors and finance. The level of enquiries about Direct Entry training was established; there were 1,996 in 1985 (some of these were multiple applications by the same person).

The recommendation is that further work should be carried out to build on this exploratory study.

Keywords: MIDWIFE TEACHERS (ATTITUDES), MIDWIFERY EDUCATION (DIRECT ENTRY), MIDWIFERY EDUCATION (MYTHS), STUDENT MIDWIVES

Downe, S. Summary of recent survey assessing midwifery training schools' attitudes to direct entry midwifery training. MIDIRS Pack 2 1986.

42. AN EVALUATION OF A MATERNITY CARE COMPONENT FOR NURSING STUDENTS
January 1985 - September 1990

Rosemary Mander, University lecturer. **Contact:** Rosemary Mander, Department of Nursing Studies, University of Edinburgh, Adam Ferguson Building, 40 George Square, Edinburgh EH8 9LL. Tel: 031 650 3896

Funded as integral or additional part of a job by employer. 6-12 hours/week of own time spent.

Abstract: This project comprised an evaluation of the implementation of a novel form of maternity care experience for nursing students, which was planned with the help of the staff of the statutory bodies and the personnel of the local Health Board. Certain anxieties had been raised during the planning phase and an evaluation was crucial to assess the extent to which these anxieties had been justified.

The research method involved the distribution of self-administered questionnaires to all involved (mothers, students, Health Board staff and general practitioners) and some personal observation. The analysis of the data was largely quantitative. The data showed that this programme caused no major difficulties for those involved. Some were unaware of the scheme and others felt that they had benefitted from being involved in it. On the basis of this on-going evaluation, it was decided that the maternity care programme was largely satisfactory to those involved and that it should continue in a slightly modified form.

Keywords: MATERNITY CARE COURSE, MATERNITY CARE EXPERIENCE, NURSE EDUCATION, NURSE EDUCATION (EVALUATION)

Mander R. What can midwives learn from the babes? Implications for midwives of a maternity care programme for nursing students. Journal of Advanced Nursing 1988;13:306-13.
Mander R. A maternity care course component and evaluation. Nurse Education Today 1989;9:227-35.

50. TEN YEARS ON: A STUDY TO INVESTIGATE THE UPTAKE OF MALE MIDWIFERY TRAINING WITHIN THE UNITED KINGDOM AND THE CAREER PATTERNS OF MALE MIDWIVES
October 1986 - October 1987

P Lewis, Midwife Teacher with clinical remit, S Robinson, Research Supervisor. **Contact:** P Lewis, St Aidan's Road, East Dulwich, London SE22 0RW.

Formed part of a course. Funded by funding agency(ies).

Abstract: The research involved an in-depth evaluation of male midwifery training and an assessment of the experiences of male midwives. Information was obtained on the numbers of men in midwifery, their status within the profession, and demographic background. The reasons for entering and leaving midwifery were also obtained as were continuing acceptability, the need for chaperonage, the mother/male midwife relationship, and the subsequent career paths of men in midwifery.

The research was carried out in three phases: Phase 1 - a short questionnaire was sent to all midwifery training schools in the UK (n=171). Phase 2 - an in-depth questionnaire was sent to all men identified as either current students or qualified male midwives. Phase 3 - interviews were carried out with practising male midwives. Analysis of the data was carried out using SPSSx.

The findings showed that a total of ninety men have entered midwifery since 1977 with a further twelve expected to take up training in 1987. Just under a quarter (21.1%) of those men entering the profession had had their training discontinued. The data showed that male student and qualified midwives were likely to be British, single, aged between twenty-five and twenty-nine years, with good educational qualifications and experience in nursing. The experience cited by the respondents suggests that the majority enter midwifery for reasons allied to nursing. Few encounter problems when applying to train and it appears that they are overwhelmingly supported by their female colleagues. The respondents' perceptions indicate that they receive favourable reactions from mothers and their partners and are acceptable to them. Refusals of care are most likely by those mothers from the ethnic minority groups. The use of chaperonage appears to be less significant than previously suggested.

The career intentions of student midwives, and qualified male midwives when students, compare favourably with those in other studies. The reason most often cited for leaving midwifery was 'the legal exclusion of men from practising outside the training hospitals prior to 1983' (41%), although others were given.

In conclusion, it appears that men have a valuable contribution to make towards midwifery and the difficulties envisaged in their training and practice are relatively few. Follow-up studies are suggested to provide further validation for these findings and to determine the continued participation and contribution of men to midwifery.

Keywords: CAREER PATHS, CHAPERONAGE, MALE MIDWIVES, MIDWIFERY EDUCATION (CESSATION), MIDWIFERY EDUCATION (RECRUITMENT)

Lewis P. Men in midwifery. Research and the Midwife Conference Proceedings 1987 1988:13-30.
Lewis P. Male midwives' training and careers. In: Wilson-Barnett J, Robinson S, eds. Directions in Nursing Research. London: Scutari Press. 1989:280-9.
Lewis P. Men in midwifery: their experiences as students and as practitioners. In: Robinson S, Thompson AM, eds. Midwives, Research and Childbirth. Vol 2. London Chapman and Hall. 1990:271-301.

52. THE HAPPY END OF NURSING: AN ETHNOGRAPHIC STUDY OF INITIAL ENCOUNTERS IN A MIDWIFERY SCHOOL
March 1987 - April 1988

R M Davies, Professional Adviser (Midwifery). **Contact:** R M Davies, Llwyn-y-Grant Place, Cyncoed, Cardiff CF3 7EX.

Formed part of a course. 2-6 hours/week of own time spent. Funded by employer: Welsh National Board.

Abstract: The study is an ethnography of initial encounters in a midwifery school. It aims to demonstrate the appropriateness of qualitative methods in midwifery educational research. An introduction to the occupation of midwifery which lays claim to professionalism is provided. The official and unofficial claims to its difference from nursing are explored.

A convenience sample of one cohort of ten students was studied using an eclectic approach. The students' construction of their world of midwifery is described and their anxieties due to role ambiguities are discussed. Some of the strategies employed for coping with these anxieties are identified and lead the reader to believe certain inappropriate nursing skills are sometimes employed. It is finally concluded that the way in which nurses become midwives is not conducive to the promotion of independent practice on qualifying, if the early socialising factors shown in this study are perpetuated throughout the course. Thus it is suggested that further research is needed in this neglected area.

Keywords: MIDWIFE'S ROLE (AMBIGUITY), MIDWIFE'S ROLE (CONFLICT), MIDWIFERY EDUCATION, MIDWIFERY PRACTICE, STUDENT MIDWIVES

Davies RM. "The happy end of nursing": an ethnographic study of initial encounters in a midwifery school. Unpublished MSc thesis, University of Wales College of Cardiff.

56. A STUDY OF THE EDUCATIONAL NEEDS OF MIDWIVES IN WALES AND HOW THEY MAY BE MET
June - August 1980
G D Maclean, International Consultant in Midwifery Education. **Contact:** G D Maclean, Maple Grove, Sketty Road, Swansea SA2 OJY.

Funded as integral or additional part of a job by employer and by funding agency(ies): Department of Health, West Glamorgan Health Authority.

Abstract: Given the limited opportunities for continuing education for midwives in Wales, this study was undertaken in order to establish the needs and possibilities. The motivation of midwives to avail themselves of continuing education was assessed along with practical issues such as availability, accessibility and acceptance of courses.

Data were collected from a 10% quasi-random sample of midwives practising in Wales by means of a questionnaire (n=149). A central core of questions was used and additional sections added for managers and tutors. Area nursing officers were interviewed using a semi-structured interview to ascertain their commitment to and the local provision of continuing education within each area of Wales. The study also took cognisance of existing facilities across the UK by observation, interview and correspondence. Literature was also reviewed.

The urgent need for a course providing the Advanced Diploma in Midwifery and Midwife Teachers Diploma in Wales was identified by Area Nursing Officers though denied by almost a quarter of midwife respondents. The need for short courses was the overwhelming need identified by the majority, the largest percentages requiring family planning, special and intensive care of the neonate and preparation for parenthood courses. The possibility of using distance learning methods was considered realistic to some. The study also briefly considered which parts of general nursing the respondents saw as essential components of midwifery, considering the possibility of the development of Direct Entry midwifery courses.

Keywords: MIDWIFERY EDUCATION (ACCESSIBILITY), MIDWIFERY EDUCATION (CONTINUING), MIDWIFERY EDUCATION (DIRECT ENTRY), MIDWIFERY OPPORTUNITIES, MIDWIFERY (WALES)

Maclean GD. A study of the educational needs of midwives in Wales and how they may be met. Research Report 1980. (Limited number published by the National Staff Committee.)

Maclean GD. It's time for a break. Nursing Mirror 1982;154:52-5.

78. CHOICE OR CHANCE? AN EXPLORATORY STUDY DESCRIBING THE CRITERIA AND PROCESSES USED TO SELECT MIDWIFERY STUDENTS
August 1987 - August 1989

Robyn Phillips, Lecturer - Education. **Contact:** Robyn Phillips, School of Education, University of Wales College of Cardiff, Senghennydd Road, Cardiff CF2 4AG. Tel: 0222 874000 Ex 5155

Formed part of a course. 6-12 hours/week of own time spent. Funded by employer and by Iolanthe Trust.

Abstract: The study was a dissertation submission for the degree of Master in Education and is a description of the key criteria and processes used in selecting students for an eighteen-month course in midwifery. The rationale for some of the criteria are also identified from the survey data.

For the study, a postal survey was preceded by initial qualitative work in order to explore the main issues involved in student midwife selection. A questionnaire was designed on the basis of this preliminary work and subsequently mailed to the senior midwife teacher responsible for each of the midwifery training schools in England and Wales, approved to conduct an eighteen-month course in midwifery for registered general nurses. One hundred and forty-two respondents (95%) returned completed questionnaires.

Analysis of the questionnaire responses identified the key characteristics/attributes/criteria which respondents believed to be important in potential midwifery recruits, in addition to some of the rationales for their inclusion. The processes through which an applicant for midwifery training may pass are also described.

The study highlights that while the methods of selection are relatively uniform throughout midwifery training institutions, the criteria believed to be important may vary, with equally diverse rationales. Thus the suggested implications for midwifery education include a possible inappropriate use of scarce resources, and unacceptable diversity of criteria and hence a need to validate both the criteria, and the processes used for their identification. Is the selection of student midwives a matter of choice, or of chance?

Keywords: MIDWIFERY EDUCATION, MIDWIFERY EDUCATION (EVALUATION), STUDENT MIDWIVES

Phillips R. Choice or chance? An exploratory study describing the criteria and process used to select midwifery students. MEd thesis, University of Wales 1989.

80. THE EVALUATION OF A POST-BASIC TRAINING COURSE FOR ANTENATAL TEACHERS
January 1982 - August 1986

Tricia Murphy-Black, Research Fellow, Ann Faulkner, Lecturer, Ann Thomson, Lecturer/Midwifery Sister. **Contact:** Tricia Murphy-Black, Research and Development Adviser, Simpson Memorial Maternity Pavilion, Lauriston Place, Edinburgh EH3 9EF. Tel: 031 229 2477 Ex 4357

Funded as integral or additional part of a job by employer: University of Manchester, Health Education Council. 2-6 hours/week of own time spent.

Abstract: The overall aim of the study was to determine if attending a post-basic antenatal teaching and group work skills course, held in two centres, would: 1) meet the expectations of the midwives and health visitors; and 2) change the teaching behaviour post-course compared with the pre-course observations. There were two studies, the first a series of seven questionnaires to sixty-five attenders to evaluate the process of the course; and the second an observation study of seventy-six antenatal classes using a pre-test post-test design, to evaluate the outcome of the course. The expectations of the midwives and health visitors attending the course were met by the training course. The antenatal classes, which were associated with an increased interaction between mothers and teachers in the post-course compared with the pre-course analysis, were those taught by a self-selected group of teachers and to a lesser extent the classes led by health visitors. The other factors analyzed demonstrated increased interaction in the classes with babies present and where the subject of discussion was breastfeeding, although these results may be related. Semi-circular seating was associated with a slight increase in interaction between mothers and teachers. There was an increased incidence of closed questions by the teachers from one of the centres and exploratory questions by the health visitors in the post-course classes. Asking 'Any questions?' did not result in the mothers asking questions in the majority of classes. Of the few questions the mothers did ask, the majority were requests for further information.

The results of the process and outcome evaluation are discussed in the publications with recommendations for the teachers, course organisers and further research.

Keywords: ANTENATAL EDUCATION, EDUCATION FOR PARENTHOOD (TEACHERS), GROUP WORK SKILLS, MIDWIFERY EDUCATION, MIDWIFERY EDUCATION (EVALUATION), TEACHING

Black PM, Faulkner A, Thomson AM. Antenatal classes: a selective review of the literature. Nurse Education Today 1984;3:130-3.

Black T, Booth K, Faulkner A. Co-operation or conflict? How midwives and health visitors view each other's contribution to antenatal education. Senior Nurse 1984;1:25-6.

Black T. Antenatal education, some aspects of the evaluation of a post basic training course. Research and the Midwife Conference Proceedings 1984:2-27.

Black PM, Faulkner A, Thomson AM. The evaluation of a post basic course for antenatal teachers: the practical problems of methodology and organisation.

In: Nursing Research - Does it Make a Difference? Proceedings of the WENR/ RCN International Conference, London 1984.

Black T, Faulkner A, Thomson AM. Interaction analysis in antenatal education: the practical applications of an academic exercise. In: Hawthorn PJ, ed. Proceedings of the RCN Research Society Annual Conference 1985. University of Nottingham 1987.

Black T, Faulkner A. Interaction analysis in antenatal education: the questioning styles of midwives and health visitors. Paper presented to the 25th Anniversary Conference "Innovations in Nursing Theory and Practice". University of Manchester Department of Nursing 1985.

Black T. Faulkner A. Improving antenatal education. Papers presented to the First International Health Education Conference for Nurses, Midwives and Health Visitors, Harrogate 1985.

Murphy-Black T. The evaluation of a post basic course for antenatal teachers. Unpublished PhD thesis, University of Manchester, 1986.

Murphy-Black T, Faulkner A. Antenatal Group Skills Training - a Manual of Guidelines. Chichester: John Wiley & Sons 1988.

Murphy-Black T, Faulkner A. Antenatal Education. In: Faulkner A, Murphy-Black T, eds. Midwifery: Excellence in Nursing, the Research Route. London: Scutari Press. 79-92.

Murphy-Black T. Antenatal education using questionnaires to evaluate a post basic training course. In: Robinson S, Thomson AM eds. Midwives, Research and Childbirth, Vol. 2. Chapman Hall, London. 1991:176-98.

Murphy-Black T. Antenatal education. In: Roch S, Alexander J, Levy V, eds. Antenatal care Midwifery Practice Series Vol 1. London: Macmillan Ltd. pp 88-104.

84. CONTINUING EDUCATION FOR NON-EMPLOYED MIDWIVES
June 1990 - August 1991
C Midgley, Course Director pre-reg Midwifery. **Contact:** C Midgley, Fairstone Hill, Oadby, Leicester LE2 5RH.

Formed part of a course. Funded by funding agency(ies): Birmingham and Solihull College of Midwifery Education and Training.

Abstract: (Not updated since 1991) The purpose of this study is to enquire whether non-employed midwives wish to continue their midwifery education whilst out of professional midwifery employment. If they do, the study will seek to identify what methods of education would be most suitable to them; to enquire from the English National Board what alternative methods of education to the present system could be used - in particular, whether individualized learning would attract credit accumulation; to identify some of the methods used by other professions, such as banks and building societies, for keeping in touch with non-employed staff; and to consider the constraints on midwives returning to employment, and how those constraints may be overcome.

Keywords: CHILDCARE FACILITIES, EMPLOYMENT (FLEXIBILITY), INDIVIDUALISED LEARNING, MIDWIFERY EDUCATION, MIDWIFERY EDUCATION (CONTINUING), MIDWIFERY EDUCATION (MOTIVATION), MIDWIVES (UNEMPLOYED)

93. MOTIVATION FOR CONTINUING EDUCATION IN MIDWIFERY IN NORTHERN IRELAND
October 1987 - April 1988

B H McCrea, Lecturer. **Contact:** B H McCrea, Department of Nursing and Health Visiting, University of Ulster, Cromore Road, Co Londonderry BT52 1SA. Tel: 0265 44141 Ex 4362

Formed part of a course. 12-20 hours/week of own time spent.

Abstract: The research was carried out to investigate whether practising midwives, working in selected hospitals in Northern Ireland, were motivated to participate in continuing education. The review of the literature discusses theories of motivation relevant to adult and continuing education, to emphasize that adults may vary in their conceptions of, and hold different values of, continuing education. Concepts of adult learning and continuing education in nursing/midwifery have been used to discuss the importance of self-directed learning and the provision of formal continuing education. Sources from the literature indicate that a motivating environment and the provision of adequate and appropriate programmes of continuing education appear to be important to motivate staff to participate in continuing education. The main tool used was a questionnaire. Data derived from questionnaires were enhanced with information from semi-structured interviews with six of the respondents. The sample of sixty midwives contained respondents of two grades, ward sister and staff midwife (response rate of 72%). A stratified random sampling technique was used to select midwives working in hospitals in one area health board in Northern Ireland.

The results indicated that respondents conceptualised continuing education as both formal and informal learning experiences. But midwives varied in the views they held of the value of continuing education to them. However, all the respondents identified continuing education as being important for professional reasons. On the basis of the findings in this study it appears that midwives lack motivation to take part in informal and formal continuing education. But the findings also imply that encouragement and support from managers, adequate provision of continuing education facilities, social responsibility and having to work night duty/part-time may influence midwives' ability to participate in available continuing education programmes.

On the basis of these findings a number of recommendations are made including the need for an effective staff appraisal system and the provision of a range of opportunities (formal and informal) for continuing education. These are emphasized as being important to motivate midwives to continue their education.

Keywords: MIDWIFERY EDUCATION (CONTINUING), MIDWIFERY EDUCATION (HIGHER), MIDWIFERY EDUCATION (MOTIVATION)

McCrea H. Motivation for continuing education in midwifery. Midwifery 1989;5:134-45.

113. THE ROLE OF THE MIDWIFE IN RELATION TO WOMENS' EARLY EXPERIENCES OF BREASTFEEDING

January 1990 - September 1991

J Billingsley, MA Student, D Stears, Senior Lecturer. **Contact:** J Billingsley, Beverley Road, Canterbury, Kent CT2 7EN.

Formed part of a course. 2-6 hours/week of own time spent.

Abstract: (Not updated since 1991) The study is concerned with the role of the midwife in supporting new mothers who have chosen to breastfeed. It recognises that 'the lost 25%' have been identified as a target group by the Department of Health sponsored 'Breastfeeding Initiative', and the project attempts to focus on the constraints which may prevent individual midwife practitioners from providing more effective health education. The study is a small qualitative piece of research which will follow through two groups of student midwives in different centres. An initial interview in the first week of training will be concerned with previous professional and life experiences considered relevant to attitudes to breastfeeding and perceptions of the midwife's role. Structured questions will explore these attitudes and perceptions specifically, and establish a base line with which to compare the results of a follow-up interview at the end of the training period, using the same or similar instruments. The input from the formal curriculum concerned with breastfeeding, the students' experience on the wards and in the community, and the influence of past experiences will be discussed and explored in some depth during the second interview. It is hoped that this will enable specific areas of difficulty to be identified. Because the sample is so small, it cannot be regarded as representative, so rigorous statistical analysis would be inappropriate.

The results will be essentially illustrative material from which tentative suggestions may be made about ways of improving the midwife's performance in this area, although some basic statistical analysis (eg t-test) may be appropriate to compare students at different centres or the same students' responses at different times.

Keywords: BREASTFEEDING, HEALTH EDUCATION, MIDWIFE'S ROLE, MIDWIFERY EDUCATION

116. A STUDY OF THE ROLE AND RESPONSIBILITIES OF THE MIDWIFE

January 1978 - December 1983

Sarah Robinson, Senior Research Fellow, Josephine Golden, Research Associate, Susan Bradley, Research Associate, Keith Jacka, Statistician. **Contact:** Sarah Robinson, Nursing Research Unit, Kings College, London University, Cornwall House Annexe, Waterloo Road, London SE1 8TX. Tel: 071 872 3063/3057

For full details see under Management Studies (Record No. 116).

119. NEWLY QUALIFIED MIDWIVES: A STUDY OF THEIR CAREER INTENTIONS AND VIEWS OF THEIR TRAINING
January 1979 - December 1984

Sarah Robinson, Senior Research Fellow, Josephine Golden, Research Associate, Keith Jacka, Statistician. **Contact:** Sarah Robinson, Nursing Research Unit, Kings College, London University, Cornwall House Annexe, Waterloo Road, London SE1 8TX. Tel: 071 872 3063/3057

Funded as integral or additional part of a job. 2-6 hours/week of own time spent.

Abstract: The purpose of this study was to ascertain whether lengthening midwifery training led to an increase in the proportion of newly qualified midwives who intended to practise midwifery and in the proportion who felt adequately prepared to do so. It was undertaken by sending a questionnaire to 930 midwives who qualified in 1979 after a 12-month course and then sending the same questionnaire to 930 midwives who qualifed in 1983 after an 18-month course. Response rates of 84% and 89% were achieved for the two groups respectively.

Findings showed that only a minority of the 18-month group embarked on the course intending to make a career in midwifery (39%) and intended to do so once qualifed (24%). Reasons cited most frequently for training were those concerned with enhancing a nursing career and these findings therefore confirmed a longstanding trend in midwifery. The 18-month group were more likely than the 12-month group to feel adequately prepared for each of the various responsibilities of the practising midwife. Findings on the relationship between career intentions and adequacy of training indicated that a course that is felt to be an adequate preparation for practice and is enjoyed may change intentions in favour of a career in midwifery.

Lack of clinical teaching was an important finding: 45% of the 18-month group said they had had insufficient teaching from midwifery tutors, 55% from hospital midwives, 68% and 71% from obstetric and paediatric medical staff respectively. Comments suggested this was due to staff shortages and, for service staff, to lack of preparation and/or a reluctance to teach students. The latter problem can be approached by continuing education for staff and better service/education liaison, whereas the former is part of the wider issue of recruitment and retention of staff. Forty two per cent of the 18-month group said that they had insufficient time for personal study; it is important that sufficient time be made available, as developing independent study skills is an important aspect of individual responsibility for continuing education.

Keywords: CAREER INTENTIONS, CAREER PATHS, CLINICAL TEACHING, MIDWIFERY EDUCATION (CONTINUING), MIDWIFERY EDUCATION (EVALUATION), MIDWIFERY EDUCATION (RECRUITMENT)

Golden J. Midwifery training; the views of newly qualified midwives. Midwives Chronicle 1980;93:190-4. Also published as: NERU Occasional Paper No.1.

Robinson S. The 18 month training: What difference has it made? Midwives Chronicle 1986;99:22-9.

Robinson S. Career intentions of newly qualified midwives. Midwifery 1986;2:25-37.

Robinson S. Midwifery training: The views of newly qualified midwives. Nurse Education Today 1986;6:49-59.

Robinson S. Preparation for practice: The educational experiences and career intentions of newly qualified midwives. In: Robinson S, Thomson A, eds. Midwives, Research and Childbirth. Vol 2. London: Chapman and Hall 1991:302-45.

120. A STUDY OF THE CAREER PATTERNS OF MIDWIVES
January 1986 - December 1992

Sarah Robinson, Senior Research Fellow, Heather Owen, Research Associate, Keith Jacka, Statistician. **Contact:** Sarah Robinson, Nursing Research Unit, Kings College, London University, Cornwall House Annexe, Waterloo Road, London SE1 8TX. Tel: 071 872 3063/3057

Funded as integral or additional part of a job by funding agency: Department of Health.

Abstract: (Not updated since 1991). This longitudinal study, begun in 1986, is following the careers of two cohorts of midwives from the time of qualification; one cohort qualified in 1979, the other in 1983. The members of the two cohorts are the midwives who took part in the King's College Nursing Research Unit's earlier study of midwives' career intentions and views of training (Record No. 119). The study was commissioned in response to concern about retention levels in midwifery and is currently funded until 1992. The main aims of the study are to ascertain: 1) the proportion of the two cohorts in practice; 2) the extent to which career intentions have been translated into practice; 3) the experience of and views about practising as a midwife; 4) perceptions about adequacy of training for practice; 5) reasons for staying in or for leaving midwifery; 6) combining family responsibilities with work as a midwife; and 7) levels of satisfaction with grades awarded under the Clinical Grading Review.

Information to date has been obtained by sending questionnaires to members of the two cohorts in 1986/87 and again in 1989. The next one will be sent out in 1992. The study has entailed tracing the two groups of midwives through a variety of professional and statutory databases and through informal networks. Response rates achieved for the two cohorts in the two follow-ups undertaken so far range from 63% to 82%. Findings from the 1986/87 questionnaire are available, and include the following. Extending training to eighteen months seems to have had little effect on retention in that three years after qualification just under half of both cohorts were practising midwifery. They displayed very similar career histories over this time, the main exception was that the 1983 group were less likely than the 1979 to have obtained a sister's post. Career intentions expressed at the time of qualification appeared to be a good indicator of careers actually followed.

Findings for the 1979 group showed that those who had only been employed in midwifery in the first three years after qualification were much more likely to have practised midwifery over the next four years than those who had undertaken other work as well as midwifery, or those who had not practised midwifery at all.

Keywords: CAREER INTENTIONS, CAREER PATHS, LONGITUDINAL STUDY, MID-WIFERY PRACTICE (CESSATION), MIDWIFERY (RETENTION LEVELS), MIDWIVES

Robinson S, Owen H, Jacka K, Dereky C. The midwives' career patterns project. Report to DHSS on Phase 2. 1988.

Robinson S, Owen H. Career intentions and career patterns of midwives. In: Wilson-Barnett J, Robinson S, eds. Directions in Nursing Research: Ten Years of Progress at London University. London: Scutari Press. 1989:265-79.

Owen H, Robinson S. Researching midwives' careers. In Research and the Midwife Conference Proceedings for 1989. Department of Nursing Studies, University of Manchester 1989:48-70.

126. TEACHING ETHICS IN MIDWIFERY EDUCATION
January 1985 - December 1987

Sr A Thompson, Senior Lecturer. **Contact:** Sr A Thompson, Uxbridge Rd, Rickmansworth, Herts WD3 2DJ.

Formed part of a course. 12-20 hours/week of own time spent. Funded by Iolanthe Trust.

Abstract: This study examines the statement that "ethics are a neglected but increasingly important element in midwifery education" and, after some discussion of the issues and values central to midwifery practice, describes one proposal for incorporating ethical reflection into the midwifery curriculum. Discussion of the need for such reflection involves consideration of changes in the nature and setting of contemporary midwifery practice. An overview of two English studies of teaching ethics in nursing is used to illustrate selected models of moral education. The current state of ethics teaching in midwifery is described with the results of research in one Thames Region Health Authority.

Since a constant comparative analytical approach is used as the research methodology, the relevant literature is interwoven with the research findings throughout the text. Issues and values in midwifery practice are identified from regional and local research and the literature. As a result, Gilligan's (1977) framework for feminine moral decision-making is examined in relation to midwifery. The particular value of covenant as a conceptual framework for the ethical delivery of care in midwifery is explored. The foregoing discussion is used as the basis for developing a proposal for facilitating ethical reflection in midwifery education. The study concludes with a description of the possible incorporation of a structural ethical component into a new curriculum for a three-year programme for Direct Entry midwifery.

Keywords: ETHICS, MIDWIFERY, MIDWIFERY EDUCATION, MIDWIFERY EDUCATION (CURRICULUM), MIDWIFERY PRACTICE

Thompson A. Conflict and covenant - ethics in midwifery education. Midwives Chronicle 1989;102:191-7.

127. DIRECT ENTRY - A PREPARATION FOR MIDWIFERY PRACTICE
April 1987 - March 1988

N Radford, Self-employed, A Thompson, Assistant Director - Midwifery Education.
Contact: A Thompson, Uxbridge Road, Rickmansworth, Herts WD3 2DJ.

Funded by funding agency: Department of Health.

Abstract: This study had four main goals: 1) to describe the national situation regarding Direct Entry midwifery training; 2) to discover the factors influencing the development of such programmes; 3) to advise on issues which should be considered by those contemplating this option; and 4) to recommend ways in which the establishment of non-nurse midwifery training could be facilitated.

Each midwifery training school, district and regional health authority was sent a questionnaire covering various aspects of Direct Entry. This survey was supplemented by visits and interviews. The excellent response rate and co-operation of all concerned ensured that a comprehensive national picture was gained. A limited survey of those enquiring about Direct Entry training was also carried out, and valuable lessons learned from this exercise. The factors inhibiting development of Direct Entry, like those encouraging it, are pragmatic, historical, and ideological. The report documents how important the various factors were in influencing decisions on Direct Entry training.

The report covers all aspects of Direct Entry training, and the chapters on each aspect can be read either in isolation, or as a part of the whole. The issues identified from the data which should be considered by schools, districts and regions contemplating the Direct Entry midwifery option are dealt with in detail.

The main recommendations involve positive action to ensure support for Direct Entry initiatives, improved information on all aspects of setting up and running courses, organised funding, independent evaluation of new projects and the development of strategic educational plans for midwifery education. The report addresses some of the practicalities associated with implementing the recommendations.

Keywords: COST EFFECTIVENESS, MIDWIFERY EDUCATION, MIDWIFERY EDUCATION (DIRECT ENTRY), MIDWIFERY EDUCATION (RECRUITMENT)

Radford N, Thompson A. Direct entry: a preparation for midwifery practice. EBN/ University of Surrey, 1988.

Radford N, Thompson A. Direct entry midwifery training. Part 1. Potential candidates. Midwives Chronicle 1988;101:167-9.

Radford N, Thompson A. Direct entry midwifery education. Part 2. Practicalities. Midwives Chronicle 1988;101:211-13.

Radford N, Thompson A. Direct entry to midwifery. Part 1. Nursing Times 1988;31:52-4.

Radford N, Thompson A. Choosing the design. Nursing Times 1988;32:42-3.

128. FACTORS AFFECTING STUDENT COMPETENCY IN MIDWIFERY
May 1988 - December 1991

M Chamberlain, Lecturer. **Contact:** M Chamberlain, Maple Crescent, Gloucester, Ontario, Canada K1B 323.

Over 20 hours/week of own time spent. Funded by Vice Chancellors of Universities of UK.

Abstract: (Not updated since 1991) The aims of this study are four-fold: 1) to identify how students acquire their midwifery skills; 2) to establish how they are taught; 3) to find out which methods are most beneficial to learning, together with those that are not; and 4) to establish who teaches them in the clinical area. The study is a qualitative case study, using an ethnographic approach of observations and interviews. Twenty-five students representing five different sets were observed in all clinical areas in the maternity hospital. Interviews were used to validate the observer's perceptions and themes arising from the data. To date, the three most important themes arising from the study include role-transition problems, communication problems and the types of teaching strategy used. The analysis for grounded theory is still in progress.

Keywords: CLINICAL TEACHING, COMMUNICATION, LEARNING ENVIRONMENT, MIDWIFERY EDUCATION (EVALUATION), MIDWIFERY SKILLS

130. FACTORS INFLUENCING MOTIVATION IN MIDWIFERY TUTORS
September 1990 - December 1991

S Taylor, Midwifery Tutor. **Contact:** S Taylor, Stawell, Bridgwater, Somerset TA7 9AD.

Formed part of a course. 6-12 hours/week of own time spent. Funded by employer: Somerset Health Authority.

Abstract: (Not updated since 1991). The aims of this ongoing study are three-fold: 1) to explore the motivation to train as a midwifery tutor; 2) to identify areas of satisfaction and dissatisfaction in the practice of midwifery education; and 3) to identify the career intentions of midwifery tutors. The study will be descriptive in method. Two regions in England will be examined, and the data gathered by means of a postal questionnaire. It is anticipated that approximately eighty tutors will take part. Preliminary data obtained from informal interviews are to form the basis of this questionnaire. A model of motivational styles will be used for analysis.

CAREER INTENTIONS, MIDWIFE TEACHERS, MIDWIFE TEACHERS (SATISFACTION), MIDWIFERY EDUCATION (CONTINUING), MIDWIFERY EDUCATION (HIGHER), MIDWIFERY EDUCATION (MOTIVATION)

137. A STUDY OF THE MENTOR-SYSTEM IN ONE MIDWIFERY INSTITUTION
November 1988 - August 1989
Sooi-Ken Too, Senior Lecturer, Practitioner. **Contact:** Sooi-Ken Too, c/o Midwifery School, Romford College of Nursing, Midwifery and Health Care, Rush Green Hospital, Dagenham Road, Romford RM7 OYA. Tel: 0708 746066 Ex 320

Formed part of a course. 12-20 hours/week of own time spent.

Abstract: The concept of mentoring has been increasingly advocated in recent years. The purpose of this descriptive study was to explore the mentor system in one particular midwifery institution. A literature search was undertaken to review studies in adult development, business, education and nursing.

Methodological triangulation techniques were used to investigate the key parameters of the mentoring system within a midwifery clinical setting. Methods used were interviews, postal questionnaires and self-completed evaluative forms. Convenience sampling was used to identify a total of seventy potential respondents. These included two groups of student midwives at different stages of training, midwives and neonatal nurses. Interviews were carried out with six newly-qualified midwives. Postal questionnaires were sent to seventy potential respondents, of whom fifty-nine (84%) returned their questionnaires. Self-completed evaluative forms were returned by sixty mentors and students.

The study brought to light the complex role and functions of the mentor. Expectations of the mentor's role varied from one student group to another, and suggested that selection of the mentors should be individualised and appropriate to the students' needs. Role-based development of the mentors, staffing levels and co-ordination of staff rotation were the key factors in the implementation of the mentor system. Self-learning and resource findings were the alternative strategies most used by the students when their mentors were absent.

The study concludes that while mentoring is a valid concept, its usefulness to this institution had not been as fully implemented as it could have been.

Keywords: MENTORS, MIDWIFERY EDUCATION, MIDWIFERY EDUCATION (EVALUATION)

143. STUDENT MIDWIVES' PERSPECTIVES ON MATERNAL SENTIMENTS DURING CHILDBIRTH
October 1989 - June 1990
M Williams, Midwife Teacher. **Contact:** M Williams, Cave Hill, Maidstone ME15 GDY.

Formed part of a course. 6-12 hours/week of own time spent. Funded by employer and by funding agency: Iolanthe Trust.

Abstract: The purpose of this investigation was to explore the maternal feelings of junior student midwives during their time on a labour ward.

The population interviewed were six volunteer female student midwives from a set of nine. Each student was an experienced registered general nurse who had completed eight weeks practical experience in the community and eight weeks in the delivery suite. A non-directive unstructured interview technique was used. The interviews which lasted between half an hour and one hour were taped, transcribed and analysed.

A dominant and common theme was that childless students were particularly affected by the emotional atmosphere of the labour rooms. Feelings were especially intense during their first allocation, when many students indicated a lack of readiness for the emotions they encounted.

The results highlight a number of gaps between theory and practice. All students acknowledged pain, anger, control and coping, noise (screaming, shouting) and fear as important in labour. Of these only pain and fear are addressed in the curriculum. Suggestions for appropriate adaptations to the curriculum are made.

Keywords: ANGER, EXPERIENCE (STUDENT MIDWIVES'), FEAR, LABOUR, MIDWIFERY EDUCATION, SCREAMING, STUDENT MIDWIVES (EMOTIONS)

148. A SURVEY OF MIDWIFERY EDUCATION IN THE UNITED KINGDOM WITH REFERENCE TO ISSUES OF PROFESSIONAL EDUCATION, ACCOUNTABILITY AND THE LOCATION OF MIDWIFERY SCHOOLS

August 1988 - May 1989

J Magill-Cureden, Senior Lecturer, Research and Development. **Contact:** J Magill-Cureden, Belgrade Rd, Hampton, Middlesex TW12 2AZ.

Formed part of a course. 12-20 hours/week of own time spent.

Abstract: Given the context of a profession that is accountable for its own education, this study reports the results of a survey of midwifery schools in the United Kingdom, which investigated where midwifery education should be sited. A literature search explored the issues of professionalism and accountability, examining the implications of both for midwifery education. A survey was undertaken by postal questionnaire to obtain information on the location of midwifery schools and their accountability. In total, 170 schools of midwifery were surveyed. Fourteen were used for testing and piloting the questionnaire, while the remaining 156 were used for the main study. Of these, there was a usable response rate of 85%.

Three main areas of investigation were used to frame the questions: 1) general information about the size and structure of the school, together with its proximity to neighbouring schools; 2) an enquiry into the present accountability of midwifery teachers for midwifery education, using component themes of accountability (ie budget responsibility, policy-making and policy-making changes, decision making, and evaluation); and 3) an enquiry into present senior midwifery teachers' views on the future location of midwifery education. The questionnaire was reviewed by an educational psychologist, a general educationalist and three midwifery teachers.

An analysis was carried out by grouping the schools in one of six categories, which were based on the structure of the schools. The responses were placed on a grid and analyzed per category using a colour coding system.

The results showed that: 1) most midwifery schools were structured within the midwifery service units of one particular Health Authority; 2) 80% of schools had less than seven midwife teachers; 3) schools that were independent or structured in more than one Health Authority tended to be larger; 4) midwifery educationalists had more autonomy and managerial accountability in larger schools; 5) midwife teachers had less control and responsibility in schools that were structured within midwifery service units. It was apparent that while midwife teachers were accountable for the educational aspects of a school, less than half of the respondents were accountable for managerial aspects. For example, only 30% of the heads of schools had budgetary control. This lack of control reduced the responsibility for decision-making. Midwife teachers indicated a preference for locating midwifery education within either Colleges of Midwifery or Institutes of Health Studies.

The study concluded that midwife teachers should be fully responsible for the management and educational aspects of professional midwifery education, and that the structures for education should be located within the larger institutions, thereby ensuring that close clinical and educational relationships be preserved.

Keywords: MIDWIFE TEACHERS (LEVELS), MIDWIFE TEACHERS (SATISFACTION), MIDWIFERY EDUCATION, MIDWIFERY EDUCATION (ACCOUNTABILITY), MIDWIFERY EDUCATION (EVALUATION), MIDWIFERY SCHOOLS (LOCATION), PROFESSIONALISM

150. AN EVALUATION OF PRE-REGISTRATION MIDWIFERY EDUCATION IN ENGLAND
December 1990 - November 1993
C Maggs, Director, J Kent, Research associate, N Mackeith, Research assistant. **Contact:** N Mackeith, Ravenscar Mount, Leeds LS8 4AX.

Funded by funding agency(ies): Department of Health.

Aims of the study: To evaluate pre-registration midwifery education with reference to the implications for the workforce and the views of the students and managers.

Ethics committee approval gained: Yes

Research design: Descriptive – Qualitative and Quantitative – Survey/Ethnography/Case Study/Historical/Focus Groups

Data collection:
    Techniques used:
        Documentary analysis
        Interviews
        Postal questionnaires
        Group interviews
        Fieldnotes
        Workshops.
    Time data were collected:
        First site introductory visit 1991.
        Stage 1 fieldwork in case study sites 1991-2.
        Stage 2 fieldwork in case study sites 1992-3.
    Testing of any tools used:
        Schedules and questionnaires piloted in one other site.
    Topics covered:
        Students: Personal circumstances and the reasons for doing midwifery courses.
        Staff: Theory and practicalities of teaching and managing the course.
    Setting for data collection:
        Midwifery education institutions.
        Hospitals.
        Higher education institutions.
        Students' homes.

Details about sample studied:
    Planned size of sample:
        Six case study sites from a list of 16.
    Rationale for planned size:
        Feasibility.
    Entry criteria:
        Institutions offering pre-registration midwifery education.
    Sample selection:
        Colleges at various points on a continuum.

Interventions, Outcomes and Analysis:
    Analysis:
        Content analysis.

Keywords: MIDWIFE TEACHERS (VIEWS), MIDWIFERY EDUCATION, MIDWIFERY EDUCATION (DIRECT ENTRY), MIDWIFERY EDUCATION (EVALUATION), MIDWIFERY EDUCATION (PRE-REGISTRATION), MIDWIFERY MANAGERS, STUDENT MIDWIVES, WORKFORCE IMPLICATIONS

160. RECRUITMENT AND MARKETING IN A SCHOOL OF MIDWIFERY
June 1990 - May 1991
V M White, Midwife Teacher. **Contact:** V M White, Grove Park, Tring, Hertfordshire HP23 5JL.

Formed part of a course. 12-20 hours/week of own time spent.

Aims of the study: To investigate the reasons why potential student midwives choose to train in a particular school and if these characteristics are the same as those perceived and marketed by the midwifery schools.

Ethics committee approval gained: No

Research design: Descriptive – Qualitative and Quantitative – Survey

Data collection:
Techniques used:
Questionnaires to potential student midwives.
Interviews of heads of midwifery education.
Time data were collected:
Questionnaires - on day of recruitment interview.
Interviews followed on from questionnaires.
Testing of any tools used:
Questionnaire was piloted the previous year.
Topics covered:
The concept of marketing.
Responsibility for marketing.
Marketing methods.
Choice of school.
Information sent to students.
Shortage of students.
Setting for data collection:
School of midwifery.

Details about sample studied:
Planned size of sample:
24 questionnaires.
6 interviews.
Rationale for planned size:
All students attending for interview on two days.
Heads of midwifery education in similar size schools.
Entry criteria:
Schools of the same size and geographical position ie outer London.
Sample selection:
Convenience.

Actual sample size:
20 questionnaires.
3 interviews.
Response rate:
Questionnaires - 70%

Interventions, Outcomes and Analysis:
Analysis:
Content analysis by hand.

Results: There was agreement that there was a shortage of students.
The midwife teachers did not see the need for any change in the "tried and tested" methods of recruitment currently in use. The potential students were more likely to live locally or know someone in training.
A friendly atmosphere and the style of education were important factors when choosing a school.

Recommendations for further research: 1. To find out why there is a high drop out rate between appointment and commencing the course.
2. To design a marketing communication programme for recruiting non-practising nurses to midwifery.

Keywords: MARKETING, MIDWIFE TEACHERS, MIDWIFERY, MIDWIFERY EDUCATION, MIDWIFERY EDUCATION (MARKETING), MIDWIFERY EDUCATION (RECRUITMENT)

191. THE HISTORY OF MIDWIFERY EDUCATION FROM 1902 TO 1936
July 1990 - August 1991
S J Ridgway, Head of Midwifery and related studies. **Contact:** S J Ridgway, Cropthorne Drive, Hollywood, Worcestershire B47 5PZ.
For full details see under Historical Studies (Record No. 191).

201. INVESTIGATING MIDWIFERY EDUCATION IN A MULTIRACIAL/ MULTICULTURAL SOCIETY
February 1992 - September 1993
E E Neile, Midwife Teacher. **Contact:** E E Neile, Wellesley Avenue, Beverley High Road, Hull HU6 7LN.

Formed part of a course. 12-20 hours/week of own time spent. Funded by employer: Humberside College of Health.

Aims of the study: To investigate:
1. What provision is made within curricula for the teaching of multiracial and multicultural education in schools and colleges of nursing and midwifery.
2. Teachers' readiness to teach multicultural education.
3. What teaching midwife teachers do about race and culture and what learning they encourage students to do.

4. What students think they should learn about race and culture in order to become effective practitioners.

5. What student midwives have learnt about race and culture in their programmes of education.

Ethics committee approval gained: No

Research design: Descriptive – Qualitative and Quantitative – Survey

> **Data collection:**
> > **Techniques used:**
> > > Interviews and questionnaires.
> > **Time data were collected:**
> > > November 1992 to March 1993.
> > **Testing of any tools used:**
> > > Pilot study: June-October 1992.
> > **Topics covered:**
> > > Understanding of multicultural issues.
> > > How much multiculturalism is learnt in initial teacher training and since.
> > > What is taught to students.
> > > What student midwives think that they should learn about race and culture, what they have learnt and how they have learnt it.
> > **Setting for data collection:**
> > > Colleges of health - a cross section selected at random.

> **Details about sample studied:**
> > **Planned size of sample:**
> > > 10% of the midwifery education population, then approximately 17 institutions.
> > **Rationale for planned size:**
> > > Approximately 1/10th of the midwifery education population in order to survey a representative cross section.
> > **Entry criteria:**
> > > Practising midwifery teachers in England.
> > > Student midwives progressing in midwifery education.
> > > Midwives qualified for up to a year.
> > **Sample selection:**
> > > Random
> > **Actual sample size:**
> > > 318 student questionnaires sent.
> > > 126 teacher questionnaires sent.
> > > 6 midwife teachers interviewed.
> > **Response rate:**
> > > 74% - student questionnaires.
> > > 71% - teacher questionnaires.

Interventions, Outcomes and Analysis:
Analysis:
Descriptive analysis.

Results: Not yet available.

Keywords: ETHNIC GROUPS, MIDWIFE TEACHERS (ATTITUDES), MIDWIFE TEACH-ERS (VIEWS), MIDWIFERY EDUCATION, MIDWIFERY EDUCATION (CURRICULUM), MIDWIFERY EDUCATION (EVALUATION), MULTICULTURAL EDUCATION, STUDENT MIDWIVES (ATTITUDES)

207. A SURVEY OF THE GROUP LEARNING EXPERIENCES OF MIDWIVES AND TEACHERS OF AN ADVANCED MIDWIFERY COURSE
November 1986 - December 1990
C A Tucker, Principal, Midwifery Education. **Contact:** C A Tucker, Sherbourne Avenue, Littlestoke, Bristol BS12 8BB.

Formed part of a course. 2-6 hours/week of own time spent. Funded by employer and by Iolanthe Trust.

Aims of the study: To examine the group dynamics of an ADM course and functional roles within it.
To explore students' views of the development of group awareness skills, group performance and group dynamics.
To elicit teachers' views on group development in this particular group of adult learners.

Ethics committee approval gained: Yes

Research design: Descriptive – Qualitative – Ethnography

Data collection:
Techniques used:
Questionnaires.
Semi-structured interviews.
Time data were collected:
January 1989 - questionnaires.
March 1989 - semi-structured interviews.
Testing of any tools used:
Tested with 6 students and 1 teacher.
Topics covered:
Group awareness.
Group dynamics.
Group processes.
Relationships.

Setting for data collection:
School of Midwifery.

Details about sample studied:
Planned size of sample:
59 students, 6 teachers
Rationale for planned size:
All students on the Bristol ADM between 1984 and 1988 inclusive. 6 teachers represent the six disciplines within the curriculum.
Entry criteria:
Students: attending ADM.
Sample selection:
Convenience.
Actual sample size:
59 students
6 teachers
Response rate:
Students 89.8%
Teachers 100%

Interventions, Outcomes and Analysis:
Analysis:
SPSSx.
Content analysis.

Results: There is a strong relationship between individuals and their group, with midwives' learning experience influenced by the group.

A recommendation is made for a sensitive, open, flexible and reciprocal approach to be adopted in such courses. The facilitator's role is that of a research person and by adopting this role the teacher enhances the likelihood of meeting the needs of the individual and the group.

Keywords: ADULT LEARNERS, ADVANCED DIPLOMA IN MIDWIFERY, GROUP DYNAMICS, LEARNING ENVIRONMENT, MIDWIFE TEACHERS (EXPERIENCES), MIDWIFERY EDUCATION, MIDWIFERY EDUCATION (CONTINUING)

212. INTERNATIONAL PERSPECTIVES IN THE ENGLISH MIDWIFERY CURRICULUM
August 1991 - March 1992
G D Barber, Midwifery Lecturer. **Contact:** G D Barber, Itchen Close, Oakley, Basingstoke, Hampshire RG23 7DL.

Formed part of a course. 6-12 hours/week of own time spent. Funded by employer: Basingstoke and North Hampshire Health Authority.

Aims of the study: Investigation of the midwifery curriculum in England in order to discover whether or not international issues were, or ought to be, addressed in the education of midwives.

Ethics committee approval gained: No

Research design: Descriptive – Qualitative and Quantitative – Survey/Case Study/ Unstructured Interviews

Data collection:
Techniques used:
Postal questionnaires.
Unstructured interviews.
Time data were collected:
October to December 1991.
Testing of any tools used:
Pilot study for questionnaires with three midwife teachers.
Interviewing techniques not tested.
Topics covered:
Questionnaire: College - type, size.
Courses provided and planned.
Present international links.
Present and future status of international issues.
Issues addressed, planned developments.
Value of international issues in curriculum.
Interviews: Perceived importance of international issues.
Present curricular approach and future developments.
Setting for data collection:
Departments of Midwifery education.

Details about sample studied:
Planned size of sample:
Census of Heads of Midwifery Education
Rationale for planned size:
Manageable size. Sampling of teachers very difficult because of non-availability of accurate lists.
Entry criteria:
Colleges/Departments currently listed by English National Board.
Sample selection:
Inclusive.
Actual sample size:
70
Response rate:
94%

Interventions, Outcomes and Analysis:
Analysis:
Descriptive analysis only.

Results: The survey of Heads of Midwifery Education strongly supported the view that international aspects were valuable and important. Existing initiatives were discovered and a determination to strengthen content. Interviews with educators who had developed more advanced ideas confirmed the survey findings and provided ideas for further development.

A need for improved resources for teachers and sharing of ideas and experience was evident. Suggested models for curriculum content were designed and explored and a comparative studies framework was developed in more depth by the author.

Recommendations for further research: Investigation of curricula in other institutions.
Research into the potential of shared learning.

Keywords: INTERNATIONAL MIDWIFERY, MIDWIFERY EDUCATION, MIDWIFERY EDUCATION (CURRICULUM)

215. AN EVALUATION OF THE NON-MIDWIFERY PLACEMENTS IN A THREE YEAR DIPLOMA IN MIDWIFERY (PRE-REGISTRATION) PROGRAMME
January 1992 - October 1994
D M Fraser, Assistant Principal/Head Faculty of Midwifery. **Contact:** D M Fraser, Seven Oaks Crescent, Bramcote Hills, Nottingham NG9 3FW. Tel: 0602 421421 Ex41279

Funded as integral or additional part of a job by employer: Mid Trent College of Nursing and Midwifery, and partially by self. Formed part of a course. 6-12 hours/week of own time spent.

Aims of the study: To evaluate the teaching and learning processes related to caring for women with medical, surgical and mental health problems with a view to improving the curriculum for current and future pre-registration student midwives.

The study seeks to address the following questions:
1. What do pre-registration student midwives need to learn to enable them to care effectively for women with medical, surgical or mental health problems?
2. How do students view the teaching processes and learning opportunities related to these aspects of care?
3. How do the views of teachers and practice placement staff compare with those of the students?
4. What factors influence the teaching and learning processes and experiences for pre-registration student midwives?

Ethics committee approval gained: No

Research design: Descriptive – Qualitative and Quantitative – Case Study/Action Research

Data collection:
  Techniques used:
    Interviews.
    Questionnaires.
    Case note review.
    Student records of achievment.
    Records of observation.
  Time data were collected:
    Case notes - retrospectively.
    Interviews - immediately after the placement.
    Observation - classroom, reflection after practice placements.
  Testing of any tools used:
    Questionnaire and interview schedules piloted.
  Topics covered:
    Theoretical and practical experience obtained.
    How and why learning was effective.
    Factors which inhibit learning. Relevance of experience to future role as a midwife.
  Setting for data collection:
    Hospital and College.

Details about sample studied:
  Planned size of sample:
    15 Students
  Rationale for planned size:
    First cohort of a new programme.
  Entry criteria:
    All students on a new programme.
  Sample selection:
    Inclusive.
  Actual sample size:
    15
  Response rate:
    100%

Interventions, Outcomes and Analysis:
  Analysis:
    Manual analysis.

Results: Not yet available.

Keywords: EXPERIENCE (STUDENT MIDWIVES'), LEARNING ENVIRONMENT, MIDWIFERY EDUCATION, MIDWIFERY EDUCATION (PRE-REGISTRATION), PLACEMENTS, TEACHING METHODS

218. EXPERIENCES OF SHARED LEARNING WITHIN A PRE-REGISTRATION DIPLOMA IN MIDWIFERY EDUCATION PROGRAMME: AN EVALUATIVE STUDY

March 1992 - January 1993

J E Marshall, Midwife Teacher. **Contact:** J E Marshall, Gripps Common, Blackberry Chase, Owthorpe Road, Cotgrave, Nottingham NG12 3TF. Tel: 0602 691169 x45196

Formed part of a course. 6-12 hours/week of own time spent. Funded by English National Board for Nursing, Midwifery and Health Visiting.

Aims of the study: To evaluate the appropriateness and value of the shared learning component that student midwives undertake in the pre-registration diploma in midwifery within the Mid Trent College of Nursing and Midwifery, and thus determine the means by which such experiences may be improved in order to be more conducive in meeting the learning needs of ALL students.

Ethics committee approval gained: No

Research design: Descriptive – Qualitative – Action Research

> **Data collection:**
> > **Techniques used:**
> > > Questionnaires (student midwives, student nurses, nurse/midwife teachers).
> > > Taped group discussions (student midwives).
> > > Extract from end of term evaluation reports.
> > **Time data were collected:**
> > > Questionnaires distributed 9 months into shared learning.
> > > In depth group discussions (beginning of 2nd year ie 13th month).
> > > End of term evaluations at 4 months, 8 months and 11 months of the 3 year programme.
> > **Testing of any tools used:**
> > > Questionnaires - piloted 18th May to 5 June 1992.
> > **Topics covered:**
> > > Interprofessional shared learning.
> > > Interprofessional relationships - students and teachers.
> > > Pre-registration midwifery/nursing diploma programme.
> > > Implications for policy, education and training.
> > > Practical problems and ethical dilemmas of action research.
> > **Setting for data collection:**
> > > Mid Trent College of Nursing and Midwifery (Nottingham and Mansfield Education Centres).

> **Details about sample studied:**
> > **Planned size of sample:**
> > > 45 (15 Student midwives, 15 student nurses, 15 nurse/midwife teachers).

Rationale for planned size:
>All student midwives undertaking the pre-registration diploma in midwifery.

Entry criteria:
>All student midwives included.
>
>Student nurses - 5 from each of the three groups in which the student midwives shared learning.
>
>Nurse/midwife teachers who had facilitated shared learning sessions.

Sample selection:
>1:4-5 of student midwives.

Actual sample size:
>45

Response rate:
>Questionnaires - 100%
>
>Student midwives group discussions - group 1: 7 student midwives, group 2: 8 student midwives - 100%.
>
>End of term evaluation: 100%

Interventions, Outcomes and Analysis:
Analysis:
>Manual.

Results: The study determined the appropriate size of a group in order to ensure adequate representation of the groups involved to maximise shared learning for all students included. The composition was made up of 25 members - 5 from each branch of nursing and midwifery.

Identified factors which enhanced students' learning in shared learning sessions and hours included continuity of teachers, small groups and being aware of group's needs. Shared learning was hindered by failures of communication, logistical problems and timetabling changes (in one of the education centres).

Shared learning was seen to be effective as a learning strategy in enabling the student midwives to achieve the required learning outcomes for each term of the programme.

Specific advantages of sharing learning with student nurses included a widening of the midwives' and nurses' understanding and appreciation of care across other fields, improved relationships and more opportunities for collaborative work. Constraints of time and logistics made putting on such sessions complicated. Practical issues which require specific attention relate to timetabling, resources (space and personnel), library facilities, and extent of travelling to the education centre for shared sessions.

Resource issues determined the extent of midwife teacher involvement in shared learning and the ways in which student midwives' learning during this component of the programme could be enhanced.

Recommendations for further research: A replication study with subsequent co-horts of students.

Keywords: MIDWIFERY EDUCATION, MIDWIFERY EDUCATION (PRE-REGISTRATION), SHARED LEARNING

224. WHY DON'T MIDWIVES PUBLISH THEIR RESEARCH?
June 1992 - December 1993
Ann Thomson, Senior Lecturer/Director. **Contact:** Ann Thomson, School of Nursing Studies, University of Manchester, Coupland III Building, Coupland Street, Manchester M13 9PL. Tel: 061 275 5342

Funded as integral or additional part of a job by employer: University of Manchester. 2-6 hours/week of own time spent.

Aims of the study: To investigate why completed research which had been registered on the MIRIAD database had not been published.

Ethics committee approval gained: No

Research design: Descriptive – Quantitative – Survey

 Data collection:
  Techniques used:
   Questionnaires
  Time data were collected:
   Retrospectively.
  Testing of any tools used:
   Panel of experts tested questionnaire.
  Topics covered:
   Why the research was undertaken.
   Funding source.
   Reasons for non publication.
   Factors which would have assisted.
  Setting for data collection:
   Postal questionnaire to researchers throughout the UK.

 Details about sample studied:
  Planned size of sample:
   All completed studies up to end of 1990 where there were no listings of publications in the 1991 MIRIAD report.
  Rationale for planned size:
   Total entries.
  Entry criteria:
   All completed studies up to end of 1990 where there were no listings of publications in the 1991 MIRIAD Report.

Sample selection:
    Inclusive.
Actual sample size:
    Not yet available.

Interventions, Outcomes and Analysis:
    Analysis: Amdahl computer SPSSx.

Keywords: MIDWIFERY RESEARCH, PUBLICATION

254. LIBRARY RESOURCES: MIDWIVES' USE DURING PERIODS OF EDUCATION
September 1993 - September 1994
V Fenerty, Librarian. **Contact:** V Fenerty, Fairholme Road, Withington, Manchester M20 4SA.

Formed part of a course. 2-6 hours/week of own time spent. Funded by employer: Manchester College of Midwifery.

Aims of the study: To establish whether the use of midwifery resources is related to the level of midwifery education being undertaken.

Ethics committee approval gained: No

Research design: Descriptive – Qualitative and Quantitative – Survey

Data collection:
    Techniques used:
        Questionnaires.
        Group interviews.
    Time data were collected:
        While students on course.
    Testing of any tools used:
        Questionnaires piloted with 21 students, 5 tutors.
    Topics covered:
        Resources.
        Age.
        Education.
        Library instruction.
    Setting for data collection:
        Hospital - college classroom.

Details about sample studied:
    Planned size of sample:
        3 complete cohorts of students (Pre-reg, Post-reg, ADM).
    Rationale for planned size:
        Total cohort for that year.

Entry criteria:
>All students having studied for 1 year.

Sample selection:
>Convenience.

Actual sample size:
>Recruitment ongoing.

Interventions, Outcomes and Analysis:
>**Analysis:**
>>SPSS

Keywords: ADVANCED DIPLOMA IN MIDWIFERY, INFORMATION SOURCES, LIBRARIES, MIDWIFERY EDUCATION, MIDWIFERY EDUCATION (POST-REGISTRATION), MIDWIFERY EDUCATION (PRE-REGISTRATION)

256. MIDWIFERY STUDENTS' PERCEPTIONS OF STUDENT CENTRED LEARNING
May 1992 - December 1993

B Grant, Course Leader - Midwifery Programmes. **Contact:** B Grant, Marywood Square, Glasgow, G41 8BJ.

Formed part of a course. Funded by employer: Glasgow College of Nursing and Midwifery.

Aims of the study: 1. To identify the nature of midwifery students' perceptions of student-centred learning.
2. To ascertain the effects of previous nursing educational experiences on those perceptions.
3. To determine whether the teaching methods and materials used in the midwifery programme bear any relationship to their perceived understanding of student-centred and teacher-centred learning and their perceived use of learning approaches and associated strategies.
4. To identify other factors that influence their use of particular learning approaches and associated strategies.
5. To determine students' views of the changes they would like to see made in the midwifery programme.

Ethics committee approval gained: No

Research design: Descriptive – Qualitative and Quantitative – Survey

Data collection:
>**Techniques used:**
>>Questionnaire.

>**Time data were collected:**
>>On specific days of the students' course.

Testing of any tools used:
Pilot study of 10 ADM students.
Topics covered:
Ways of learning.
Educational tools used by students.
Influence of previous nursing experience.
Improvements or modifications in programme.
Setting for data collection:
Colleges of Nursing and Midwifery.

Details about sample studied:
Planned size of sample:
30-40
Rationale for planned size:
Statistical basis.
Entry criteria:
Available classes.
Sample selection:
Convenience.
Actual sample size:
27 questionnaires distributed.
20 completed.
Response rate:
74%

Interventions, Outcomes and Analysis:
Analysis:
Content analysis.

Results: Findings for this group of students showed a tendency to prefer more teacher-centred methods. All would have liked more study time and found working shifts interfered with study patterns.

Keywords: STUDENT CENTRED LEARNING, STUDENT MIDWIVES, TEACHING METHODS

258. WITH WOMEN: A REFLEXIVE PROJECT
September 1991 - January 1995
Julie Kent, Research Associate/Project Manager. **Contact:** Julie Kent, Department of Sociology, University of Bristol, 12 Woodland Road, Bristol BS8 1UQ.

Funded as integral or additional part of a job by Department of Health and Maggs Research Associates. Subsequently funded by ESRC as postgraduate studentship award.

Aims of the study: This research addresses two questions:
1) How is the experience of being a student midwife socially constructed? The educational experiences of pre-registration student midwives will be examined in order to develop an understanding of what "becoming a midwife" means.

2) What are the implications of a reflexive approach to social research? The research considers how an understanding of "the reflexive project" might inform social and midwifery research practice and examines the potential of participatory research methods.

Ethics committee approval gained: No

Research design: Descriptive – Qualitative – Participatory Research/Group Inquiry

Data collection:
Techniques used:
Group workshops tape recorded - notes taken, short critical incidents written.
Time data were collected:
At three monthly intervals over 18 months (September 1991 - June 1993).
Topics covered:
Students' educational experiences.
Setting for data collection:
A College of Midwifery and Nursing and a College of Health Studies.

Details about sample studied:
Planned size of sample:
Group size between 8-16 students
Rationale for planned size:
All students in September 1991 cohort at two colleges invited to participate.
Entry criteria:
Student midwives.
Sample selection:
Convenience.
Actual sample size:
Between 8-14 at 3 monthly meetings.
Response rate:
100%

Interventions, Outcomes and Analysis:
Analysis:
Critical analysis in collaboration with group participants.

Keywords: EXPERIENCE (STUDENT MIDWIVES'), MIDWIFERY EDUCATION (PRE-REGISTRATION), STUDENT MIDWIVES

Kent J, Maggs C. An evaluation of pre-registration midwifery education in England. 1992 Working paper 1: Research design: (Bath:Maggs Research Associates)
Kent J. What are your views of pre-registration midwifery education? MIDIRS Midwifery Digest 1992;2:15-16.

Kent J. An evaluation of pre-registration midwifery education in England. Research Design : A case study approach. Midwifery 1992;8:69-75.

Kent J. Midwives - No need to be a nurse? Nursing Times 1994 (in press).

259. AN INVESTIGATIVE STUDY TO EXPLORE THE EXTENT TO WHICH ANDRAGOGY AND EXPERIENTIAL LEARNING ARE APPLIED IN MIDWIFERY EDUCATION

March - July 1992

Theo Kwansa, Midwifery Teacher. **Contact:** Theo Kwansa, Glasgow College of Nursing and Midwifery, East Division, 110 St James Road, Glasgow G4 OPS. Tel: 041 552 1562

Formed part of a course. Over 20 hours/week of own time spent. Funded by employer: Glasgow College of Nursing and Midwifery.

Aims of the study: To establish the views of educationists about the principles of pedagogy and andragogy.

To establish the extent to which course participants are acknowledged as adult learners with a rich reserve of prior experiences that can be utilised as a worthwhile resource for collaborative learning.

To investigate midwife teachers' willingness to make a commitment to the notion that as adult learners, student midwives can be entrusted with their own learning and that they can be given more responsibility for relevant aspects of their own education.

To determine teachers' awareness of a need for more flexibility, more creativity and more learner participation in the planning and implementation of the teaching/learning activities and evaluate components of their own educational programmes.

Ethics committee approval gained: Yes

Research design: Descriptive – Qualitative – Survey

   Data collection:
   Techniques used:
   Questionnaire.
   Interviews.
   Time data were collected:
   March - June 1992.
   Testing of any tools used:
   Questionnaires and interview schedules; tested with 10 people.
   Topics covered:
   Educator practices related to the principles of andragogy and experiential learning.
   Setting for data collection:
   Colleges of Nursing and Midwifery.

Details about sample studied:
   Planned size of sample:
      60-80
   Rationale for planned size:
      Sufficient to obtain substantially generalisable findings.
   Entry criteria:
      Midwifery educationists.
      In current practice.
   Sample selection:
      Convenience.
   Actual sample size:
      40
   Response rate:
      87.5%

Interventions, Outcomes and Analysis:
   Analysis:
      Content analysis based on Glaser and Strauss (1969) notion of
      theory/hypothesis generating strategies for qualitative research.

Results: The findings from the study indicate varied educators' perceptions of the concepts of andragogy and pedagogy, with lack of familiarity and misconception about progressive pedagogy. Variations in educator practices indicate that a pedagogic approach is more commonly applied than the andragogic approach.

Perceptions of the concept of experiential learning were varied, as were the educators' assessment of the benefits of experiential learning.

Although most educators relate experiential learning to active student interaction with the learning environment, some appear to specifically contextualise this within the controlled environment of the practical demonstration laboratories.

There is evidence suggesting that not all educators keep up to date with expert knowledge about the theories, concepts and practical implications of current adult educational approaches.

Recommendations for further research: Replication of the study when most Colleges of Nursing and Midwifery have fully implemented the Project 2000 proposals for Nurse Education. A larger study might use combined observational and taped interviewing procedures to generate more generalisable hypotheses, and involve all groups of teachers in Nursing/Midwifery Education to obtain comparable findings.

Keywords: ANDRAGOGY, EXPERIENTIAL LEARNING, MIDWIFERY EDUCATION, PEDADOGY

263. TEACHING STYLES AND TEACHING STRATEGIES: AN INTERVIEW STUDY OF MIDWIFERY TEACHERS
October 1991 - May 1993
M M Michie, Midwifery Tutor. **Contact:** M M Michie, Esmond Street, Glasgow G3 8SL.

Formed part of a course. 12-20 hours/week of own time spent. Funded by employer: Glasgow College of Nursing & Midwifery.

Aims of the study: To determine how teaching style is conceptualised by midwifery teachers, the strategies which they employ and factors influencing these, and to what extent teaching style is consistent or variable.

Ethics committee approval gained: No

Research design: Descriptive – Qualitative – Ethnography

Data collection:
Techniques used:
Semi-structured interviews.
Time data were collected:
October - November 1991
Testing of any tools used:
Interview schedule - piloted with two tutors.
Topics covered:
Teaching experience.
Strategies.
Influencing factors.
Setting for data collection:
Colleges of Nursing and Midwifery.

Details about sample studied:
Planned size of sample:
10
Rationale for planned size:
Time factor.
Entry criteria:
Inclusion: 5 years' experience (or more) as a midwifery tutor.
Exclusion: Senior tutors.
Sample selection:
Convenience.
Actual sample size:
13 midwifery tutors approached; 10 participated (from 5 Health Boards in Scotland).
Response rate:
77%

Interventions, Outcomes and Analysis:
Analysis:
Constant comparison.

Results: Five themes emerged revealing a developmental pattern of style, reflecting progress from novice to expert teacher and reflective practitioner. The study concluded that, within the context of midwifery education, teaching style can be conceptualised as a manifestation of the teacher's professional development. This enables her to employ appropriate strategies to overcome her learning preferences and limitations in order to respond appropriately to the needs of learners.

A flexible style allows the teacher to adapt her teaching to the needs of individual classes and circumstances as they arise. A rigid teaching style may reflect inexperience or failure to develop the self-confidence to respond flexibly within teaching situations. Versatility does not appear to be dependent on the length of teaching experience but is suggestive of a qualitative dimension of the experiential learning outcomes of the teacher.

Recommendations for further research: A longitudinal study to determine whether there are identifiable stages in teacher development.

Comparative studies:

a) Between midwifery and nursing teachers

b) Between teachers in midwifery, post-16, and higher education.

Keywords: MIDWIFERY EDUCATION, TEACHING METHODS, TEACHING STYLES

265. AN EXPLORATORY STUDY OF THE PERCEPTIONS, EXPECTATIONS AND EXPERIENCES OF STUDENTS ON UNDERGRADUATE MIDWIFERY PROGRAMMES
October 1992 - April 1993

M Panchal, Midwife. **Contact:** M Panchal, Allenby Road, Southall, Middlesex UB1 2HG.

Funded as integral or additional part of a job by King's College. Formed part of a course. 12-20 hours/week of own time spent.

Aims of the study: 1. An investigation of student midwives':

a) perceptions of the role of the midwife.

b) expectations of how they want to practice, once qualified.

c) experience of an undergraduate midwifery programme.

2. A comparison of those who had taken a direct entry route with those who had taken the post nursing registration route.

Ethics committee approval gained: No

Research design: Descriptive – Qualitative and Quantitative – Survey

Data collection:
    Techniques used:
        Interviews with midwifery educators.
        Postal questionnaires with student midwives.
    Time data were collected:
        February 1993 - Students' data.
        (To tap second semester of all 3 years of training).
        December 1992 - January 1993 - Tutors' data.
    Testing of any tools used:
        Questionnaires - Piloted with 3 students.
        Interviews - Piloted with 1 tutor.
    Topics covered:
        Age and background.
        Professional affiliations.
        Educational background.
        Reasons for undertaking BSc/RM course.
        Perceptions of midwife's role.
        Reasons for restrictions of midwife's role.
        Expectations of practice.
        Career intentions.
        Experiences:
        - of move into higher education.
        - supernumerary status.
        - mentorship.
        - clinical and class room teaching.
        - enjoyment of course.
        - transition from staff nurse to student midwife.
    Setting for data collection:
        University.

Details about sample studied:
    Planned size of sample:
        47 students.
        5 tutors.
    Rationale for planned size:
        Total number of students in both groups.
        Tutors - sufficient for small exploratory study.
    Entry criteria:
        Students on an undergraduate midwifery programme.
        Tutors intensively involved in undergraduate midwifery programme.
    Sample selection:
        Convenience.
    Actual sample size:
        Students 42. Tutors 5
    Response rate:
        Students 89%. Tutors 100%

Interventions, Outcomes and Analysis:
Analysis:
Pre-coded questionnaires:
Fox pro computer programme.
Chi-square.
Open questions:
Content analysis.

Results:
The post-nursing registration group:
- were more professionally active and involved.
- were relatively more clear as to why they had chosen to train as a midwife.
- were very critical of their course and the role and responsibilities of midwives.
- since starting the course had changed their career intentions in many instances towards independent practice.
- had long term career intentions of working in the community as independent practitioners or in education.
The direct entry group:
- did not fit the characteristics of direct entry students found in the literature ie they were not young and were not professionally active, but they did wish to remain in midwifery. They were not very critical of their course or of midwifery.
- their long term career intentions were to work in hospitals and in management.
The expectations of the students reflected those of their tutors.

Recommendations for further research: 1. A follow up study to see what the students actually end up doing and whether "expectations" were realised.
2. A study of performance outcomes and different expectations of students from different educational backgrounds - direct entry, diploma, degree.

Keywords: EXPECTATIONS (STUDENT'S), MIDWIFE'S ROLE, MIDWIFERY EDUCATION, MIDWIFERY EDUCATION (POST-REGISTRATION), MIDWIFERY EDUCATION (PRE-REGISTRATION), STUDENT MIDWIVES

276. DELIVERING THE PRE-REGISTRATION MIDWIFERY STUDENT: RECRUITMENT AND SELECTION FOR PRE-REGISTRATION MIDWIFERY EDUCATION IN ENGLAND
September 1991 - July 1994
N Mackeith, Midwife Research Assistant. **Contact:** N Mackeith, Ravenscar Mount, Leeds LS8 4AX.

Funded as integral or additional part of a job by employer: Maggs Research Associates. 6-12 hours/week of own time spent.

Aims of the study: To explore policy and practice of recruitment and selection for the new pre-registration courses at five sites in England.

Ethics committee approval gained: Yes

Research design: Descriptive – Qualitative and Quantitative – Ethnography/Case Study

Data collection:
Techniques used:
Questionnaires.

Interviews.

Observations.

Documentary analysis.
Time data were collected:
During two visits to each site: one to discuss policy and the second to observe practice.
Testing of any tools used:
Interview schedule and observation tools piloted at another site.
Topics covered:
Policy on recruitment and selection.

Equal opportunities.

Criteria used in interviewing.
Setting for data collection:
Midwifery education settings - institutions of higher education and hospitals.

Details about sample studied:
Planned size of sample:
5 midwifery education institutions.
Rationale for planned size:
Maximum practicable.
Entry criteria:
All those not involved in an additional case study MRA project.
Sample selection:
From existing statistics on student populations.
Actual sample size:
5 sites.
Response rate:
100%

Interventions, Outcomes and Analysis:
Analysis:
SPSS

Content analysis.

Results: Not yet available.

Keywords: MIDWIFERY EDUCATION, MIDWIFERY EDUCATION (PRE-REGISTRATION), MIDWIFERY, (RECRUITMENT AND SELECTION)

289. GENDER SOCIALISATION AND GENDER OCCUPATIONS WITH REFERENCE TO TEACHING, NURSING AND MIDWIFERY
March 1991 - November 1992
G Edwards, Regional Co-ordinator. **Contact:** G Edwards, Ravenmeols Lane, Formby, Merseyside L37 4DG.

Formed part of a course. 2-6 hours/week of own time spent.

Aims of the study: To demonstrate the relationship between gender identity and socialisation in childhood and the career prospects of women in female dominated occupations especially teaching, nursing and midwifery.

Ethics committee approval gained: No

Research design: Descriptive – Qualitative – Review of Literature

Data collection:
Techniques used:
Literature search and review.
Time data were collected:
Literature search undertaken from 1990-1992 (mainly from 1975, after the Sex Discrimination Act).
Topics covered:
Gender identity and socialisation.
Socialisation at home and school.
Vertical and horizontal segregation.
Gendered jobs.

Interventions, Outcomes and Analysis:
Analysis:
Content analysis.

Results: Women are socialised throughout their lives to expect and to achieve a lower professional status than men, even within those professions which comprise mainly women ie teaching, nursing and midwifery.

Keywords: GENDER, MIDWIFERY, SOCIALISATION

291. HELPING THEM TO BE WISE: THE PREPARATION OF STUDENT MIDWIVES FOR AUTONOMOUS PRACTICE
February · December 1993
S M Currie, Midwifery Teacher. **Contact:** S M Currie, Ardness Place, Inverness IV2 44J.

Formed part of a course. 12-20 hours/week of own time spent. Funded by employer.

Aims of the study: An investigation of how the student midwife is prepared for autonomous practice and some of the factors which might influence this, including the relationship between the student midwife and the supervising midwife.

Ethics committee approval gained: No

Research design: Descriptive – Qualitative – Grounded theory

> **Data collection:**
> > **Techniques used:**
> > > Interviews.
> > **Time data were collected:**
> > > 9-15 months into students' training.
> > **Testing of any tools used:**
> > > No.
> > **Topics covered:**
> > > Decision making.
> > > Assertiveness.
> > > Interpersonal behaviour.
> > > Mentorship.
> > > Socialisation processes.
> > > Teaching/learning strategies.
> > > Professional judgement.
> > > Restrictions on clinical practice.
> > **Setting for data collection:**
> > > College.
> > > Maternity Unit.

> **Details about sample studied:**
> > **Planned size of sample:**
> > > Approximately 6-8 student/staff midwife 'pairs'.
> > **Rationale for planned size:**
> > > Constraints of degree and time.
> > **Entry criteria:**
> > > Students working in a variety of clinical areas.
> > > Midwives with whom they had the most interaction in these clinical settings
> > **Sample selection:**
> > > Purposive.

Actual sample size:
    7 students and the 7 supervising midwives, plus 4 midwives working on night duty.

Interventions, Outcomes and Analysis:
    Analysis:
        Grounded theory.

Results: The results suggest that students exhibit a fear of independent action through non-assertive behaviour, passive learning and subsequent compliance. Students are observing role conflict as the midwives in the hospital environment aim to provide women centred care whilst juggling with the restrictions on their practice (including hierarchies and related to policies). The status quo may be accepted or, at times, challenged by the students. Thus the rhetoric of midwifery as an autonomous profession was not confirmed by this study.

Keywords: MENTORS, MIDWIFERY EDUCATION, STUDENT MIDWIVES

Management Studies

6. A COMPARATIVE STUDY OF THE DUTCH AND BRITISH ORGANISATION OF MATERNITY CARE

August 1986 - January 1994

Edwin van Teijlingen, Researcher. **Contact:** Edwin van Teijlingen, Chads, Ward 14A, City Hospital, Edinburgh EH10 5SB. Tel: 031 447 1001 Ex 3595

Formed part of a course. Over 20 hours/week of own time spent. Funded by University of Aberdeen and Campaign for Maternity Unit in Moray.

Aims of the study: To compare the organisation of the Dutch and British maternity services with particular reference to what is regarded as "low risk" and "high risk".

Ethics committee approval gained: No

Research design: Descriptive – Qualitative – Survey

> **Data collection:**
> > **Techniques used:**
> > > Documentary review
> > > Interviews
> > **Time data were collected:**
> > > July 1986 to November 1989 (plus one interview - June 1993).
> > **Testing of any tools used:**
> > > Tested on colleagues.
> > **Topics covered:**
> > > Perceptions of low and high risk.
> > > Responsibility of midwives.
> > > Factors which influence choice of place of birth.
> > > Policies.
> > **Setting for data collection:**
> > > Hospital and community.

> **Details about sample studied:**
> > **Planned size of sample:**
> > > 40-50 professional people in each group (in Netherlands and Scotland) - GPs, midwives, Health Board officials, obstetricians, researchers, maternity home helps.
> > **Rationale for planned size:**
> > > Time and resource constraints.

Entry criteria:
>Netherlands - anyone who wrote in English on policies or organisation of maternity care.
>
>Scotland - anyone who had written in the media between 1987-1988 on the closure of units in Grampian, or individuals they nominated.

Sample selection:
>Opportunistic.

Actual sample size:
>Scotland - 23
>
>Netherlands - 24

Response rate:
>Scotland - 60%
>
>Netherlands - 60%

Interventions, Outcomes and Analysis:
>**Analysis:**
>>Content analysis.
>>
>>Categorisation by themes.

Results: The organisation of maternity care in Scotland and the Netherlands can both be analysed by reference to the social and medical models of childbirth. One of the main characteristics of each model is centred on the question of the nature of risk in childbirth and its acceptability.

The concepts of 'patriarchy' and 'medicalisation' as possible bases for explaining the differences between the Dutch and Scottish/British organisation of maternity care seem inappropriate. The level of state intervention in the organisation of maternity care, ie limiting the professional competition, is an important difference between the Netherlands and Scotland/Britain. In order to incorporate state intervention in the interprofessional competition between midwives and doctors it is suggested that Andrew Abbott's (1988) theory of 'systems of professions' throws some light on the problem. [Abbott A. 1988. The system of professions: An essay on the division of expert labour. Chicago: University of Chicago Press.]

Recommendations for further research: More theoretical research is needed regarding the role and position of semi-professions.

Further research into cultural differences in the perception of pain and expectations in different cultures with regard to acceptable and/or avoidable pain levels in labour.

Keywords: BRITAIN, HIGH TECHNOLOGY, LOW TECHNOLOGY, MATERNITY SERVICES, MEDICALISATION, MIDWIVES, NETHERLANDS, PLACE OF BIRTH

Teijlingen van ER. Een vertaling in het Engels voor "kraamverzorgende". Tijdschrift voor Verloskundigen 1987;11:353-6.

Teijlingen van ER, McCaffery P. The profession of midwife in the Netherlands. Midwifery 1987;3:178-86.

Teijlingen van ER. Going Dutch? Midwife, Health Visitor and Community Nurse 1989;4:146-7.

Teijlinjen van ER. The profession of maternity home-care assistant and its significance for the Dutch midwifery profession. International Journal of Nursing Studies 1990;27:355-66.

Teijlinjen van ER. Maternity home-care assistant: a unique occupation. In: Abraham-Van der Mark E ed. Successful Home Birth and Midwifery: The Dutch Model, Westport, Connecticut: Bergin and Garvey 1993:161-71.

7. A STUDY OF THE INTRODUCTION OF THE NURSING PROCESS IN A MATERNITY UNIT
October 1979 - September 1982

R Bryar, Senior Lecturer in Nursing. **Contact:** R Bryar, Newtown, Eaton Road, Brynhyfryd, Swansea SA5 9JN.

Funded as integral or additional part of a job by employer and by funding agency(ies): CONFIDENTIAL, Edwina Mountbatten Trust.

Abstract: This study provides a description of the introduction of the nursing process and an assessment of its use in a particular organisation. The longitudinal study of the introduction of the nursing process (with 'patient' allocation) was initiated by senior midwives at the research hospital. Midwives had become increasingly dissatisfied with their role and this study is an example of the initiatives being made by midwives to re-establish their role. Consumer dissatisfaction also suggested to the midwives that they should aim to individualise care and provide more continuity of care. The nursing process, widely introduced in general nursing, had had limited application in midwifery in the United Kingdom at the start of the project. Change was introduced into the practice of midwifery staff via a programme of in-service education. Two-and-a-half years after the start of the longitudinal study, a cross-sectional study was undertaken to assess the extent of the changes introduced.

Data were collected using a variety of research methods to provide a description of midwifery care from a number of perspectives. The data were analyzed in the context of the action framework of organisational activity (Silverman, 1972). The action of midwifery staff (midwifery care) was considered in relation to: 1) the knowledge of the nursing process held by midwives and nurses; 2) the models of pregnancy in the wider society; 3) the individual midwife's knowledge of and attitudes towards these areas; and 4) the structure of the organisation and relationships between different role occupants in the organisation.

The results of the cross-sectional study indicated that although midwifery staff valued individualised care and had developed some understanding of the nursing process, care was routinised. It was concluded that the education programme aimed at the individual members of the midwifery staff produced little change in care and that such changes could only be achieved by attention to, and changes in, wider societal and organisational factors influencing midwifery care.

Keywords: INDIVIDUALISED CARE, MIDWIFERY PRACTICE, NURSING PROCESS, ORGANISATIONAL CHANGE

Bryar R. The midwifery process. In: Faulkner A, Murphy-Black T, eds. Midwifery Research. London: Scutari Press. 1990:53-68.

Bryar R. The midwifery process. In: Robinson S, Thomson AN, eds. Research in Midwifery and Childbirth. Vol 2. London: Chapman and Hall. 1991:48-71.

Adams M, Armstrong-Esther C, Bryar R, Duberley J, Strong G, Ward E. The nursing process in midwifery: trial run. Nursing Mirror 1981;153:32-5.

Bryar R, Strong G. Trial run-continued. Nursing Mirror 1983;157:45-8.

Bryar R. Introduction of change. The Midwifery Process. Proceedings of the Research and the Midwife Conference. Glasgow 1986.

Bryar R. The nursing process: a literature review. Midwifery 1987;3:109-16

Bryar R. Midwifery and models of care. Midwifery 1988;4:111-7.

9. THE POLICY AND PRACTICE IN MIDWIFERY STUDY
January 1983 - December 1988

Jo Garcia, Social Scientist, Sarah Ayers, Administrator, Sally Garforth, Research Midwife. **Contact:** Jo Garcia, National Perinatal Epidemiology Unit, Radcliffe Infirmary, Oxford OX2 6HE. Tel: 0865 224170

For full details see under Clinical Studies (Record No. 9).

10. POSTNATAL CARE IN GRAMPIAN - OBJECTIVES, EFFECTIVENESS AND RESOURCE USE
July 1988 - July 1992

Charis Glazener, Wellcome Research Fellow Postnatal Care. **Contact:** Charis Glazener, University of Aberdeen, Health Services Research Unit, Drew Kay Wing, Polwarth Building, Foresterhill, Aberdeen AB9 2ZD. Tel: 0224 681818 Ex 53732.

For full details see under Clinical Studies (Record No. 10).

14. RHONDDA KNOW YOUR MIDWIVES EVALUATION STUDY
September 1987 - June 1989

Carolyn Lester, Research Officer, Stephen Farrow, Senior Lecturer. **Contact:** Carolyn Lester, Research Team (UWCM), Ward 17, St David's Hospital, Cardiff CF1 9TZ. Tel: 0222 374818

Formed an integral or additional part of a job. Funded by employer and by funding agency(ies): University of Wales College of Medicine, Mid Glamorgan Health Authority.

Abstract: The purpose of the study was to evaluate a 'Know Your Midwives' (KYM) scheme compared with conventional maternity care. The scheme was introduced for women of one GP practice in the Rhondda, where women receive antenatal care at their local hospital, but are delivered by midwives they have not met at the district general hospital.

The method of research was a case control study where each woman in KYM care was matched with a woman of similar age and parity receiving conventional care. Information was collected by means of a booking form completed by the midwife, antenatal and postnatal fieldworker interviews, and a post delivery form completed by the midwife for 223 matched pairs. Analysis was carried out using SPSSx.

KYM women had fewer admissions for false labour and fewer episiotomies. They also had a slightly lower Caesarean rate than Rhondda women in the pre KYM year. KYM women spent a shorter time in labour at the hospital before delivery, and the babies of KYM women and controls had similar Apgar scores and rates of admission to S.C.B.U. The KYM scheme achieved its primary aim of having a known midwife at delivery in the majority of cases. KYM women showed higher attendance at antenatal classes, better understanding of information from the midwife, and more KYM women had found their antenatal care pleasant. KYM women made more positive and fewer adverse comments on intrapartum care, and more KYM women found the birth an emotionally satisfying experience. The relationship with the midwife at delivery was better for KYM women and KYM midwives showed greater professional satisfaction. Follow-up of study births has shown that more KYM women than controls accepted both triple and polio injections at their first immunisation.

Recommendations include shorter clinic waiting times, improvement in health education on smoking and breastfeeding, and enquiring into the availability and efficacy of epidural anaesthesia. Implications include a need to follow-up episiotomy and non-episiotomy subjects to determine the long- term effects, and an investigation into knowledge, provision and uptake of family planning services. The KYM scheme is a considerable improvement in the care of pregnant women.

Keywords: ADMISSIONS, COMPLAINTS, EPISIOTOMY, IMMUNISATION, KNOW YOUR MIDWIVES, LABOUR (SATISFACTION), PAIN

Lester CA, Farrow SC. An evaluation of the Rhondda Know Your Midwives Scheme. The first year's deliveries. Report to Mid Glamorgan Health Authority 1989.

18. THE ROLE OF THE INTERPRETER/LINKWORKER IN THE MATERNITY SERVICE
September 1987 - September 1989
L Hayes, Midwifery Tutor. **Contact:** L Hayes, Rectory Close, Drayton Bassett, Tamworth, Staffordshire B79 3UH.

Funded as integral or additional part of a job by employer: West Midlands Health Authority. Done in own time. Formed part of a course. 6-12 hours/week of own time spent.

Abstract: This paper describes the findings of a study conducted within the West Midlands Region in 1989. The study addressed the extent of interpreting provision available to Asian women who use the maternity services.

Twenty-two health districts that constitute the West Midlands Regional Health Authority were surveyed to collect information about this service. In addition, twenty interviews were conducted amongst interpreters/linkworkers who were working within the region. The hypothesis being tested was that 'there was insufficient provision of interpreting facilities available for non-English-speaking Asian women who use the maternity services'. The results from the survey of the health districts identified that of the seventeen health districts who had indicated that there were women who were likely to need the help of interpreters/linkworkers, only nine of them actually provided this service. The study also showed that the majority of interpreters/linkworkers (17, 85%) did not think non-English-speaking women were given as much information as English-speaking women about their care in pregnancy. The hypothesis was therefore proven.

Having a first baby, an overwhelming experience for every mother, can be a frightening one too when it happens in a country where the culture and language are both unfamiliar. Asian women in Britain face specific problems which health professionals need to understand if they are to provide the best care. This can only be achieved with the assistance of someone with knowledge and experience of Asian culture and language. A group of lay people have from necessity evolved (interpreters/linkworkers) who are multi-lingual and of similar culture. Whilst this would seem of positive benefit in providing better health care for Asian women, this group is nevertheless a scarce resource within the maternity service at present. Pregnancy care remains strongly service-orientated amongst the health professionals. Little attempt is made to build on or, indeed, acknowledge the lay competence of interpreters/linkworkers, which could add to a better cultural understanding between health professionals and the expectant Asian women in their care. This was manifestly evident in this study.

Keywords: ASIAN WOMEN, COMMUNICATION PROBLEMS, ETHNIC GROUPS, INTERPRETERS, LINKWORKERS, MATERNITY SERVICES

21. EARLY POSTNATAL TRANSFER: DOES IT PROVIDE MOTHER AND BABY THE BEST START TOGETHER?
October 1989 - April 1991

Joanne Whelton, Regional Co-ordinator CESDI. **Contact:** Joanne Whelton, Department of Epidemiology and Medical Statistics, London Hospital Medical College (at QMW), Mile End Road, London E1 4NS. Tel: 071 982 6979
For full details see under Clinical Studies (Record No. 21).

33. THE EMPLOYMENT DECISIONS OF NEWLY QUALIFIED MIDWIVES
April 1980 - April 1987

Rosemary Mander, University Lecturer. **Contact:** Rosemary Mander, Department of Nursing Studies, University of Edinburgh, Adam Ferguson Building, 40 George Square, Edinburgh EH8 9LL. Tel: 031 650 3896

Funded as integral or additional part of a job by employer: University of Edinburgh. 2-6 hours/week of own time spent. Additional funding by Scottish Home and Health Department, Gardner Bequest.

Abstract: The problem of non-retention of newly-qualified midwives is well recognised in the literature. This study comprised an attempt to provide midwifery managers with data which would help them to control the problem. An evaluation of the effects of the extension of midwifery training in the UK to eighteen months was incorporated. The research approach resembled two natural experiments running concurrently. Two self-administered postal questionnaires were distributed to 700 student midwives in Scotland, one prior to the beginning of midwifery training and one on completion. These instruments sought views about midwifery, about employment intentions and some demographic data.

The analysis of the data used predominantly quantitative approaches. The interpretation of the data was complicated by a deteriorating economic climate, and this may have influenced respondents' perceptions of the midwifery employment market and their employment decisions. A model of midwifery employment decision-making was drawn up comprising descriptive and potentially predictive elements. Conclusions were drawn concerning the short-term and non-durable nature of student midwives' employment decisions. Attitudes to midwifery and to midwifery training were found to be largely positive.

Recommendations were made relating to testing the model and to the role of the midwife. The implications for first level nurse training were considered.

Keywords: CAREER PLANNING, EMPLOYMENT, MANPOWER/WASTAGE, MIDWIFERY EDUCATION (EVALUATION), MIDWIVES, OCCUPATIONS

Mander R. Stop and consider: student midwife wastage in training. Research and the Midwife Conference Proceedings 1983.

Mander R. The employment decisions of newly qualified midwives. Unpublished PhD thesis, University of Edinburgh.

Mander R. Change in employment plans. Midwifery 1987;3:62-71.

Mander R. Who needs Midwifery? Nursing Times 1987;83:26.

Mander R. Why choose Midwifery? Nursing Times 1987;83:27.

Mander R. A discrete perception? An examination of the impressions of midwifery employment among newly qualified midwives. Senior Nurse 1988;8:15-18.

Mander R. Carers' careers - contingencies and crises. Midwives Chronicle 1989;102:3-8.

Mander R. 'The best laid schemes....': an evaluation of the extension of midwifery training in Scotland. International Journal of Nursing Studies 1989;26:27-41.

Mander R. Who continue?: A preliminary examination of data on continuence of employment in midwifery. Midwifery 1989;5:26-35.

Mander R. Short Report: Which new midwives choose to practise? Nursing Times 1989;85:62.

Mander R. Employment patterns among midwives. Health Services Manpower Review 1989;14:20-3.

Mander R. Midwifery training and the years after qualification. In: Robinson S, Thomson AM, eds. Midwives, Research and Childbirth, Vol 3. London: Chapman and Hall (in press).

34. THE EFFECT OF THE PRESENT PATTERNS OF MATERNITY CARE UPON THE EMOTIONAL NEEDS OF MOTHERS, WITH PARTICULAR REFERENCE TO THE POST-NATAL PERIOD
October 1980 - December 1982

J A Ball, Lecturer/Self-employed consultant. **Contact:** J A Ball, Elm Close, Saxilby, Lincolnshire LN1 2QH.

For full details see under Clinical Studies (Record No. 34).

49. MATERNITY SERVICES IN LOTHIAN - A SURVEY OF USERS' OPINIONS
January 1987 - June 1988

Claudia Martin, Senior Research Fellow, Lyn Jones, Senior Lecturer, Amanda Amos, Lecturer. **Contact:** Claudia Martin, The Local Government Centre, University of Warwick, Coventry CV4 7AL. Tel: 0203 524109

For full details see under Clinical Studies (Record No. 49).

64. CONTINUITY AND FRAGMENTATION IN MATERNITY CARE
October 1979 - June 1985

R Currell, Research Midwife. **Contact:** R Currell, St. Thomas's Way, Great Whelnetham, Bury St Edmunds, Suffolk IP30 0TP.

Formed part of a course. 6-12 hours/week of own time spent. Funded by funding agency(ies): Department of Health.

Abstract: A recurrent theme in the literature of the maternity services was found to be the need for a more humanised service and for individualised patient care. Continuity of care was frequently suggested as a means to improve the service. This study aimed to investigate continuity and fragmentation of care within different organisational patterns of maternity care. The hypothesis tested was that maternity care would be found along a continuum with continuity at one end and fragmentation at the other. It was postulated that women receiving the greatest degree of continuity of care would be the most satisfied with their care, and those who received the most fragmented care would be the least satisfied. It was also postulated that the midwives who gave the most fragmented care would be the least satisfied with their work and those who gave the greatest degree of continuity of care would be the most satisfied.

Two areas of the country were chosen for the study: shared care in consultant units, general practitioner unit care and home delivery care were studied in both areas. The methods of investigation used were non-participant observation and semi-structured interviews with 117 mothers and ninety-five midwives. The interviews were analyzed using categories developed during the pilot stage of the work, and others that emerged during the study, from the open-ended questions and the free answers given by the midwives and the mothers. Chi-square tests were applied where appropriate. In the observational episodes, all mother-staff contacts were counted and coded according to pre-defined categories.

The study showed considerable fragmentation in all the patterns of care, except for a very small number of the women who had home deliveries. Satisfaction with care, for both mothers and midwives, in all groups, appeared to be related to successful problem solving and the giving of 'focussed care' (Kratz 1978). Neither the use of technology nor organisation size appeared to have a direct effect on women's experience of care. Midwives appeared to find difficulty in reconciling the medical cure aspects of maternity care with the less specific 'care' aspects of midwifery. They appeared to be able to combine cure and care most successfully with women in labour and least successfully in antenatal care. It is suggested that the concept of continuity of care should be replaced by a concept of unity in care, with care centred on each woman rather than on the organisation or the providers of the service.

Keywords: CONSUMER SATISFACTION, CONTINUITY OF CARE, EXPERIENCE (WOMEN'S), MATERNITY SERVICES, MIDWIVES' SATISFACTION

Currell RA. Continuity and fragmentation in maternity care. Unpublished M. Phil. thesis. University of Exeter 1985.

Currell RA. The organisation of midwifery care. In: Alexander J, Levy V, Roch S, eds. Antenatal care. Midwifery Practice Series. London: Macmillan. 1990:20-41.

68. TREATMENT OF UMBILICAL CORDS: A RANDOMISED CONTROLLED TRIAL TO ASSESS THE EFFECT OF TREATMENT METHODS ON THE WORK OF MIDWIVES
April 1983 - July 1986
Isobel Waterhouse, Director of Nursing Services (Midwifery), Ann Medd, Trial Clerk (part-time), Malinee Somchiwong, British Council Research Fellow (NPEU). **Contact:** Miranda Mugford, National Perinatal Epidemiology Unit, Radcliffe Infirmary, Oxford OX2 6HE. Tel: 0865 224187
For full details see under Clinical Studies (Record No. 68).

72. TANGLED WEBS: FAMILY NETWORKS AND ACTIVITY EXAMINED IN ONE INNER-CITY AREA OF NEWCASTLE UPON TYNE
October 1987 - October 1989
J M Davies, Community Midwife. **Contact:** J M Davies, Rectory Terrace, Newcastle Upon Tyne NE3 1YB.
For full details see under Clinical Studies (Record No. 72).

76. STUDY OF THE LIFE AND WORK OF DISTRICT MIDWIVES IN NOTTINGHAM 1948-1973
January 1990 - December 1993
J Allison, Senior Midwife Advisor. **Contact:** J Allison, Edwards Lane, Nottingham NG5 6EQ.
For full details see under Historical Studies (Record No. 76).

77. PSYCHOLOGICAL AND SOCIAL ASPECTS OF SCREENING DURING ROUTINE ANTENATAL CARE
March 1989 - February 1992

J M Green, Senior Research Associate, Martin Richards, Reader in Human Development, Helen Statham, Research Associate, Claire Snowdon, Research Associate. **Contact:** J M Green, Maternity Services Research Group, Child Care and Development Group, University of Cambridge, Free School Lane, Cambridge CB2 3RF. Tel: 0223 334512

For full details see under Clinical Studies (Record No. 77)

81. COMPARISON OF MANAGEMENT AND OUTCOME OF LABOUR UNDER TWO SYSTEMS OF CARE
January - December 1986

D Walsh, Staff Midwife Postnatal & Antenatal ward. **Contact:** D Walsh, Darthorpe Avenue, Western Park, Leicester LE3 0UQ.

2-6 hours/week of own time spent.

Abstract: The purpose of the project was to compare the management and outcome of labour in two similar low-risk groups (primigravid women only) booked either under the consultant unit or under the GP scheme at our hospital.

The method chosen was a retrospective comparative study. One hundred women were studied, fifty in the GP scheme and fifty under consultant care. The consultant group comprised the first fifty women who delivered in the consultant unit and who met pre-selected risk criteria, after 1st January 1986. The GP scheme group comprised the first fifty women who met the same pre-selected risk criteria and who delivered in the GP unit attached to the consultant unit from September 1984, when the scheme started. A questionnaire was designed and piloted.

Other information required was gained from the women's obstetric and midwifery records. Numbers and percentages were calculated from completed data, and comparisons made. Since statistical tests were not applied, levels of significant difference could not be calculated.

Results showed that low-risk primigravid women booked under the GP Scheme: 1) were admitted later in labour and spent less time on the labour ward; 2) experienced more continuity of care while in labour - ie more were looked after by the same midwife throughout labour; 3) required epidural anaesthesia less frequently; 4) had less intervention in labour - ie less fetal monitoring and syntocinon augmentation; and 5) had a fetal outcome no worse than a similar group of low-risk primigravid women booked under the consultant unit.

These findings underline the argument for retention and even expansion of GP schemes and emphasise the need to evaluate obstetric outcome of the schemes before decisions are taken to close them.

Keywords: CARE COMPARISONS, CONSULTANT UNITS, FIRST STAGE (MANAGEMENT), GENERAL PRACTITIONER UNITS, LABOUR, MATERNITY SERVICES, OUTCOMES, SECOND STAGE (MANAGEMENT)

Walsh D. Comparison of management and outcome of labour under two systems of care. Midwives Chronicle 1989;270-3.

82. DEVELOPING A MODEL FOR MANPOWER PLANNING AND QUALITY REVIEW IN THE DELIVERY SUITE
January 1986 - December 1988
J A Ball, Lecturer. **Contact:** J A Ball, Elm Close, Saxilby, Lincolnshire LN1 2QH.

Funded as integral or additional part of a job by employer: Trent Regional Health Authority. Own time spent.

Abstract: Although there have been a number of manpower models developed for general nursing in the United Kingdom, little or no development has taken place within the midwifery services.

There are a number of logistical problems with any study of staff time needed to provide an acceptable quality of care, notably that of the basis for study - ie an observation study of actual time given to women will depend upon the current staffing of a delivery suite and the variable day-to-day workload. This study began, therefore, with a basis for staffing based upon the recommendations of the Short Report (1980) and the Maternity Service Advisory Committee Report on Postnatal Care (1983). Both state that a woman should have the attention of a midwife throughout labour.

A method of retrospective classification of women at the close of labour and delivery was developed and tested for validity and reliability in Lincoln County Hospital. The validity was further tested at three other hospitals, all of which reported satisfactory results. The mean time spent by the mother and baby per category in the delivery suite was recorded to provide a basis for staffing which matched the patterns of referral, volume of numbers and policy factors in any maternity hospital. The method has now been tested upon over 20,000 cases in Trent Region and a consistent pattern of manpower needs has been developed.

Keywords: DELIVERY SUITE, MANPOWER PLANNING, MIDWIFERY, MIDWIFERY STAFFING, OUTCOMES (MATERNAL), OUTCOMES (NEONATAL), PERFORMANCE INDICATORS, WORKLOAD

Ball JA. Dependency levels in the delivery suite. Research and the Midwife Conference Proceedings 1988:2-24.

Ball JA. Birthrate. A method for outcome review and manpower planning for delivery suites. Nuffield Institute for Health Service Studies. University of Leeds, Fairbairn House 71-75 Clarendon Road Leeds LS2 9P1: Manual 1989.

83. A SURVEY OF TRANSITIONAL CARE
January 1984 - February 1989

C A Whitby, Midwife Manager, Jean F Boxall, Hon Research Fellow University of Exeter, Clive Lawrence, Lecturer, University of Exeter, John Tripp, Senior Lecturer, University of Exeter. **Contact:** C A Whitby, Neonatal Unit, Rosie Maternity Hospital, Robinson Way, Cambridge CB2 2SW. Tel: 0223 245151

2 hours/week of own time spent. Funded as integral or additional part of a job by employer and by funding agency(ies): Iolanthe Trust.

Abstract: A survey of neonatal units has been undertaken to establish how many maternity units have to separate mothers from their well, low birthweight babies or low dependency special care babies.

A questionnaire was sent to the nurse in charge of 351 British neonatal units. Two hundred and fifty-one were returned. The study also looked at some differences in the hospitals practising transitional care, or shared care with the mother, and a group of maternity wards looking after babies down to 1.8kg on normal maternity wards. Too few well pre-term babies, or low dependency special care babies, were nursed at their mother's bedside. The establishment of transitional care areas, either in a separate ward or using the neonatal unit mothers' rooms and/or adjacent maternity beds would facilitate this initiative. Normal wards caring for infants down to 1.8kg do not provide the same neonatal nursing care, and do not allow mothers as much involvement in baby care or personal activity as units practising transitional care, but do prevent some unnecessary separation of mother and baby.

It is recommended that: 1) transitional care or shared care with the mother be made available to all UK mothers with well pre-term or low dependency special care babies; 2) midwives be encouraged to participate in this care in collaboration with the neonatal nurses and paediatricians; 3) this initiative should not be used just as a means of releasing staff for intensive care or delivery suites; and 4) the goal should be to involve mothers in their own infants' care as soon after the birth as possible, preferably at the bedside. In doing this mothers should take over total infant care earlier, and as a result they will be ready for home sooner and be more confident.

Keywords: LOW BIRTHWEIGHT, NEONATAL UNITS, ROOMING IN, TRANSITIONAL CARE

Boxall J, Whitby C, Lawrence C, Tripp J. Who is holding the baby? Midwives Chronicle 1989;34-6.
Teaching video on transitional care called "Being together".

87. PATTERN ANALYSIS OF MIDWIFERY CARE
June - September 1988
Susan Williams, Mary Thomson Research Fellow. **Contact:** Susan Williams, Glasgow College, Cowcaddens, Glasgow G4 OBA. Tel: 041 332 3731 Ex 4

Funded as integral or additional part of a job by employer.

Abstract: (Not updated since 1991) CONFIDENTIAL.

Keywords: HOLISTIC CARE, MIDWIFE'S CARE, MIDWIFERY PRACTICE, MIDWIFERY SERVICES, PATTERN ANALYSIS, ROUTINES, WORKLOAD

88. MATERNITY SURVEY
February - April 1988
Susan Williams, Mary Thomson Research Fellow. **Contact:** Susan Williams, Glasgow College, Cowcaddens, Glasgow G4 OBA. Tel: 041 332 3731 Ex 4

Funded as integral or additional part of a job. Funded by employer. Ayrshire and Arran Health Board.

Abstract: (Not updated since 1991) CONFIDENTIAL.

Keywords: COMMUNICATION PROBLEMS, CONSUMER SATISFACTION, HOSPITAL FOOD, MATERNITY SERVICES

Williams S. Maternity Survey 1988. Unpublished.

94. ASIAN ANTENATAL CARE PROGRAMME
November 1989 - March 1992
Judy Dance, Research Nurse, Shams Un Nihar, Linkworker, Ratna Alom, Linkworker, Nasim Altaf, Linkworker, Farah Diba, Linkworker, Rekha Sarkar, Linkworker. **Contact:** Judy Dance, Room 06 : Community Offices, Yardley Green Unit, East Birmingham Hospital, Yardley Green Road, Birmingham B9 5PX. Tel: 021 766 6611 Ex 2306 For full details see under Clinical Studies (Record No. 94).

96. WHY DO MIDWIVES LEAVE?
November 1987 - April 1988
S M Sauter, General Manager, Maternity and Gynaecology. Contact: S M Sauter, Albany Close, Bexley, Kent DA5 3ES. Tel: 081 302 2678 Ex 4111

Formed part of a course. 2-6 hours/week of own time spent.

Abstract: The aim of this project was to look at the recruitment and retention of midwives. A majority of the research was carried out in the South East Thames Regional Health Authority. A total of 140 questionnaires were sent to: student midwives (60) and midwives who were leaving the service and managers (80). The response rate was 73% from qualified midwives and 1% from students. The question-naires were sent to four teaching units within the South East Thames Region, repre-senting a wide range of catchment areas, population mix and housing availability. All these units were training schools for midwives and offered post-graduate employ-ment.

As a midwifery manager, my own instincts led me to feel that although the media gave low pay as the reason for many midwives leaving, I did not feel that this was necessar-ily the case. In some instances, the questionnaires lend credence to this: 95.6% of the midwives were SRN and RM, while only 4.4% were RMs only. Of the RMs, a total of 69.6% were staff midwives and 30.4% were sisters.

The question of recruitment and retention within the European Community as a whole was also examined with questionnaires being sent to the twelve EEC countries. The response rate was 75%. The various European-based organisations were extremely helpful in their replies and gave a very encouraging picture for the midwifery profes-sion on the Continent. Why then do we seem to have such a problem in England? The answer seems to lie in: 1) the way the Health Service organises midwifery training; and 2) the pay scales, which are among the lowest in Europe. Almost all of the midwives in Europe work independently of the health care system, which may give them a greater feeling of being practitioners in their own right.

Keywords: HEALTH VISITORS (TRAINING), MIDWIFERY EDUCATION, MIDWIFERY EDUCATION (RECRUITMENT), MIDWIFERY PRACTICE (CESSATION), MIDWIFERY (RECRUITMENT IN EUROPE)

97. THE DIVISION OF LABOUR: IMPLICATIONS OF MEDICAL STAFFING STRUCTURES FOR MIDWIVES AND DOCTORS ON THE LABOUR WARD
March 1985 - October 1986

J M Green, Senior Research Associate, Vanessa Coupland, Research Assistant, Jenny Kitzinger, Research Assistant. **Contact:** J M Green, Maternity Services Research Group, Child Care and Development Group, University of Cambridge, Free School Lane, Cambridge CB2 3RF. Tel: 0223 334512

Funded as integral or additional part of a job by funding agency(ies): Health Promotion Research Trust.

Abstract: This study was designed to look at the implications for midwives and doc-tors of working without registrars on the labour ward, as recommended by the 1981 Short Report on medical education. Six maternity units were studied, three working with registrars and three without. There were a number of differences between units, although often not related to staffing structures. Units without registrars tended to have consultants who saw themselves as 'practitioners' rather than 'managers', and who had a positive attitude towards midwives. Midwives working without registrars tended to be much more satisfied with their role, although there was more likely to be a conflict with SHOs.

Keywords: DOCTORS' SKILLS, LABOUR, MATERNITY SERVICES, MIDWIFE'S ROLE, MIDWIFERY STAFFING (STRUCTURES), MIDWIVES' SATISFACTION, REGISTRARS, STAFF ATTITUDES

Green JM, Kitzinger, J Coupland V. The division of labour: implications of medical staffing structures for midwives and doctors on the labour ward. Child Care and Development Group Cambridge 1986.

Coupland V, Green JM, Kitzinger JV, Richards M. Obstetricians on the labour ward: implications of medical staffing structures. British Medical Journal 1987;295:1077-9.

Green JM, Kitzinger JV, Coupland VA. The implications of medical staffing for midwives on the labour ward. Research and the Midwife Conference Proceedings Manchester 1987.

Green JM, Coupland VA, Kitzinger JV, Harvey JD, Hare MJ. Observations on obstetric staffing: the myth of the 3-tier norm. Journal of Obstetrics and Gynaecology 1989;9:289-92.

Coupland VA, Green JM, Kitzinger JV. Implications of medical staffing structure for doctors and midwives on the labour ward. In: The Needs of Parents and Infants: A Symposium on the Health Needs of Parents and Infants. Health Promotion Research Trust Cambridge 1989.

Kitzinger JV, Green JM, Coupland VA. Labour relations: Doctors and midwives on the labour ward. In: Garcia J, Kilpatrick R, Richards M, eds. The Politics of Maternity Care. Oxford: Oxford University Press. 1990.

Green JM, Kitzinger JV, Coupland VA. Midwives' responsibilities, medical staffing structures and women's choice on childbirth. In: Robinson S, Thomson A, eds. Midwives, Research and Childbirth. Vol 3. London: Chapman & Hall

106. AN EXPERIMENTAL APPROACH TO HOME SUPPORT FOR THE BREASTFEEDING MOTHER
January 1979 - December 1980

Mary J Houston, Midwife Researcher, Peter W Howie, Consultant Obstetrician, Ann Cook, Research Sister, Alan S McNeilly, Research Scientist. **Contact:** Mary J Renfrew, National Perinatal Epidemiology Unit, Radcliffe Infirmary, Oxford OX2 6HE. Tel: 0865 224876

Funded as integral or additional part of a job by employer MRC Reproductive Biology Unit. Formed part of a course. 2 hours/week of own time spent.

Abstract: The purpose of the study was to examine the effect of a system of postnatal support at home for breastfeeding women. This was seen to be important as almost half of the women who chose to start breastfeeding stopped as a result of problems, by four to six weeks after delivery.

The study group of twenty-eight women were recruited from one hospital in Edinburgh: they were selected on the basis of fulfilling the entry criteria (resident in Edinburgh, delivery of mature, normal birth weight babies, leaving hospital breastfeeding) over the ten-week study period. The matched control group of fifty-two women met the same criteria but were recruited over the subsequent twenty weeks. Women in the experimental group were visited at home by appointment every fortnight until the cessation of breastfeeding, by the same midwife. At these visits, women were given the opportunity to raise problems; these were discussed, and general support was given. Women in the control group received only normal postnatal care. Control group women were interviewed at home twenty-four weeks postpartum.

Mothers in the experimental group had a significantly longer duration of breastfeeding (100% still feeding at twelve weeks, and 86% at twenty-four weeks; 78% of the control group were still feeding at twelve weeks, 64% at twenty-four weeks) and a significantly later introduction of artificial milk or solid food. None of the women in the experimental group stopped breastfeeding because of 'insufficient milk' compared with 19% of women in the control group. Women in the experimental group reported that the important factors in the system of support were that the support was given by the same midwife and on a regular, predictable basis.

Keywords: BREASTFEEDING, SUPPORT (HOME), SUPPORT (PROFESSIONAL)

Houston MJ. Successful breastfeeding: the need for support. Proceedings of the Research and the Midwife Conference 1980: London and Glasgow.

Houston MJ, Howie PW, Cook A, McNeilly AS. Do breastfeeding mothers get the home support they need? Health Bulletin 1981;166-72.

Houston MJ. Breastfeeding: Success or failure. Journal of Advanced Nursing. 1981;6:447-54.

Houston MJ. Home support for the breastfeeding mother. In: Houston MJ, ed. Maternal & Infant Health Care: Recent Advances in Nursing Series. Edinburgh: Churchill Livingstone. 1984.

Houston MJ. Supporting breastfeeding at home. Midwives Chronicle 1984;97:42-4.

Houston MJ, Howie PW. Home support for the breastfeeding mother. Midwife, Health Visitor and Community Nurse 1981;17:378-82.

Houston MJ, Howie PW. The importance of support for the breastfeeding mother at home. Health Visitor 1981;54:243-4.

Houston MJ. Requirements for successful breastfeeding. Unpublished PhD thesis 1982 MRC Reproductive Biology Unit/CNAA/University of Edinburgh.

115. REPORT ON THE KIDLINGTON TEAM MIDWIFERY SCHEME
April - November 1989

Pamela Watson, Not presently working, Alison Kitson, Head Research and Evaluation, Lesley Page, Director of Midwifery. **Contact:** Alison Kitson, Institute of Nursing, Radcliffe Infirmary, Oxford OX2 6HE. Tel: 0865 816667

Funded as integral or additional part of a job by employer: Institute of Nursing.

Abstract: The purpose of this study was to examine the implementation of a team midwifery scheme based in the community with particular reference to: 1) the experience of midwives and women under their care; 2) the impact of the scheme on other health care workers; and 3) associated financial costs.

The method used was a survey. Fifty mothers who had been cared for by the team and fifty who had experienced the normal service provision were interviewed. The experimental and control group were matched on a range of demographic and obstetric factors. The main findings were that there was a noticeable downward trend in the use of analgesia during labour in the experimental group, together with descriptions of more positive experiences of labour by these same women.

Recommendations arising from the study were that there should be replication of the study with more teams and for a longer period of time.

Keywords: CONTINUITY OF CARE, EXPERIENCE (WOMEN'S), MIDWIFERY SERVICES (EVALUATION), PAIN RELIEF (LABOUR), TEAM MIDWIFERY

Kitson A. The Kidlington team midwifery project. In Focus 1990;3:4-5
Watson P. Report on the Kidlington team midwifery scheme. Institute of Nursing. Oxford 1990.

116. A STUDY OF THE ROLE AND RESPONSIBILITIES OF THE MIDWIFE
January 1978 - December 1983

Sarah Robinson, Senior Research Fellow, Josephine Golden, Research Associate, Susan Bradley, Research Associate, Keith Jacka, Statistician. **Contact:** Sarah Robinson, Nursing Research Unit, Kings College, London University, Cornwall House Annexe, Waterloo Road, London SE1 8TX. Tel: 071 872 3063/3057

Funded as integral or additional part of a job by funding agency(ies): Department of Health.

Abstract: Commissioned in 1979 in response to growing concern that certain developments in maternity care were preventing midwives from fulfilling the role for which they were qualified, this study comprised an analysis of many aspects of that role. These included procedures and activities undertaken, responsibility for and views about decision-making, staffing levels, time to give women support and advice, career plans and job satisfaction. The main focus of the study was the degree of responsibility midwives were able to exercise for decision-making and the inter-relationship of these responsibilities with those of medical staff.

Questionnaires were sent to nationally drawn samples of midwives, health visitors, general practitioners and medical staff in obstetrics. Response rates of 78% (4248), 89% (1177), 67% (1232) and 55% (333) were achieved for these groups respectively. Health visitors and medical staff were included to ascertain whether views differed about who was responsible and who should be responsible for making specified decisions.

Findings showed that although midwives carried out a major part of the care provided for women, a substantial proportion were not able to exercise the degree of clinical responsibility for which they were trained and qualified, as they worked in situations in which medical staff had assumed this responsibility. For example, a substantial majority of the community midwives were not required to take responsibility for the overall assessment of pregnancy, in that they worked in clinics in which the abdominal examination was usually carried out by the doctor, or was carried out by the midwife but then repeated by the doctor. A substantial proportion of midwives worked in units in which certain decisions basic to the management of a normal labour were made by medical staff, or were determined by unit policy and in which medical staff also examined normal postnatal women either once or twice during their stay or daily.

Medical involvement of the kind demonstrated by this research has several implications for maternity care: midwifery skills are often wasted in that they are either not used or they are duplicated; opportunities for midwives to develop and maintain confidence in skills and in decision-making ability are limited; the fragmentation of care entailed limits opportunities for midwives to provide women with support, and midwives are likely to experience frustration and lack of job satisfaction if they are unable to fulfil the role for which they are qualified. In the absence of any evidence to indicate that medical staff provide better care than midwives in terms of either perinatal outcome or satisfaction with care, it is recommended that the maternity services are organised in a way that facilitates the full deployment of midwifery skills.

Keywords: MATERNITY SERVICES, MEDICAL STAFF, MIDWIFE'S ROLE, MIDWIFE'S ROLE (CONFLICT), MIDWIFERY PRACTICE (CHANGES), MIDWIFERY PROCEDURES

Robinson S. Are there enough midwives? Nursing Times 1980;76:726-30.

Robinson S. Midwifery manpower. NERU ocasional paper No 4 Nursing Education Research Unit, King's College, London University 1980.

Robinson S. Midwifery manpower. Social Services Committee: Perinatal and Neonatal Mortality. Vol 5. London: HMSO. 1980.

Robinson S, Golden J, Bradley S. Preliminary report on the project on the role and responsibilities of the midwife: Part 1 - Antenatal care. Midwives Chronicle 1981;94:11-5.

Robinson S, Golden J, Bradley S. Preliminary report on the project on the role and responsibilities of the midwife: Part 2 - Labour and delivery. Midwives Chronicle 1981;94:49-53.

Robinson S, Golden J, Bradley S. Preliminary report on the project on the role and responsibilities of the midwife: Part 3 - Postnatal care. Midwives Chronicle 1981;94:74-6.

Robinson S. The midwife's role in maternity care. In: Providers and alternative patterns of maternity. Proceedings of the 1981 Conference on Human Relations in Obstetric Practice. University of Glasgow. 1981;pp 30-50.

Robinson S, Golden J, Bradley S. The midwife: A developing or diminishing role? In: Robinson S, ed. Research and the Midwife -proceedings for the 1979 and 1980 Conferences. Nursing Education Research Unit, King's College, London University 1981.

Robinson S, Golden J, Bradley S. The role of the midwife in the provision of antenatal care. In: Enkin M and Chalmers I, eds. Effectiveness and Satisfaction in Antenatal Care. Spastics International Medical Publications, William Heinemann Ltd. 1982;234-46.

Robinson S, Golden J, Bradley S. A study of the role and responsibilities of the Midwife. NERU Report No. 1. Nursing Education Research Unit, Kings College, London University 1983.

Robinson S. Normal maternity care: whose responsibility? British Journal of Obstetrics and Gynaecology 1985;92:1-3.

Robinson S. Caring for childbearing women: Some factors restricting the midwife's contribution. Nursing Times 1985;81:28-31.

Robinson S. Responsibilities of midwives and medical staff: Findings from national survey. Midwives Chronicle 1985;98:64-71.

Robinson S. Midwives, obstetricians and general practitioners: The need for role clarification. Midwifery 1985;1:102-13.

Robinson S. Maternity care: A duplication of resources. Journal of the Royal College of General Practitioners 1985;35:346-7.

Robinson S. Providing maternity care in the community: Some aspects of the role of the midwife. Part 1. Midwife, Health Visitor and Community Nurse 1985;21:222-8.

Robinson S. Providing maternity care in the community: Some aspects of the role of the midwife. Part 2. Midwife, Health Visitor and Community Nurse 1985;21:274-9.

Robinson S. Midwives and their role. In: Gretton A, Harrison A, eds. Health Care UK 1987. An Economic, Social and Policy Audit. Policy Journals, Berkshire 1988.

Robinson S. Caring for childbearing women: The inter-relationship of midwifery and medical responsibilities. In: Robinson S, Thomson AM, eds. Midwives, Research and Childbirth. Vol 1. Chapman and Hall 1988;8-41.

Robinson S. The role of the midwife; opportunities and constraints. In: Chalmers I, Enkin M, Keirse M, eds. Effective Care in Pregnancy and Childbirth. Oxford: Oxford University Press. 1989:162-80.

Robinson S. Midwives' responsibilities for decision making. In: Wilson-Barnett J, Robinson S, eds. Directions in Nursing Research: Ten Years of Progress at London University. Scutari Press. 1989:66-75.

Robinson S. Maintaining the independence of the midwifery profession: A continuing struggle. In: Garcia J, Kilpatrick R, Richards M, eds. The Politics of Maternity Care. Oxford: Oxford University Press. 1990:61-91.

119. NEWLY QUALIFIED MIDWIVES: A STUDY OF THEIR CAREER INTENTIONS AND VIEWS OF THEIR TRAINING
January 1979 - December 1984

Sarah Robinson, Senior Research Fellow, Josephine Golden, Research Associate, Keith Jacka, Statistician. **Contact:** Sarah Robinson, Nursing Research Unit, Kings College, London University, Cornwall House Annexe, Waterloo Road, London SE1 8TX. Tel: 071 872 3063/3057

For full details see under Educational Studies (Record No. 119)

120. A STUDY OF THE CAREER PATTERNS OF MIDWIVES
January 1986 - December 1992

Sarah Robinson, Senior Research Fellow, Heather Owen, Research Associate, Keith Jacka, Statistician. **Contact:** Sarah Robinson, Nursing Research Unit, Kings College, London University, Cornwall House Annexe, Waterloo Road, London SE1 8TX. Tel: 071 872 3063/3057.

For full details see under Educational Studies (Record No. 120).

133. ANTENATAL SURVEY TO DEFINE THE QUALITY OF CARE IN THE WINCHESTER HEALTH AUTHORITY
October - October 1989

G Fairclough, Midwife Teacher. **Contact:** G Fairclough, Monnow Gardens, West End, Southampton SO3 3QD.

Formed part of a course. 12-20 hours/week of own time spent. Funded by employer: Winchester Health Authority.

Abstract: The objectives of this study were twofold: 1) to define what is meant by a 'quality' antenatal service; and 2) to examine if a quality service is provided in Winchester Health Authority. The method used was a questionnaire survey whose design followed the recommendations of the Royal College of Obstetricians and Gynaecologists (1982), and the Maternity Services Advisory Committee. Fifty women were randomly selected by the midwives who were present at their confinement, the women placing the completed questionnaires in a box for collection. Thirty-two of the questionnaires were returned.

An analysis of the results showed that 29% of the women were 'satisfied' with their care, while the remaining 71% were 'very satisfied'; twenty-two (68.7%) sought medical advice before the thirteenth week of pregnancy; 67.7% attended eleven-plus antenatal clinics; and 59.4% attended parentcraft classes. Of those who did not attend, only two were primigravidae. Criticisms of the service included the appointments system and communications, which were felt to be inadequate. Overall, the survey has provided a basis for improving the quality of antenatal services in the Winchester Health Authority.

Keywords: ANTENATAL CARE, ANTENATAL CARE (EVALUATION), COMMUNICATION PROBLEMS, CONSUMER SATISFACTION, MATERNITY SERVICES (QUALITY)

135. INTERPROFESSIONAL COMMUNICATION: A STUDY OF COMMUNITY MIDWIVES AND HEALTH VISITORS IN GLOUCESTER HEALTH DISTRICT
August 1989 - April 1990

T J McGrath, Midwife Teacher. **Contact:** T J McGrath, Lawn Rd, Ashleworth, Gloucester GL19 4JL.

Formed part of a course. 6-12 hours/week of own time spent. Funded by employer and by funding agency(ies): Iolanthe Trust.

Abstract: The purpose of the study was to assess the extent of inter-professional communication between community midwives and health visitors working within Gloucester Health District. The limited amount of research that has been done in the field of communication between the health professionals is reviewed. Relevant theoretical perspectives are also considered, including role issues, the influence of power and status, and models of collaboration.

An initial exploratory phase, consisting of focussed interviews with key staff, preceded the main study. The experience of fifteen midwives and eighteen health visitors, from an original sample of forty-five, was examined using a prospective record which logged all forms of contact over a two-week period. Supplementary information from a questionnaire assisted with interpretation of the logged data, and the use of a rating scale determined the level of collaboration as perceived by the respondents. Most recorded contacts were concerned with individual clients, while difficulties of liaison were mainly related to the unavailability of staff due to different patterns of working. Variables such as length of time in post and location of staff (rural or city locality) were highlighted as important.

The results show that community midwives and health visitors in Gloucester Health District are communicating and not working in isolation. Some failures were revealed in communications and the level of interaction generally comprised the simple exchange of information. Joint working and collaboration which goes beyond this type of exchange, though evident in some staff, is not the usual pattern of practice.

Some recommendations are made with implications for practice, management, education and research.

Keywords: COMMUNICATION, COMMUNICATION (INTERPROFESSIONAL), COMMUNITY CARE, COMMUNITY MIDWIVES, HEALTH VISITORS, MIDWIFE'S ROLE (AMBIGUITY), POSTNATAL CARE

McGrath TJ. Interprofessional communication: a study of community midwives and health visitors in Gloucester Health District 1990. Unpublished dissertation. Held in University of Wales College of Medicine, and the National Library of Wales.

136. STUDY OF UMBILICAL CORD SEPARATION
March - December 1985
Y Stone, Community Services Manager, Maternity. **Contact:** Y Stone, Waverley Way, Carshalton Beeches, Surrey SM5 3LQ.

Funded as integral or additional part of a job by employer: Merton and Sutton Health Authority. 2 hours/week of own time spent.

Abstract: In a community midwifery service, it became apparent that because of late separation of the umbilical cord, midwives were spending a significant amount of their time visiting women after the tenth postnatal day.

A retrospective study was begun of all babies seen between March and September 1984 (in total 1503). Of these, 256 babies were excluded as the day of cord separation was not stated in the community records. It was found that community midwives made 331 visits after the tenth day to examine or treat the cord or stump. In 11% of cases, the cord had separated by the sixth day, while a further 20% did not separate until after the tenth day. We found that one midwife always recorded the cord off before the sixth postnatal day. Further investigation revealed that her treatment was no different from the other midwives, although we did notice that a majority of her babies were delivered at a particular District General Hospital. We looked into the cord care of each local hospital, and found it to be similar in all but one respect: babies delivered at our hospital had their cords sprayed with Polybactrin at delivery. It was decided to discontinue this practice for six months, then to make a follow-up survey of the effects on cord separation time and any potential effects on umbilical cord infection.

Community records for the months July to September 1985 were then studied in a second retrospective study. We found that a total of 1097 babies had been attended by midwives. Of these, ninety-eight were excluded from the study as the date of cord separation was not stated. The midwives made ninety-two visits after the tenth day to treat the umbilical cord, which was a 50% reduction on the previous study's visits. During the period of the second study, 42% of the cords had separated by the sixth day, while only 6% had not separated by the tenth day. There were no cases of umbilical cord infection.

We believe this study supports previous work, and appears to confirm that applying Polybactrin spray to the cord at delivery causes a delay in separation, with no noticeable benefits in reduction of umbilical infection. Polybactrin spray was not reintroduced into the hospital delivery practice.

Keywords: COMMUNITY CARE, CORD CARE, CORD SEPARATION, MIDWIFERY PROCEDURES, NEONATAL CARE, POLYBACTRIN SPRAY, POSTNATAL VISITS

141. A STUDY OF THE INTERPERSONAL ASPECTS OF COLLEGIAL RELATIONSHIPS AND OTHER RELATED THEMES OCCURRING BETWEEN MIDWIVES WORKING IN A MATERNITY UNIT
August 1990 - April 1991

Frances Black, Worker: Primary Nursing Network. **Contact:** Frances Black, School of Nursing Studies, U.W.C.M., Heath Park, Cardiff CF4 4XW. Tel: 0222 761628

Funded as integral or additional part of a job funded by employer and by funding agency(ies). Formed part of a course. 6-12 hours/week of own time spent.

Abstract: The purpose of this study was to investigate collegial relationships between midwives working on a maternity unit.

A period of non-participant observation in the unit was followed by interviews with nine of the midwives previously observed. An analysis of the resulting data was carried out by noting how many times eighteen categories of collegial interactions occurred. In the course of this analysis, a number of themes came to light, which included tension, catharsis, communication and midwives' perceptions of team midwifery; these, too, were analyzed.

These findings generated the following recommendations: management of the environment should be undertaken by staff other than midwives; and the presence of tension and the occurrence of cathartic mechanisms should be noted and supported by managers. Team midwifery was seen by the midwives as instrumental in developing themselves and their practice. It was also noted that where the policy of mutual support and help between midwives is followed through, it could encourage more creativity, fulfilment and job satisfaction.

Keywords: CATHARSIS, COLLEGIALITY, COMMUNICATION, INTRAPROFESSIONAL SUPPORT, STAFF ATTITUDES, TEAM MIDWIFERY, TENSION

Black F. MN Dissertation 1991. Held in University of Wales College of Medicine.

153. WOMEN-CENTRED CARE: A MIDWIFERY-BASED SCHEME WHICH PROVIDES WOMEN WITH INCREASED CHOICES AND CONTROL
April 1989 - October 1990
Charlette Middlemiss, Midwife Researcher, Paul A Atkinson, Supervisor. **Contact:** Charlette Middlemiss, Princess of Wales Hospital, Coity Road, Bridgend, Mid-Glamorgan, S Wales CS31 1RQ. Tel: 0656 662166 blp 2308

Formed part of a course. 6-12 hours/week of own time spent. Funded by employer.

Abstract: This century has seen extensive changes in maternity care. These changes are due primarily to improvements in maternal and perinatal mortality rates, the woman's place in society and the expectations of women using the maternity services. For the feminist, childbirth represents one of the many fronts on which the struggle for women's control of their lives is taking place. An important aspect of that struggle is the medical profession, which has established itself as the legitimate authority on all matters relating to maternal and fetal health. The effects of traditional hospital-centred care have had dramatic consequences on the choices available to women and on the role and status of the midwife.

This study reports on a midwifery-based scheme developed principally to give childbearing women improved continuity of care. The philosophy is based on the midwifery model, which adopts a women-centred approach to care. Ethnographic-style interviews were conducted with fifteen women who had recently received care via the midwifery scheme. The subjective experiences of the women suggest that the midwives played a prominent role in their care, which resulted in improved continuity of care. Women's descriptions indicate that greater choice and control are available when a women-centred, midwifery-based approach is provided. However, although doctors accept the midwifery scheme in principle, the study highlights how most of them continue to involve themselves to some degree in the provision of care. The data revealed how medical involvement often limited women's choices and control at various stages of pregnancy.

Keywords: CHILDBIRTH (CHOICES), CHILDBIRTH (CONTROL OF), CONTINUITY OF CARE, EXPERIENCE (WOMEN'S), FEMINISM, INDIVIDUALISED CARE, MATERNITY SERVICES, MIDWIFERY

158. SURVEY OF DISTRICT MIDWIFERY POLICIES - ANTENATAL AND POSTNATAL CARE
October 1990 - October 1991
Jo Garcia, Social Scientist, Mary J Renfrew, Director, Midwifery Research Programme, Pam Hughes, Project Secretary, Hazel Ashurst, Computer Co-ordinator. **Contact:** Jo Garcia, National Perinatal Epidemiology Unit, Radcliffe Infirmary, Oxford OX2 6HE. Tel: 0865 224170

Funded as integral or additional part of a job by employer: Department of Health.

Aims of the study: To document district policies in respect of:
1. the selection of pregnant women for different patterns of antenatal care on the basis of estimated risk;
2. postnatal transfer to the care of community-based midwives.

Ethics committee approval gained: No

Research design: Descriptive – Quantitative – Survey

> **Data collection:**
> > **Techniques used:**
> > > Postal questionnaire.
> > **Time data were collected:**
> > > April - May 1991.
> > **Testing of any tools used:**
> > > Study piloted in one region.
> > **Topics covered:**
> > > Antenatal care policies.
> > > Postnatal care policies.
> > **Setting for data collection:**
> > > All directors of midwifery in England.

> **Details about sample studied:**
> > **Planned size of sample:**
> > > 189
> > **Rationale for planned size:**
> > > Total population.

Entry criteria:
Directors of midwifery service in England.
Sample selection:
Inclusive.
Actual sample size:
167 out of 189
Response rate:
88%

Interventions, Outcomes and Analysis:
Analysis:
SPSS
Simple cross tabulations.

Results: The main finding: policies on postnatal home visiting by midwives had changed to be selective, as opposed to routine, up to the 10th postnatal day, in all but 20% of districts.

Other findings: respondents reported that agreed, district-wide, antenatal care policies existed in about half the districts.

Recommendations for further research: Evaluation of different approaches to selective postnatal home visiting would be desirable.

Keywords: CARE COMPARISONS, COMMUNITY CARE, DISTRICT POLICIES, HOSPITAL POLICY, HOSPITAL POLICY (ANTENATAL CARE), HOSPITAL POLICY (POSTNATAL CARE), MATERNITY SERVICES, MIDWIFERY POLICIES

Garcia J, Renfrew M, Marchant S. Postnatal home visiting by midwives. Midwifery 1994;10:40-3.

159. THE NPEU POSTNATAL CARE PROJECT
February 1990 - December 1993
Jo Garcia, Social Scientist, Sally Marchant, Research Midwife, Pam Hughes, Secretary.
Contact: Jo Garcia, National Perinatal Epidemiology Unit, Radcliffe Infirmary, Oxford OX2 6HE. Tel: 0865 224170

Funded as integral or additional part of a job by Department of Health and by funding agency: Wolfson Foundation.

Aims of the study: To investigate the provision of care in the early postpartum period by carrying out a descriptive survey of postnatal care in two districts within one English Health Region.

Ethics committee approval gained: Yes

Research design: Descriptive – Qualitative and Quantitative – Survey

Data collection:
Techniques used:
Case note and register review.

Mothers:
- interviews,
- diaries and calendars,
- questionnaires.

Midwives and Health Visitors:
- questionnaires.

Time data were collected:
Interviews - within 48 hours post delivery.

Diaries - on 4 specified days during first 12 postnatal days.

Daily calendar - from 1st to 14th postnatal day.

Questionnaire - 8 weeks post delivery.

Case notes/records - contemporaneously.

Testing of any tools used:
All methods were piloted outside and within study districts.

Topics covered:
Maternal morbidity.

Maternal provision of support.

Views of midwives and health visitors.

Satisfaction of mothers with provision of care.

Midwives' views of purpose of postnatal care.

Setting for data collection:
Two English Health Districts to cover postnatal care in hospital and in the community.

Details about sample studied:
Planned size of sample:
200 postnatal mothers (100 from each of two District Health Authorities).

Rationale for planned size:
Practicality within time scale.

Entry criteria:
Inclusion:

All postnatal women regardless of type of delivery or parity.

Exclusion:

Maternal illness

Neonatal illness.

Sample selection:
Total population in study period.

Actual sample size:
192 total (100 from District 1, 92 from District 2).

Response rate:
District 1 - 92%

District 2 - 68%

Interventions, Outcomes and Analysis:
    Analysis:
        Computer analysis for main data.
        Content analysis.

Keywords: CONSUMER OPINION, CONSUMER SATISFACTION, EXPERIENCE (WOMEN'S), POSTNATAL CARE, POSTNATAL CARE (EVALUATION), PUERPERIUM

Marchant S, Garcia J. The NPEU Postnatal Care Project. In: International Confederation of Midwives 23rd Triennial Congress Proceedings 1993;111:1171-80.
Garcia J, Marchant S. Back to normal? Postpartum Health and Illness. Research and the Midwife Conference Proceedings 1993:2-9.

165. A STUDY TO DETERMINE IF DIRECT CARE REDUCES WITH INCREASING GRADE OF MIDWIFE
October 1990 - March 1991
M M Heggie, Midwifery Lecturer. **Contact:** M M Heggie, Gleneldon Rd, Streatham, London SW16 2BZ.

Formed part of a course. Funded by employer: Camberwell Health Authority, and by funding agency: Iolanthe Trust.

Aims of the study: To determine whether direct care by midwives in hospital postnatal areas reduced with increasing grade in order to increase standards of care for mothers and babies and provide role modelling for learners, increased job satisfaction and 'client' satisfaction.

Ethics committee approval gained: Yes

Research design: Descriptive – Qualitative – Ethnography

    Data collection technique:
        Techniques used:
            Diary sheets for whole population.
            Semi-structured interviews with a sub-sample
        Time data were collected:
            8 week period for return of diary sheets.
            Interviews completed during last 3 weeks of above 8 week period.
        Testing of any tools used: Expert review.
            Interview schedule piloted with one midwife.
        Topics covered:
            Diary sheets: all activities and breaks.
            Demographic details.
            Interview Schedule:
            Reasons for becoming a midwife.
            Current role.

Preparation for job.
Satisfaction.
Perceptions of grade limits.
Time allocations.
Importance of mothers' views.
Setting for data collection:
Hospital.

Details about sample studied:
Planned size of sample:
Diary sheets - 31
Interviews - 6
Rationale for planned size:
Diary sheets - total population.
Interviews - first two of each grade.
Entry criteria:
Diary sheets - all midwives working on combined antenatal/post-natal wards in one midwifery unit.
Interviews - 2 x grades G, F and E.
Sample selection:
Convenience.
Actual sample size:
Diary sheets - 31
Interviews - 6
Response rate:
Diary sheets - 61.3%
Interviews - 100%

Interventions, Outcomes and Analysis:
Analysis:
Content analysis.
Categorisation by themes.

Results: All midwives felt they should have provided more direct care.
Analysis of data showed little difference between time spent in direct care given by the E and F Grade midwives whose work was considered similar by the sample. G Grade midwives, however, undertook less direct care due to administrative responsibilities.
The study identified a need to examine methods of managing and delivering maternity care in order to increase the amount of time available for midwives to give direct care. Expeditious use of support staff was recommended. Clarification of the overlap between midwives and medical staff's work; re-organisation of clinical areas to increase continuity and reduce handover time; and an increase in establishment, to reduce the use of agency staff, were all perceived as ways in which improvements could be made.
Where midwives are valued and involved in decision making, morale is raised, so efforts should be made to foster such an environment.

Recommendations for further research: Repeat the study with the addition of non-participant observation and involving a senior midwife manager to eliminate any bias towards education.

Assess satisfaction levels of mothers, staff and students before and after changes in management implemented.

Comparisons between wards and other units related to direct care giving.

Keywords: CARE COMPARISONS, LEARNING ENVIRONMENT, MIDWIFE'S CARE, MIDWIFE'S ROLE, MIDWIFERY GRADES, MIDWIFERY SERVICES (EVALUATION), MIDWIVES' SATISFACTION

188. MIDWIFE MANAGED DELIVERY UNIT: A CLINICAL, SOCIAL AND ECONOMIC EVALUATION
December 1991 - December 1993

Fiona M Cruickshank, Research Sister, Labour Ward, Gordon D Lang, Consultant Obstetrician, Joan M Milne, Clinical Midwifery Manager, Dana Blyth, Research Assistant, Moira Turner, Project Assistant, Vanora Hundley, Research Fellow, Charis Glazener, Wellcome Research Fellow. **Contact:** Vanora Hundley, Aberdeen Maternity Hospital, Cornhill Road, Aberdeen AB9 2ZA. Tel: 0224 681818 Ex 53875

For full details see under Clinical Studies (Record No. 188).

189. A SURVEY OF SYSTEMS OF MIDWIFERY CARE IN SCOTLAND
November 1990 - October 1991

Tricia Murphy-Black, Research Fellow. **Contact:** Tricia Murphy-Black, Research and Development Adviser, Simpson Memorial Maternity Pavilion, Lauriston Place, Edinburgh EH3 9EF. Tel: 031 229 2477 Ex 4357

Funded as integral or additional part of a job. Funded by funding agency(ies): Scottish Office Home and Health Department.

Aims of the study: To obtain a national picture of systems of care offered to childbearing women in Scotland.

Ethics committee approval gained: No

Research design: Descriptive – Qualitative and Quantitative – Survey

> **Data collection:**
> > **Techniques used:**
> > > Questionnaires.
> > **Time data were collected:**
> > > May 1991.
> > **Testing of any tools used:**
> > > Pre-testing of questionnaire.

Topics covered:
Systems of care.
Quality assurance/standard setting schemes.
Continuity of care.
Setting for data collection:
Hospital and community.
All maternity units in Scotland.

Details about sample studied:
Planned size of sample:
All 55 supervisors of midwives appointed at that time.
Rationale for planned size:
National coverage.
Entry criteria:
All units in Scotland providing maternity care.
Sample selection:
All units.
Actual sample size:
53 units.
Response rate:
90%

Interventions, Outcomes and Analysis:
Analysis:
Quantitative data - frequencies and cross tabulation.
Qualitative data - content analysis.

Results: Integrated units (with hospital and community midwives under the same management) are more likely to have implemented new systems of care to reduce fragmentation than non-integrated units. The most frequently used system is individualised care plans (88% of units). Birth plans, patient allocation, nursing/midwifery process or model, and the domino scheme are operating in over 60% of units. Team midwifery is the least used system, in use in 21% of units, but planned for a further 30%.

A system of standard setting is in operation in 57% of units of the formal packages for quality assurance, Midwifery Monitor and Quest Maternity are in most frequent use.

It was concluded that midwives in Scotland are aware of the problems of fragmented care and are using various methods to improve consumer satisfaction. Systems are adapted to suit needs or to take account of local and organisational constraints.

Recommendations for further research: Investigations of the impact of different systems of care on the consumers: An evaluation study.

Keywords: CONTINUITY OF CARE, MATERNITY SERVICES, MIDWIFE'S CARE, SCOTLAND

Murphy-Black T. Midwifery care in Scotland. Nursing Times 1992;88:55.

Murphy-Black T. A survey of systems of midwifery care in Scotland. Nursing Research Unit Report. Dept of Nursing Studies, University of Edinburgh 1992.

Murphy-Black T. Using the nursing process and models in midwifery. Journal of Clinical Nursing 1992;1:167-8.

Murphy-Black T. The use of systems of midwifery care in Scotland. Midwifery 1992;8:113-24.

194. JOB SATISFACTION AND DISSATISFACTION AMONGST NEONATAL NURSES
October 1988 - June 1990

S Williamson, Research Midwife. **Contact:** S Williamson, Hazelhurst Road, Worsley, Manchester M28 4SW.

Funded as integral or additional part of a job and by funding agency: Special Care Baby Unit Fund Raising Society. Formed part of a course.

Aims of the study: To identify which aspects of the work on a Neonatal Intensive Care Unit contribute to job satisfaction or dissatisfaction.

To determine what if any effect the clinical regrading has had on attitudes to work and job satisfaction.

To identify factors which might contribute to the retention of trained neonatal nurses.

To identify which aspects of Neonatal Nursing attract potential recruits.

To identify factors which might contribute to staff turnover in a Neonatal Intensive Care course.

Ethics committee approval gained: No

Research design: Descriptive – Qualitative – Survey

    Data collection:
        Techniques used:
            Semi-structured interviews.
        Time data were collected:
            August - October 1989.
        Testing of any tools used:
            Pre-tested on colleagues.
            Piloted with 15 nurses.
        Topics covered:
            Job satisfaction and dissatisfaction.
            Sources of limitation at work.
            Working environment.
            Upsetting events.
            Inter-personal relationships.
            Recruitment and retention.
            Clinical regrading.
            Demographic data.

Setting for data collection:
A hospital Neonatal Intensive Care Unit.

Details about sample studied:
Planned size of sample:
All of the 60 staff.
Rationale for planned size:
Total population.
Entry criteria:
Permanent staff in this NNIC Unit.
Sample selection:
Convenience.
Actual sample size:
50 neonatal nurses. (10 were not interviewed because of constraints on time).
Response rate:
83%

Interventions, Outcomes and Analysis:
Analysis:
Content analysis.
SPSSx.
Mann-Whitney U test.
Kruskal- Wallace.
Chi-square.

Results: The majority of respondents found their work stimulating and rewarding. However, the over-riding factor which exerted a negative influence, was the perceived under-valuing of their individual contribution at work by senior medical and nursing colleagues.

The factors which staff saw as important for retention (ie. pay, promotion prospects, staff development, off-duty being better organised) also influenced satisfaction. The nature of the work itself caused most satisfaction and recruitment problems. It did not seem to affect individual attitudes towards work, inasmuch as they all found the work rewarding. It affected them in a personal way: they felt undervalued by management and morale was low.

Recommendations for further research: Effect of regrading needs to be studied in broader terms than those of job satisfaction or dissatisfaction.
Relationship between nursing and medical staff.

Keywords: INTERPERSONAL RELATIONSHIPS, JOB SATISFACTION, MIDWIFERY (RECRUITMENT AND SELECTION), NEONATAL NURSES (RETENTION), NURSES (NEONATAL), REGRADING

Williamson S. Job satisfaction and dissatisfaction amongst neonatal nurses. Report submitted to the Special Care Baby Unit Fund Raising Society, Hope Hospital, Salford and to the Chief Nursing Officer, Salford 1990 (Unpublished).

Williamson S. Job satisfaction and dissatisfaction amongst neonatal nurses. Midwifery 1993;8:85-95.

Williamson S. Job satisfaction and dissatisfaction amongst neonatal nurses. Nursing Times 1993;89:11.

205. BIRTH OUTCOMES IN BRADFORD PAKISTANIS: INFLUENCE OF SOCIOECONOMIC AND CULTURAL FACTORS AND IMPLICATIONS FOR HEALTH SERVICES
December 1991 - December 1993

Iain Smith, Project Manager, Health Care Needs Assessment, Sue Proctor, Research Midwife, Waqar Ahmad, Lecturer, Asian Studies, Alison Macfarlane, Medical Statistician, Gulshan Karbani, Genetic Counsellor (Leeds General Infirmary). **Contact:** Sue Proctor, Clinical Epidemiology Research Unit, New Mill, Victoria Road, Saltaire BD18 3LD. Tel: 0274 366128/366026

For full details see under Clinical Studies (Record No. 205).

210. THE PROVISION OF CARE AT A MIDWIVES' ANTENATAL CLINIC
January 1982 - January 1984

Ann Thomson, Senior Lecturer. **Contact:** Ann Thomson, School of Nursing Studies, University of Manchester, Coupland III Building, Coupland Street, Manchester M13 9PL. Tel: 061 275 5342

For full details see under Clinical Studies (Record No. 210).

214. WOMEN'S EXPERIENCE OF MATERNITY CARE IN MID SURREY
April 1990 - February 1991

R Coppen, Midwifery Lecturer, P Kolodij, Computer Student Postgraduate, A Coppen, Consultant Psychiatrist, P Wilson, Quality Assurance Manager. **Contact:** R Coppen, Tattenham Crescent, Epsom Downs, Surrey KT18 5NY.

For full details see under Clinical Studies (Record No. 214).

225. THE MIDWIFERY DEVELOPMENT UNIT (MDU); A RANDOMIZED CONTROLLED TRIAL
July 1992 - July 1995

Deborah Turnbull, Project Manager, Mary McGinley, Head of Midwifery Services, Barbara Maclennan, Area Nurse, Midwifery, Ian Greer, Professor of Obstetrics and Gynaecology, Gillian M McIlwaine, Consultant Public Health Women's Health. **Contact:** Deborah Turnbull, Midwifery Development Unit, Glasgow Royal Maternity Hospital, Rottenrow, Glasgow G4 ONA. Tel: 041 552 3400

For full details see under Clinical Studies (Record No. 225).

230. THE RESOURCE IMPLICATIONS OF DIFFERENT APPROACHES TO THE MANAGEMENT OF PERINEAL TRAUMA
November 1991 - October 1994

Sarah Howard, Health Economics Researcher, Miranda Mugford, Economist, Denise Mickell, Student. **Contact:** Sarah Howard, National Perinatal Epidemiology Unit, Radcliffe Infirmary, Oxford OX2 6HE. Tel: 0865 224126
For full details see under Clinical Studies (Record No. 230).

234. ECONOMIC ASPECTS OF CARE OF WOMEN DURING NORMAL LABOUR
September 1986 - October 1994

Miranda Mugford, Economist, Gerard Breart, Director, Inserm, James Thornton, Senior Lecturer in Obstetrics, Ethel Burns, Midwifery Lecturer Practitioner, Najoua Mlika-Cabanne, Epidemiology Researcher, Shane Kavanagh, Student. **Contact:** Miranda Mugford, National Perinatal Epidemiology Unit, Radcliffe Infirmary, Oxford OX2 6HE. Tel: 0865 224187
For full details see under Clinical Studies (Record No. 234).

236. FOREST HEALTHCARE: EVALUATION OF MIDWIFERY GROUP PRACTICE
January 1993 - April 1994

B Bryans, Care Group Director (Women and Children), W Sykes, Research Consultant, B Lynch, Midwife Manager. **Contact:** W Sykes, Midhurst Avenue, London N10 3EP.
For full details see under Clinical Studies (Record No. 236).

245. EVALUATION OF ONE TO ONE MIDWIFERY PRACTICE
October 1993 - September 1996

Lesley Page, Professor of Midwifery, Agneta S Bridges, Midwifery Research Fellow, Richard Lilford, Professor of Obstetrics and Gynaecology, James Piercy, Research Fellow, Ruth Wilkins, Research Adviser, Trudy Stevens, Research Associate, Sarah Beake, Project Assistant. **Contact:** Agneta S Bridges, Queen Charlotte's and Chelsea Hospital, Goldhawk Road, London W6 OXG. Tel: 081 748 4666 Ex 5131

Funded as integral or additional part of a job by employer: North West Thames Regional Health Authority.

Aims of the study: 1. To compare one-to-one midwifery with conventional maternity care with regard to safety.
2. To compare one-to-one midwifery with conventional maternity care with regard to cost.
3. To assess the organisational and professional impact of implementing one-to-one midwifery care.

4. To assess whether and to what extent one-to-one midwifery care:
    - increases client satisfaction with maternity care and/or pregnancy,
    - reduces physical morbidity,
    - reduces medical and surgical intervention,
    - improves psychological outcomes.
5. To assess the extent to which organisational targets are met.

Ethics committee approval gained: No

Research design: Descriptive/Experimental – Qualitative and Quantitative – Survey/Ethnography/Historical

Data collection:
Techniques used:
Interviews.
Participant observation.
Survey questionnaires.
Clinical audit.
Economic audit from obstetric case notes.
Project diaries kept by midwives.
Time data were collected:
From obstetric notes retrospectively.
Survey questionnaire - late antenatal, early postnatal, three months postnatal.
Testing of any tools used:
Piloted between October 1993 and January 1994.
Topics covered:
Continuity of care.
Satisfaction with particular aspects of care.
Psychological and physical well being.
Mother and baby relationship.
Self-esteem.
Postnatal depression.
Intervention rates - costs.
Setting for data collection:
Hospital and community setting.
Urban.

Details about sample studied:
Planned size of sample:
For historical study 500 from existing system.
For one-to-one care - subsamples of women from the geographical areas.
For economic evaluation - all women (1000).
Rationale for planned size:
Based on power calculation.
Entry criteria:
All women receiving one-to-one midwifery care within the Centre for Midwifery Practice (women in W3 & W12).

For Cohort study: Sample of 500 women from two similar geographical areas who share similar socio-economic characteristics.

Sample selection:
> Convenience.
> Random subsamples.

Actual sample size:
> Recruitment ongoing.

Interventions, Outcomes and Analysis:

Interventions used:
> Introduction of one-to-one midwifery care.

Main outcomes measured:
> Satisfaction with care.
> Breastfeeding rates.
> Operative and medical intervention.
> Rates of postnatal depression.
> Physical and emotional wellbeing.
> Costs.

Follow up:
> Not applicable

Analysis:
> Quantative data:
> Summary statistics.
> Chi-square.
> T-tests.
> Non-parametric tests.
> Descriptive statistics.
> Qualitative data:
> Content analysis.
> Ethnograph.

Keywords: BREASTFEEDING (INCIDENCE), CONSUMER SATISFACTION, CONTINUITY OF CARE, INTERVENTIONS, OUTCOMES (MATERNAL), POSTNATAL DEPRESSION, POSTNATAL HEALTH, RELATIONSHIPS

262. STAFFING REQUIREMENTS FOR SCOTLAND TO MEET CHANGING DEMANDS FOR MATERNITY SERVICES: MODELS TO AID DECISION MAKING

March 1993 - August 1994

Sara Twaddle, Health Economist, Patricia Purton, Director of Royal College of Midwives (Scotland), Barbara Maclennan, Area Nursing Officer, Patricia Meldrum, Researcher. **Contact:** Patricia Meldrum, Department of Public Health, Greater Glasgow Health Board, Glasgow Royal Maternity Hospital, Rottenrow, Glasgow G4 ONA. Tel: 041 552 3400

Funded as integral part of a job by funding agency: Scottish Office Home and Health Department.

Aims of the study: To develop a flexible computer based model of staffing for maternity services in mainland Scotland, to meet the needs of women, taking account of demographic and social factors, and statutory responsibilities.

Ethics committee approval gained: No

Research design: Descriptive – Quantitative – Survey/Survey Modelling

Data collection:
    Techniques used:
        Questionnaires.
        Literature Reviews.
        Interviews.
        Observation.
    Time data were collected:
        March 1993 to August 1994.
    Testing of any tools used:
        Advised by Steering Group, no pilot necessary.
    Topics covered:
        Current organisation and provision of services.
        Planned changes.
        Barriers to change.
        Possible methods of care and their feasibility.
        Implications of these on staffing.
        Role of health care assistants.
        Budget limitations.
    Setting for data collection:
        Consultant maternity units in all mainland Scottish Health Board areas.

Details about sample studied:
    Planned size of sample:
        22 consultant units in Scotland.
    Rationale for planned size:
        Total population.
    Entry criteria:
        Exclusion: The islands (contact by telephone only).
    Sample selection:
        Comprehensive coverage of Scotland.
    Actual sample size:
        Recruitment ongoing.

Interventions, Outcomes and Analysis:
    Analysis:
        Computer spreadsheets for modelling.
        SPSS/PC for other analysis.

Keywords: MATERNITY SERVICES, MIDWIFERY STAFFING (MODELS), SCOTLAND

269. MAPPING TEAM MIDWIFERY
October 1991 - November 1992
Ian Seccombe, Research Fellow, Ann Wraight, Research Midwife, Jane Ball, Research Officer, John Stock, Research Fellow. **Contact:** Ann Wraight, Department of Obstetrics and Gynaecology, St George's Hospital Medical School, London SW17 ORE. Tel: 081 672 9944 Ex53670

Funded as integral or additional part of a job and by funding agency: Department of Health.

Aims of the study: To identify, through a descriptive mapping exercise, what midwifery staff management practices are being carried out in England and Wales in the name of "Team Midwifery".
To identify how the different "Team Midwifery" models function, and what, in the opinions of the service providers and managers, facilitates or hinders their midwifery services.

Ethics committee approval gained: No

Research design: Descriptive – Qualitative and Quantitative – Survey/Case Study

> **Data collection technique:**
> > **Techniques used:**
> > > 1. Postal questionnaire survey.
> > > 2. Semi-structured interviews.
> > **Time data were collected:**
> > > Spring 1992.
> > **Testing of any tools used:**
> > > Questionnaires tested by 10 heads of midwifery services.
> > **Topics covered:**
> > > Team midwifery models.
> > > Management structures.
> > > Staffing levels, grade mix.
> > > Views of managers.
> > **Setting for data collection:**
> > > All units providing maternity care in England and Wales.

> **Details about sample studied:**
> > **Planned size of sample:**
> > > 283 units.
> > **Rationale for planned size:**
> > > All units in England and Wales.
> > **Entry criteria:**
> > > Offering maternity care.
> > **Sample selection:**
> > > Inclusive.
> > **Actual sample size:**
> > > 269 units.

Response rate:
95%

Interventions, Outcomes and Analysis:
Analysis:
SPSS

Results: The concept of team midwifery has a broad range of definitions and wide variety of working practices.
The majority of respondents (86%) gave improving continuity of care as one reason for introducing a team scheme.
37% reported that they have an established team scheme.
Regional distribution is uneven.
Overall, only a third of units with teams could identify the proportion of women delivered by a known midwife.
Every team scheme needs to be "home grown" to meet needs of local population.
There is lack of information on the relative costs of different patterns of care, therefore, assessment of costs is difficult in comparing team midwifery with other systems of care.

Keywords: CONTINUITY OF CARE, MIDWIFERY MAPPING, MIDWIFERY MODELS, TEAM MIDWIFERY

Wraight A, Ball J, Seccombe I, Stock J. Mapping Team Midwifery. IMS Report Series 242. 1993.

270. INDUSTRIAL RELATIONS AND PROFESSIONAL ISSUES IN TEAM MIDWIFERY
March - August 1993
John Stock, Research Fellow, Ann Wraight, Research Fellow. **Contact:** Ann Wraight, Department of Obstetrics and Gynaecology, St George's Hospital Medical School, London SW17 ORE. Tel: 081 672 9944 Ex 53670

Funded as integral or additional part of a job and by funding agency: Royal College of Midwives.

Aims of the study: To identify and explore key professional and industrial relations issues pertaining to team midwifery.
To identify processes involved in the introduction of team midwifery including an examination of the appropriateness of the current grading structure.

Ethics committee approval gained: No

Research design: Descriptive – Qualitative – Case Study

Data collection:
    Techniques used:
        Semi-structured interviews.
    Time data were collected:
        May and August 1993.
    Testing of any tools used:
        No.
    Topics covered:
        Implications to midwives of team midwifery:
        - flexible work patterns,
        - on call,
        - unsocial hours,
        - professional development,
        - part time midwives,
        - clinical grading.
    Setting for data collection: Hospital and community (team midwives).

Details about sample studied:
    Planned size of sample:
        Seven sites (minimum 1 manager in each: to include one midwife representing each team).
    Rationale for planned size:
        Team midwifery in operation.
        Different locations and populations.
        Different approaches to team midwifery.
    Entry criteria:
        Exclusion: small GP units.
    Sample selection:
        Identified from list of units known to operate team midwifery based on IMS previous work (mapping team midwifery).
    Actual sample size:
        Seven sites with 1-2 managers and 4-8 team midwives in each site.
    Response rate:
        100%

Interventions, Outcomes and Analysis:
    Analysis:
        Content analysis.

Results: Responsibilities and roles were changed in line with the grades of the midwives in the teams. Support was given to junior staff.

Advantages to midwives working in teams include ability to use all skills, high level of peer support, improved status, increased job satisfaction.

Disadvantages include the need to work more flexible hours, inability to work in chosen areas, total responsibility, poorly differentiated roles.

Costs depend on the model of team midwifery adopted.

Team midwifery does not suit all midwives.

Process of change represents a large organisational and cultural move.

Keywords: HOURS OF WORK, INDUSTRIAL RELATIONS, MIDWIFE'S ROLE, TEAM MIDWIFERY

272. RECENT DEVELOPMENTS IN MATERNITY CARE IN BRITAIN: TOWARDS A SOCIOLOGICAL PERSPECTIVE
September 1990 - September 1991

Jane Sandall, Postgraduate researcher. **Contact:** Jane Sandall, Department of Sociology, University of Surrey, Guildford, Surrey GU2 5XH. Tel: 0483 300800 Ex 2804

Formed part of a course. Over 20 hours/week of own time spent. Funded by Kings Fund Institute.

Aims of the study: To explore whether the current proposals to reorganise midwifery care should be understood as part of a coherent occupational strategy of professionalization, by midwives reasserting their autonomy and control over birth or the beginning of a powerful alliance between midwives and women.

Ethics committee approval gained: No

Research design: Descriptive – Qualitative – Historical

>**Data collection:**
>>**Techniques used:**
>>>Review of historical documents.
>>**Time data were collected:**
>>>1990-1991.
>>**Testing of any tools used:**
>>>No.
>>**Topics covered:**
>>>Historical changes.
>>>Continuity of care.
>>>Sociological analysis.
>>>Economic conditions.
>>>Autonomy.
>>>Female professional project.
>>**Setting for data collection:**
>>>Information sources: archives, socio-historical journals, sociological journals and midwifery journals and policy documents.

>**Interventions, Outcomes and Analysis:**
>>**Analysis:**
>>>Content analysis.

Results: This socio-historical study argues that independent midwifery emerged under specific social and economic conditions, which united the provision of a cheap service to the poor with the desire of some middle class women to establish female control over childbirth. This alliance kept the ideology of a midwife as an independent practitioner alive during the 20th century, whilst in practice her economic and clinical autonomy was being eroded.

Feminist writers such as Witz (1990) describe the strategy pursued by midwives in the 19th century to achieve registration in 1902 as a 'female professional project' using a strategy of dual closure. This includes the two way exercise of power, upwards as a form of usurpation and downwards as a form of exclusion.

Partly in response to a redefinition of normality and abnormality, but also informed by feminism and unhappiness about the organisation of maternity care, midwives began to develop their new 'professional project'. This study suggests that the ideology of continuity of care reasserts control over the heart of midwifery practice. Initially spearheaded by a few politically active radical midwives, a campaign to develop midwives' autonomy included the strategies already described by Witz. Now, as in 1902, midwives are tightly constrained by three sets of power relations which are challenged by the proposals in the 'Vision' (ARM 1986). By proposing group practices and contracting their labour to the new purchaser health authorities, they challenge their traditional employers. By electing their supervisors of midwives, they challenge the traditional disciplinary machinery that has always controlled 'errant' midwives. By providing continuity of care to all women regardless of complications, they challenge the traditional demarcationary boundaries of the medical profession. Thus midwives are claiming a discrete sphere of knowledge and expertise, legitimated by a desire for a more equal partnership with women in an area where medical care has been criticised.

This strategy as in 1902, looks to the state to sponsor their project and current attempts to develop professional status are dependent on state mandate, funding and political expediency. The interest shown by the British government in the cost effectiveness of midwife care and the alliance that has been forged with consumers may well enable this particular female professional project to be successful. The key question is whether female dominated occupations can avoid the criticisms that male dominated professions such as medicine have endured or whether midwives can develop a new model of a profession in partnership with the women they work with.

Recommendations for further research: Greater evaluation of continuity of care by midwives including process as well as outcome.

Keywords: AUTONOMY, CONTINUITY OF CARE, INDEPENDENT MIDWIFERY, MATERNITY SERVICES, MIDWIFE'S CARE

Sandall J. Choice, continuity and control? Recent developments in maternity care in Britain. In: Soothill K, MacKay L, Webb C, eds. Interprofessional Relations in Health Care. Edward Arnold (in press).

275. CONTINUITY OF CARE FROM COMMUNITY MIDWIVES: A STUDY INTO THE PRESENT SATISFACTION AND FUTURE NEEDS OF WOMEN IN THE AMMAN VALLEY AREA
June 1992 - August 1993

Rose Marx, Community Midwife, Gwyneth R Isaac, Community Midwife, Ann D Jones, Community Midwife, Meinir Rowland, Community Midwife, Rosamund Bryar, Senior Lecturer Teamcare Valleys, Graham Clark, Health Sector Research. **Contact:** Rose Marx, Amman Valley Midwives, c/o Antenatal Clinic, Amman Valley Hospital, Glanamman, Ammanford, Dyfed SA18 2BQ. Tel: 0269 822226

For full details see under Clinical Studies (Record No. 275).

278. COMMUNITY TEAM MIDWIFERY CARE: AN ASSESSMENT OF ITS VALUE AND MEANING FOR WOMEN AND MIDWIVES
December 1992 - August 1993

G Lee, Part time staff midwife. **Contact:** G Lee, Kirkstall Road, London SW2 4HF.

For full details see under Clinical Studies (Record No. 278).

279. AUTONOMY - WHO WANTS IT? AN EVALUATION OF MIDWIFERY LED CARE
July 1992 - June 1994

A Laverty, Midwife. **Contact:** A Laverty, Carter Lane, Mansfield, Notts NG18 3DQ.

Formed part of a course. 6-12 hours/week of own time spent. Funded by employer: North Notts Health Authority.

Aims of the study: 1. To ascertain midwives' perceptions and opinions of the 'genesis scheme' of midwifery led care (Study A).
2. To identify reasons for midwives' referral of women in labour to consultant care (Study B).
3. To examine delivery outcomes of women booked under the 'genesis scheme' of midwifery led care.

Ethics committee approval gained: Yes

Research design: Descriptive – Qualitative and Quantitative – Survey/Retrospective Examination of case notes

>   **Data collection:**
>   **Techniques used:**
>   Study A: Questionnaire based on Likert scale to midwives.
>   Study B: Newly designed checklist.
>   **Time data were collected:**
>   Study A: Over 8 week period.
>   Study B: Retrospectively postnatally.
>   **Testing of any tools used:**
>   Expert review.
>   Questionnaires piloted.

Topics covered:

Study A: Midwives' perceptions of:

- autonomy.
- genesis scheme of midwifery led care, its implementation; basic concept.
- team midwifery and peer support.

Study B: Outcomes such as blood loss, length of labour, perineal trauma, Apgar scores, admission to special care, interventions, reasons for referral.

Setting for data collection:

Study A: Hospital and community.

Study B: Consultant led maternity unit.

Details about sample studied:

Planned size of sample:

Study A: All midwives involved in midwifery led care (N=109).

Study B: All women booked for midwifery led care admitted in labour or with SRM.

Rationale for planned size:

Study A: Total population.

Study B: Total population.

Entry criteria:

Study A: *Exclusion:*

students;

midwives above 'G' grade;

midwives not practising clinical midwifery (tutors etc);

midwives on maternity leave or long term sick leave.

Study B: *Exclusion:*

Women referred to consultant care from midwifery led care prior to onset of labour.

Sample selection:

Study A: convenience.

Study B: convenience.

Actual sample size:

Study A: 65 returns

Study B: recruitment ongoing

Response rate:

Study A: 60%

Interventions, Outcomes and Analysis:

Analysis:

Study A:

- frequencies.
- Chi-square.
- trend analysis.
- content analysis.

Study B:

–Not yet decided.

Results: Study A: Midwives view the scheme and midwifery led care positively, believing themselves to be independent autonomous practitioners adequately educated to care for low-risk women with no obstetric intervention.

Results suggest that midwives are still content to hide behind the consultant and a few are still reluctant to whole heartedly grasp accountability and responsibility.

Study B: Not yet available.

Keywords: AUTONOMY, MIDWIFE'S CARE, MIDWIFERY MANAGED CARE, OUTCOMES

Historical Studies

76. STUDY OF THE LIFE AND WORK OF DISTRICT MIDWIVES IN NOTTINGHAM 1948-1973
January 1990 - December 1993
J Allison, Senior Midwife Advisor. **Contact:** J Allison, Edwards Lane, Nottingham NG5 6EQ.

Formed part of a course. Over 20 hours/week of own time spent. Funded by employer.

Abstract: (Not updated since 1991) Statistical data for this ethnographic study are being obtained from midwives' district and personal registers, old diaries, work sheets, letters and personal memorabilia. Other sources included Medical Officer of Health Reports, hospital registers, and obstetric archives. Lengthy taped interviews with retired midwives and District Supervisors of midwives have also been carried out.

Keywords: COMMUNITY CARE, COMMUNITY MIDWIVES, HOME BIRTHS, MATERNITY SERVICES, MIDWIFE'S ROLE, MIDWIFERY (HISTORY), PLACE OF BIRTH

A description of the management of low birthweight babies born at home in the City of Nottingham (UK) 1952-1966. Encyclopedia of childbearing. New York (details not confirmed).

191. THE HISTORY OF MIDWIFERY EDUCATION FROM 1902 TO 1936
July 1990 - August 1991
S J Ridgway, Head of Midwifery and related studies. **Contact:** S J Ridgway, Cropthorne Drive, Hollywood, Worcestershire B47 5PZ.

Formed part of a course. 6-12 hours/week of own time spent. Funded by employer: Birmingham and Solihull College of Midwifery Education and Training.

Aims of the study: 1. To identify changes in midwifery education prior to the 1902 Midwives Act.
2. To determine the reasons for change, change agents and opposition to change prior to 1902 and up to 1936.
3. To examine the socio-political climate from 1902 to 1936 and investigate correlations between midwifery education and change in mortality statistics.
4. To analyse the educational strategies of other caring professions and their influence in relation to midwifery education.
5. To identify intrinsic or extrinsic factors which have either a positive or negative effect on legislative control of midwifery education.

Ethics committee approval gained: No

Research design: Descriptive – Qualitative – Historical

> **Data collection:**
> > **Techniques used:**
> > > Historical records.
> > > Journals.
> > > Interviews with midwives.
> > **Time data were collected:**
> > > January 1990 - June 1991.
> > **Topics covered:**
> > > Change-agents, mechanisms, opposition to change.
> > > Medico-socio-political influences.
> > > Midwifery education.
> > **Setting for data collection:**
> > > Archives, historical records.

> **Details about sample studied:**
> > **Planned size of sample:**
> > > 2 midwives were interviewed.
> > **Rationale for planned size:**
> > > Any midwives available.
> > **Entry criteria:**
> > > Midwives who trained prior to 1936.
> > **Sample selection:**
> > > Opportunistic.
> > **Actual sample size:**
> > > 3
> > **Response rate:**
> > > 67%

> **Interventions, Outcomes and Analysis:**
> > **Analysis:** Content analysis.

Results: The main change agents initially were bishops who helped to influence Acts of Parliament. Doctors supported the bishops. As midwives became better educated they gathered mortality statistics to support the need for a Midwives Act. After the 1902 Act was passed, the change agents remained the same but grew in number. Opposition to change came originally from the doctors who feared an influx of under-educated women would jeopardise their status. This opposition decreased following passing of the 1902 Act.

A number of factors helped to influence Government-mortality statistics: poor midwifery care, social awareness, employment/unemployment, housing and nutrition. Despite various Acts and reports, however, the crude maternal mortality rate hardly changed from 1902 to 1936.

Keywords: CHANGE AGENTS, HISTORY, MIDWIFERY EDUCATION

Studies which will not be completed

Some studies listed in previous reports will not now be completed. It would have been surprising if there had not been some unfinished studies. The work involved between generating an idea for a study and completing it is often unpredictable, and greater than might have been anticipated. In addition, people's circumstances may change - such as their place of work, or where they live - and this accounts for a number of the studies which have not come to fruition. Researchers have told us of four such studies.

In addition, we have been unable to contact the researchers for full information about another nine studies for which preliminary details only were listed in previous reports. So as not to lose the important questions which they asked, we have listed their titles and study numbers here. Details about the plans for these studies can be found in the two previous MIRIAD reports (1990 and 1991).

STUDIES WHICH WILL NOT BE COMPLETED

16. The incidence and distribution of spontaneous abortions, stillbirths, neonatal deaths and congenital abnormalities within the Dumfries and Galloway area during 1980-1990: identifying common factors
22. Do we provide adequate support during the antenatal period to parents whose babies require admission to the Neonatal Unit?
62. The possible correlation between striae gravidarum and perineal trauma
156. Domiciliary confinement in Manchester from 1960-1985

STUDIES WHERE FULL DETAILS ARE NOT AVAILABLE

91. Quality assurance - maternity services
129. The health-care needs of the disabled women during pregnancy
132. Assessing the quality of postnatal care in hospital
139. The development and de-skilling of midwives
147. Psychological self-assessment by pregnant women
157. Maternal perception of fetal well-being: the maternal/fetal relationship and the influence of and on antenatal care
161. An exploratory study in self-acceptance and self-perception in ADM students
164. The role of the midwife in the fetal assessment centre
166. The Bloomsbury breastfeeding workshop evaluation project

Sources of funding for MIRIAD studies

The sources and amounts of funding for studies varied considerably; for example, one study received £20 from hospital funds, while another received £50,000 from a large funding agency. Many studies received no formal funding, and researchers themselves provided the resources for others, both in time and money.

Sources of funding are listed here in alphabetical order. The studies to which they have contributed are listed below their name. All sources of funding are listed, whether large or small. Sources of funding are listed if they contributed at all to a study; they may not have supported the whole study.

Association of Radical Midwives
Assessment of attitudes relating to direct entry midwifery training among clinical and tutorial staff in twelve health authorities.

Ayrshire & Arran Health Board
Innovations for antenatal booking

Basingstoke and North Hampshire Health Authority
International perspectives in the English midwifery curriculum

Birmingham & Solihull College of Midwifery Education & Training
Continuing education for non-employed midwives
The history of midwifery education from 1902 to 1936

Birthright
The policy and practice in midwifery study
Oxytocin infusion during second stage of labour in primiparous women using epidural analgesia: a randomised double blind placebo controlled trial

Bradford NHS Hospitals Trust
Health behaviour in pregnancy: roles and responsibilities in antenatal care

British Council Fellowship
Treatment of umbilical cords: a randomised controlled trial to assess the effect of treatment methods on the work of midwives

British Telecom
The role of the midwife in the domiciliary care of women with high-risk pregnancies

Camberwell Health Authority
A study to determine if direct care reduces with increasing grade of midwife

Campaign for Maternity Unit in Moray
A comparative study of the Dutch and British organisation of maternity care

Chiesi - Farmaceutici, Milan, Italy
A study of single administration Pro-Piroxicam in post-episiotomy pain relief

City Hospital NHS Trust
Midwives' and obstetricians' perceptions of waterbirths

Community Health Council
Women's experience of maternity care in mid Surrey

Confidential
A study of the introduction of the nursing process in a maternity unit

Coombe Hospital Research and Development Trust Fund
Comparative studies in the third stage of labour

Cornwall and Isles of Scilly Health Authority
Factors associated with and predictive of postnatal depression

Crawley Hospital
To examine the use of chlorhexidine acetate as a swabbing lotion on labouring women

Department of Health (England)
A study of the educational needs of midwives in Wales and how they may be met
An examination of the content and process of the antenatal booking interview
Basic supportive care in labour : interaction with and around labouring women
Continuity and fragmentation in maternity care
Treatment of umbilical cords: a randomised controlled trial to assess the effect of treatment methods on the work of midwives
The policy and practice in midwifery study
The multicentre randomised controlled trial of alternative treatments for inverted and non-protractile nipples in pregnancy
Social support and pregnancy outcome
A study of the role and responsibilities of the midwife
A study of the career patterns of midwives
An evaluation of pre-registration midwifery education in England
Survey of district midwifery policies - antenatal and postnatal care
Characterisation of long-term postpartum health problems.
A national study of labour and birth in water
The resource implications of different approaches to the management of perineal trauma
Economic aspects of care of women during normal labour
Mapping team midwifery
The NPEU postnatal care project

DHSS Nursing Research Scholarship
The effect of the present patterns of maternity care upon the emotional needs of mothers, with particular reference to the post-natal period

Directorate of Public Health Medicine
Ipswich childbirth study

District Councils within the Lothian Region
Maternity services in Lothian - a survey of users' opinions

District Health Authority
Assessment of analgesic and laxative use on two postnatal wards at Princess Mary Maternity Hospital, Newcastle Upon Tyne

Doncaster Royal Infirmary and Montagu NHS Trust
Routine postnatal haemoglobin estimations

Dorset Institute of Higher Education
Bowel care in the puerperium

East Anglian Regional Health Authority
Bath additive trial
Third trimester placental grading by ultrasonography as a test of fetal well being

East Birmingham Hospital
Asian antenatal care programme

East Dorset Health Authority
Artificial rupture of membranes in spontaneous labour at term: some factors which may affect the decision

Eastern Health & Social Services Board
To swab or not to swab!

Economic & Social Research Council (ESRC)
Sociological aspects of the mother/community midwife relationship

Edwina Mountbatten Trust
A study of the introduction of the nursing process in a maternity unit

Elizabeth Clark Trust
Conflicting advice on breastfeeding. What are we saying now?

English National Board for Nursing
Experiences of shared learning within a pre-registration diploma in midwifery education programme: An evaluative study

Ethicon UK Ltd
A randomised controlled trial comparing vicryl with black silk in perineal skin suturing following childbirth

Frances Harrison College of Healthcare
Research or ritual? A survey of the midwife's management of the second stage of labour

Gardner Bequest, University of Edinburgh
The employment decisions of newly qualified midwives

Glasgow College
Long term recall of labour pain
Attachment in mothers of pre-term babies

Glasgow College of Nursing & Midwifery
Midwifery students' perceptions of student centred learning
An investigative study to explore the extent to which andragogy and experiential learning are applied in midwifery education
Teaching styles and teaching strategies: an interview study of midwifery teachers

Glasgow Royal Maternity Hospital
A preliminary study of neonatal nurses'/midwives' perceptions of neonatal pain with particular reference to the low birthweight infant

Greater Glasgow Health Board
A randomised study to assess the benefits and hazards of delivery in a birthing chair
The unripe cervix: management with vaginal or extra-amniotic prostaglandin E2
A comparative assessment of an automated blood microprocessor for fetal blood PH measurements in the labour ward
Induction of labour: a comparison of a single prostaglandin E2 vaginal tablet with amniotomy and intravenous oxytocin

Health Education Council
The evaluation of a post-basic training course for antenatal teachers

Health Promotion Research Trust
Psychological and social aspects of screening during routine antenatal care
The division of labour: implications of medical staffing structures for midwives and doctors on the labour ward

Hinchingbrooke Hospital
Birth - Hospital or home?

Hospital Savings Association Scholarship
A comparative study on treatment versus non treatment of the umbilical cord.

Hull Maternity Hospital
Absent friends in Hull - a study of attendance at parentcraft classes

Humberside College of Health
Investigating midwifery education in a multiracial / multicultural society

ICI
Pelvic floor exercises in postnatal care

Institute of Education, University of London
Social support and pregnancy outcome

Institute of Nursing, Oxford
Report on the Kidlington Team Midwifery Scheme

Iolanthe Trust
The role of the midwife in the domiciliary care of women with high-risk pregnancies
Factors associated with and predictive of postnatal depression
Artificial rupture of membranes in spontaneous labour at term: some factors which may affect the decision
The policy and practice in midwifery study

Assessment of attitudes relating to direct entry midwifery training among clinical and tutorial staff in twelve health authorities.

The Southampton study of the prevalence of inverted and non-protractile nipples amongst antenatal women who intend to breastfeed

The Southampton randomized controlled trial of alternative treatments for inverted and non-protractile nipples during pregnancy

Social support and pregnancy outcome

A survey of transitional care

Midwives' care of the birth mother: a qualitative study of the care of mothers placing their babies for adoption

Student midwives' perspectives on maternal sentiments during childbirth

Teaching ethics in midwifery education

Interprofessional communication: a study of community midwives and health visitors in Gloucester Health District.

A study to determine if direct care reduces with increasing grade of midwife

Choice or chance? An exploratory study describing the criteria and processes used to select midwifery students.

An investigation into midwives' attitudes to midwifery practice and the role of women

A survey of the group learning experiences of midwives and teachers of an advanced midwifery course

Community midwives' views and experiences of home birth

J Scarborough and Sons
An observational study on the effect of the technique "moxibustion for breech presentation" on mother and fetus

Jane Hodge Foundation
The role of the midwife in the domiciliary care of women with high-risk pregnancies

Jannsen Pharmaceuticals, Dublin
Comparative studies in the third stage of labour

John Radcliffe Hospital, Oxford
Aromatherapy in labour

King's College, London
Primigavidae's experience of the antenatal booking interview

An exploratory study of the perceptions, expectations and experiences of students on undergraduate midwifery programmes

Kings Fund Institute
Recent developments in maternity care in Britain: towards a sociological perspective.

Young mothers' learning through group work : a descriptive study

Knapton Trust Fund for Research
The effects of a low haemoglobin on postnatal women

Lambeth Southwark and Lewisham FHSA
The antenatal care project: A randomized controlled trial of a reduction in the number of routine antenatal visits for low risk women

Locally organised research scheme

The midwife's management of the third stage of labour

Lothian Health Board
Evaluation of a new parenthood programme available for Primigravidae
Influencing breastfeeding success
Maternity services in Lothian - a survey of users' opinions

Maggs Research Associates
With women : a reflexive project
Delivering the pre-registration midwifery student: Recruitment and selection for
pre-registration midwifery education in England

Maidstone Hospital
Preliminary evaluation of hydrotherapy in labour, using hard indicators

Manchester College of Midwifery
Library resources: midwives' use during periods of education

Maws/RCM Research Scholarship
Some facets of social interaction surrounding the midwife's decision to rupture the membranes.
Uptake of six weeks postnatal examination by puerperal women in Oldham
Early postnatal transfer: Does it provide mother and baby the best start together?
Third trimester placental grading by ultrasonography as a test of fetal well being.
The Southampton study of the prevalence of inverted and non-protractile nipples amongst
antenatal women who intend to breastfeed
The Southampton randomized controlled trial of alternative treatments for inverted and
non-protractile nipples during pregnancy
Deliveries - Mothers or Midwives? - A study of communication styles in midwifery
The West Berkshire perineal management trial
A randomised comparison of glycerol-impregnated chromic catgut with untreated chromic
catgut for repair of perineal trauma
"They know what they're doing!"
A randomized controlled trial of aerobic and pelvic floor exercises in pregnancy

Medical Audit Committee
Borough of Barnet, study of breastfeeding uptake and its' continuation

Medical Research Council of Canada
Perceptions of first time mothers during the first three postpartum months

Medway Health Authority
Randomized controlled trial measuring the effects on labour of offering a light, low fat diet

Merton and Sutton Health Authority
Study of umbilical cord separation

Mid Glamorgan Health Authority
Rhondda Know Your Midwives evaluation study

Mid Trent College of Nursing and Midwifery
An evaluation of the non-midwifery placements in a three year diploma in midwifery
(pre-registration) programme
Investigation of ethical decision making by midwives

MRC Reproductive Biology Unit
How long should a breastfeed last?
The measurement of breast milk intake
Examination of the problems encountered by, & care offered to, breastfeeding women
Extra fluid intake by the breastfed baby and duration of breastfeeding
An experimental approach to home support for the breastfeeding mother
Early milk transfer and the duration of breastfeeding

National Birthday Trust
Ipswich childbirth study
A confidential enquiry into the relief of pain in labour

National Board for Nursing, Midwifery and Health Visiting
Midwives' personal experience of breastfeeding

Newcastle Health Authority
Tangled webs: family networks and activity examined in one inner-city area of Newcastle
Upon Tyne

NHS Management Executive
Choice, continuity and control? : sociological aspects of continuity of midwifery care in
England and Wales

Norfork and Norwich Hospital
Evaluation of preparation for parenthood classes for couples adopting a baby

North Nottinghamshire Health Authority
Autonomy - who wants it? An evaluation of midwifery led care

North West Regional Health Authority
Smoking in pregnancy: the effects of the tar, nicotine and carbon monoxide yields of ciga-
rettes on the fetus in labour, at birth and in the newborn period
Saliva and blood pethidine concentrations in the mother and the newborn baby
A study of infant growth in relation to the type of feeding
Psychological aspects of fetal monitoring: maternal reaction to the position of the monitor
and staff

North West Thames Regional Health Authority
Evaluation of one to one midwifery practice

Northcott Devon Medical Foundation
A comparative study of hand and mechanically expressed human milk - nutritional content
and effect on babies weight and growth

Northern Health and Social Services Board
Iron supplementation during pregnancy

Nottingham City Hospital
Influences upon and duration of breastfeeding

Nottingham Community Health
Young mothers' learning through group work : a descriptive study

Nottingham Health Authority
Is natural childbirth going out of fashion?

Nuffield Foundation
Factors affecting labour pain

Nuffield Provincial Hospitals Trust
Great expectations: a prospective study of women's expectations and experiences of childbirth

Nurses War Memorial Fund
Uptake of six weeks postnatal examination by puerperal women in Oldham

Nursing Research Training Fellowship
Why don't women breastfeed?

Osterfeed
Influences upon and duration of breastfeeding

Oxford District Health Authority
Survey of infant feeding practices

Oxford Regional Health Authority
Pelvic floor exercises in postnatal care
The West Berkshire perineal management trial
Relief of perineal pain following childbirth: A survey of midwifery practice
Effects of salt and Savlon bath concentrate post partum
Ultrasound and pulsed electromagnetic energy treatment for perineal trauma. A randomised placebo-controlled trial
Dyspareunia associated with the use of glycerol-impregnated catgut to repair perineal trauma. Report of a three year follow up study
A randomised comparison of glycerol-impregnated chromic catgut with untreated chromic catgut for repair of perineal trauma
A randomized controlled trial to compare three types of fetal scalp electrode
Diastasis of the symphysis pubis - its diagnosis and longer term sequelae in a cohort of child bearing women in West Berkshire
Cleansing and lubricating prior to vaginal examination and vaginal procedures in labour. A comparison of the use of chlorhexidine based solutions and creams, lubricating jelly and sterile water.

Primary Care Development Fund
A randomized controlled trial of aerobic and pelvic floor exercises in pregnancy
The antenatal care project: A randomized controlled trial of a reduction in the number of routine antenatal visits for low risk women

Public Health and Operational Research Award
The Hinchingbrooke third stage trial

Queen Charlotte's and Chelsea Hospital
Breast feeding support group in hospitals

Regional Health Authority
Forest Healthcare: Evaluation of midwifery group practice

Rocket of London Ltd
A randomized study of the sitting position for delivery using a newly designed obstetric chair

Royal College of Midwives
Industrial relations and professional issues in team midwifery

Scotia Pharmaceuticals Ltd
Double blind prospective study of the effect of gamma linolenic acid in the management of postnatal depression

Scottish Home and Health Department/Scottish Office Home and Health Department
A prospective study to identify critical factors which indicate mothers' readiness to care for their very low birthweight baby at home
Breastfeeding in Aberdeen
Postnatal care at home: a descriptive study of mothers' needs and the maternity services
Acquiring parentcraft skills in Aberdeen
The Scottish Low Birthweight Study
Why don't women breastfeed?
The employment decisions of newly qualified midwives
The Midwifery Development Unit (MDU); A randomized controlled trial
Development of feeding behaviour in breast- and bottle-fed infants
A study of support for families with a very low birthweight baby
Caesarean section versus vaginal delivery: A comparison of outcomes
Midwife managed delivery unit: a clinical, social and economic evaluation
A survey of systems of midwifery care in Scotland
Identifying the key features of continuity of care in midwifery
Staffing requirements for Scotland to meet changing demands for maternity services : models to aid decision making
Outcomes of caesarean delivery

SDHA Nurses and Midwives Research Funds
Epidural analgesia and position in the passive second stage of labour: Outcomes for nulliparous women

Sheffield District School of Midwifery
A randomised controlled trial to evaluate the use of spontaneous bearing down efforts in the second stage of labour

Sheffield Health Authority
A randomised controlled trial to evaluate the use of spontaneous bearing down efforts in the second stage of labour

Smith and Nephew Foundation
Facilitating informed choice in childbirth: A study of midwives and their clients

Somerset Health Authority
Factors influencing motivation in midwifery tutors
Survey of postnatal recovery following perineal repair by midwife

South West Thames Regional Health Authority
To examine the use of chlorhexidine acetate as a swabbing lotion on labouring women

357

Southern Derbyshire Health Authority
Assessment of attitudes relating to direct entry midwifery training among clinical and tutorial staff in twelve health authorities.

Spastics Society
The role of the midwife in the domiciliary care of women with high-risk pregnancies

Special Care Baby Unit Fund Raising Society
Job satisfaction and dissatisfaction amongst neonatal nurses

Special Trustees, St Thomas's Hospital
A randomized controlled trial of aerobic and pelvic floor exercises in pregnancy

St Bartholomews Hospital
Parentcraft as education
A comparative study on treatment versus non treatment of the umbilical cord.

Staff Enterprise Fund, Royal Devon and Exeter Hospital
Conflicting advice on breastfeeding. What are we saying now?

Stirling University Studentship
Factors affecting labour pain

Teamcare Valleys
Continuity of care from community midwives: A study into the present satisfaction and future needs of women in the Amman Valley area.

The Hospital for Sick Children Foundation, Toronto
The multicentre randomised controlled trial of alternative treatments for inverted and non-protractile nipples in pregnancy

The Jean Boxall Memorial Trust Fund
Feeding and growth patterns of infants in a neonatal unit

The Royal Free Hospital
Parentcraft as education

Tower Hamlets Education Trust
The triple test for spina bifida and Down's syndrome - How women choose whether or not to have the test

Trent Regional Health Authority
A randomized study of the sitting position for delivery using a newly designed obstetric chair
Developing a model for manpower planning and quality review in the delivery suite

UK Universities overseas research student award
Perceptions of first time mothers during the first three postpartum months

University Hospital
Midwives' and obstetricians' perceptions of waterbirths

University of Aberdeen
A comparative study of the Dutch and British organisation of maternity care

University of Edinburgh
Maternity services in Lothian - a survey of users' opinions

University of Glasgow
The unripe cervix: management with vaginal or extra-amniotic prostaglandin E2
Induction of labour: a comparison of a single prostaglandin E2 vaginal tablet with amniotomy and intravenous oxytocin

University of Manchester
The evaluation of a post-basic training course for antenatal teachers
A pilot study of a randomised controlled trial of pushing techniques in the second stage of labour
The provision of care at a midwives' antenatal clinic
An investigation of the effects of admission to hospital on pregnant women's smoking behaviour
Why don't midwives publish their research?

University of Sheffield Medical School
Community team midwifery care: An assessment of its value and meaning for women and midwives

University of Ulster, Faculty Research Committee
Midwives' perceptions of their relationship with clients

University of Wales College of Medicine
Rhondda Know Your Midwives evaluation study

University of Wales School of Nursing Studies
An evaluation of a new undergraduate preparation for midwives

Vice Chancellors of Universities of UK
Factors affecting student competency in midwifery

Wandsworth Health Authority
To assess the effect of increased appropriate intervention and support among pregnant cigarette smokers and their families

Wellcome Trust
Breastfeeding in Aberdeen
Postnatal care in Grampian - objectives, effectiveness and resource use

Welsh National Board
The happy end of nursing: an ethnographic study of initial encounters in a midwifery school

Welsh Scheme for Development of Health and Social Research
The role of the midwife in the domiciliary care of women with high-risk pregnancies

West Birmingham Health Authority
Some facets of social interaction surrounding the midwife's decision to rupture the membranes

West Glamorgan Health Authority
Report of a survey made into the content of advice given to mothers regarding infant feeding

by midwives and health visitors working within the West Glamorgan Health Authority, Swansea Health District
A study of the educational needs of midwives in Wales and how they may be met

West Midlands Health Authority
The role of the interpreter/linkworker in the maternity service.

Whittington Hospital Trust
Are you sitting comfortably? The development of a perineal audit system enabling midwives to follow their perineal management up to 13 months following delivery.

Winchester Health Authority
Antenatal survey to define the quality of care in the Winchester Health Authority

Wolfson Foundation
The NPEU postnatal care project

WomansChoice
An assessment of antenatal care in Tower Hamlets

World Health Organisation
The Bristol Third Stage Trial: Active versus physiological management of third stage of labour

Yorkshire Regional Health Authority
Birth outcomes in Bradford Pakistanis: Influence of socioeconomic and cultural factors and implications for health services

Author Index

Keyword Index